# Foot and Ankle Imaging

*Guest Editor*

HILARY UMANS, MD

## RADIOLOGIC CLINICS OF NORTH AMERICA

www.radiologic.theclinics.com

November 2008 • Volume 46 • Number 6

SAUNDERS an imprint of ELSEVIER, Inc.

**W.B. SAUNDERS COMPANY**
*A Division of Elsevier Inc.*

1600 John F. Kennedy Boulevard • Suite 1800 • Philadelphia, Pennsylvania 19103-2899

http://www.theclinics.com

**RADIOLOGIC CLINICS OF NORTH AMERICA Volume 46, Number 6**
**November 2008 ISSN 0033-8389, ISBN 13: 978-1-4160-6601-9, ISBN 10: 1-4160-6601-2**

Editor: Barton Dudlick

*Radiologic Clinics of North America* (ISSN 0033-8389) is published bimonthly in January, March, May, July, September, and November by Elsevier Inc., 360 Park Avenue South, New York, NY 10010-1710. Business and Editorial Offices: 1600 John F. Kennedy Boulevard., Suite 1800, Philadelphia, PA 19103-2899. Customer Service Office: 11830 Westline Industrial Drive, St. Louis, MO 63146. Periodicals postage paid at New York, NY and additional mailing offices. Subscription prices are USD 328 per year for US individuals, USD 487 per year for US institutions, USD 160 per year for US students and residents, USD 383 per year for Canadian individuals, USD 611 per year for Canadian institutions, USD 473 per year for international individuals, USD 611 per year for international institutions, and USD 230 per year for Canadian and foreign students/residents. To receive student and resident rate, orders must be accompanied by name of affiliated institution, date of term and the signature of program/residency coordinatior on institution letterhead. Orders will be billed at individual rate until proof of status is received. Foreign air speed delivery is included in all *Clinics* subscription prices. All prices are subject to change without notice. **POSTMASTER:** Send address changes to *Radiologic Clinics of North America*, Elsevier Journals Customer Service, 11830 Westline Industrial Drive, St. Louis, MO 63146. **Customer Service: 1-800-654-2452 (US and Canada). From outside of the United States and Canada, call 1-314-453-7041. Fax: 1-314-453-5170. E-mail: JournalsCustomerService-usa@elsevier.com (for print support) and JournalsOnlineSupport-usa@elsevier. com (for online support).**

*Reprints.* For copies of 100 or more of articles in this publication, please contact the Commercial Reprints Department, Elsevier Inc., 360 Park Avenue South, New York, New York 10010-1710. Tel.: (+1) 212-633-3812; Fax: (+1) 212-462-1935; E-mail: reprints@elsevier.com.

*Radiologic Clinics of North America* also published in Greek Paschalidis Medical Publications, Athens, Greece.

*Radiologic Clinics of North America* is covered in *MEDLINE/PubMed (Index Medicus), EMBASE/Excerpta Medica, Current Contents/Life Sciences, Current Contents/Clinical Medicine, RSNA Index to Imaging Literature, BIOSIS, Science Citation Index,* and *ISI/BIOMED.*

Printed in the United States of America.

# Contributors

## GUEST EDITOR

**HILARY UMANS, MD**
Associate Professor of Radiology, Director
of Musculoskeletal Radiology, Jacobi Medical
Center, Albert Einstein College of Medicine, Bronx,
New York

## AUTHORS

**LAURA W. BANCROFT, MD**
Professor of Radiology, University of Central
Florida, Florida Hospital, Orlando, Florida; and
Associate Professor of Radiology, Mayo Clinic
College of Medicine, Rochester, Minnesota

**JOSEPH M. BESTIC, MD**
Musculoskeletal Fellow, Department of Radiology,
Mayo Clinic, Jacksonville, Florida

**ANA CANGA, MD**
Radiology Department, Hospital Universitario
Marqués de Valdecilla, Avenida de Valdecilla sn,
Santander, Cantabria, Spain

**LUIS CEREZAL, MD**
Radiology Department, Instituto Radiologico
Cantabro, Clínica Mompía, Avenida de los Condes
sn, Mompía, Cantabria, Spain

**JULIA CRIM, MD**
Professor and Chief of Musculoskeletal Imaging,
Department of Radiology, University of Utah
School of Medicine, Salt Lake City, Utah.

**ANDREA DONOVAN, MD**
Department of Radiology, Sunnybrook Health
Sciences Centre, Toronto, Ontario, Canada

**DAVID P. FESSELL, MD**
Department of Radiology, University of Michigan
Hospitals and Health Centers, Taubman Center,
Ann Arbor, Michigan

**JULIE M. GREGG, GDU, PhD**
Senior Sonographer, Symbion Imaging, Vaucluse
Hospital, Brunswick, Victoria, Australia

**STEPHEN F. HATEM, MD**
Staff Radiologist, Musculoskeletal and Emergency
Radiology, Cleveland Clinic, Cleveland, Ohio

**MELANIE A. HOPPER, MBChB, MRCS, FRCR**
Leeds Teaching Hospitals, Leeds, UK

**JON A. JACOBSON, MD**
University of Michigan, Ann Arbor, Michigan

**MARK J. KRANSDORF, MD**
Professor of Radiology, Mayo Clinic College of
Medicine, Jacksonville, Florida; and Department
of Radiologic Pathology, Armed Forces Institute of
Pathology, Washington, District of Columbia

**EVA LLOPIS, MD**
Radiology Department, Hospital de la Ribera,
Carretera de Corbera km1, Alzira, Valencia, Spain

**PAUL MARKS, MD**
Supervising Radiologist, Symbion Imaging, The
Avenue Hospital, Windsor, Victoria, Australia

**KETAN N. NARAN, MD**
Musculoskeletal Radiology Fellow, Thomas
Jefferson University Hospital, Philadelphia,
Pennsylvania

**JEFFREY J. PETERSON, MD**
Associate Professor of Radiology, Mayo Clinic
College of Medicine, Jacksonville, Florida

**SHARIK KABIR RATHUR, MD**
Department of Diagnostic Radiology, University
of Miami, Jackson Memorial Hospital, Miami,
Florida

**PHILIP ROBINSON, MBChB, MRCP, FRCR**
Leeds Teaching Hospitals; and Musculoskeletal
Centre X-Ray Department, Chapel Allerton
Hospital, Beckett Street, Leeds, UK

**ALEJANDRO ROLÓN, MD**
Radiology Department, Centro de Diagnóstico
Dr. Enrique Rossi, Arenales, Buenos Aires,
Argentina

**TIMOTHY G. SANDERS, MD**
Professor (visiting, part-time), Department of
Diagnostic Radiology, College of Medicine,
University of Kentucky, Lexington, Kentucky;
and National Musculoskeletal Imaging, Weston,
Florida

**TIMOTHY SCHNEIDER, MD**
Surgeon, Melbourne Orthopaedic Group,
Windsor, Victoria, Australia

**MARK E. SCHWEITZER, MD**
Department of Radiology, The Ottawa Hospital,
Ottawa Ontario, Canada

**ADAM C. ZOGA, MD**
Assistant Professor of Radiology, Director of
Ambulatory Imaging Centers and Musculoskeletal
MRI, Thomas Jefferson University Hospital,
Philadelphia, Pennsylvania

# Contents

**Preface**                                                                                          xi

Hilary Umans

**Ankle Impingement Syndromes**                                                                      957

Melanie A. Hopper and Philip Robinson

Acute or repetitive trauma to the ankle can result in painful restriction of movement caused by impingement of soft tissue and osseous structures. Ankle impingement syndromes are classified according to their anatomic relationship to the tibiotalar joint. This article reviews the relevant anatomy, etiology, and clinical features of ankle impingement syndromes, and demonstrates the potential imaging findings and discusses management of each for these conditions.

**MR Arthrography of the Ankle: Indications and Technique**                                          973

Luis Cerezal, Eva Llopis, Ana Canga, and Alejandro Rolón

MR arthrography has become an important tool for the assessment of a variety of ankle disorders. MR arthrography permits more sensitive imaging of suspected intra-articular pathology in cases in which conventional MR imaging is either insufficient or inadequate for diagnosis or treatment planning. The main indications for MR arthrography are the evaluation of ligamentous injuries, impingement syndromes, cartilage lesions, osteochondral lesions of the talus, loose bodies, and several synovial joint disorders. Indirect MR arthrography can be a useful adjunct to conventional MR imaging and may be preferable to direct MR arthrography in those cases in which an invasive procedure is contraindicated or image guidance is not available.

**Osteochondral Lesions About the Ankle**                                                            995

Ketan N. Naran and Adam C. Zoga

Osteochondral lesions (OCLs) about the foot and ankle often manifest clinically as prolonged joint pain after trauma, often an ankle sprain, which is refractory to conventional, conservative therapeutic treatment. Noncontrast MR imaging is the standard of care imaging modality for diagnosing and classifying osteochondral lesions, but equivocal or difficult lesions can be assessed more specifically with direct MR arthrography or in conjunction with multidetector CT. Once an OCL has been identified, the imager should make every effort to determine whether it is stable or potentially unstable.

**Postoperative Imaging of the Total Ankle Arthroplasty**                                            1003

Joseph M. Bestic, Laura W. Bancroft, Jeffrey J. Peterson, and Mark J. Kransdorf

Promising results reported with currently available total ankle arthroplasty designs have led to an increased use of such devices as an alternative to ankle arthrodesis.

Despite recent improvements in implant design and surgical technique, complications associated total ankle arthroplasty devices continue to be reported. Postoperative evaluation of total ankle arthroplasties relies on a combination of clinical and radiologic assessment. Familiarity with commonly used current total ankle arthroplasty devices and appropriate postoperative imaging techniques is imperative for effective characterization of the expected postoperative imaging appearances of such devices and facilitating detection of potential postoperative complications.

## Imaging of Tarsal Coalition                                                                     1017

Julia Crim

A coalition is a congenital bony, cartilaginous, or fibrous connection (called a bar) between two or more bones. Coalitions are clinically significant because they prevent normal joint motion. Tarsal coalition may be difficult to identify on clinical and imaging evaluation. Given the high prevalence of coalition, radiologists must be alert to the often subtle imaging findings.

## Ultrasound of the Hindfoot and Midfoot                                                          1027

David P. Fessell and Jon A. Jacobson

Ultrasound has demonstrated great utility and accuracy for imaging the hindfoot and midfoot. Its advantages include its capacity to allow evaluation during dynamic maneuvers, imaging of patients who cannot undergo MR imaging, and real-time evaluation of the symptomatic site. It can also reveal abnormalities that are not apparent during static imaging. This article makes the case that radiologists should continue to be experts in all aspects of musculoskeletal imaging, including ultrasound or the business will be taken over by other specialties. If musculoskeletal ultrasound is lost, additional modalities such as MR imaging may be lost as well. Radiologists, with their expertise and years of training, are uniquely suited to apply this versatile modality to foot and ankle pathology.

## Imaging of Lisfranc Injury and Midfoot Sprain                                                   1045

Stephen Hatem

Injuries to the tarsometatarsal joint and of the Lisfranc ligament present a challenge. They are difficult to diagnose and outcomes worsen as diagnosis is delayed. As a result, radiologists and clinicians must have a clear understanding of the relevant nomenclature, anatomy, injury mechanisms, and imaging findings.

## MR Imaging and Ultrasound of Metatarsalgia—The Lesser Metatarsals                               1061

Julie M. Gregg, Timothy Schneider, and Paul Marks

Metatarsalgia is a common problem for many in the community. The condition includes many different entities, such as interdigital neuroma, synovitis or metatarsophalangeal joint instability, Freiberg infarction, stress fractures, and systemic disorders. Many patients presenting with metatarsalgia have a combination of diagnostic abnormalities. The key is to establish the principal pathology and from there construct an appropriate treatment regimen.

**Imaging of Painful Conditions of the Hallucal Sesamoid Complex and Plantar Capsular Structures of the First Metatarsophalangeal Joint**     1079

Timothy G. Sanders and Sharik Kabir Rathur

Numerous injuries and pathologic conditions can involve the hallucal sesamoidal complex and plantar capsular structures of the first metatarsophalangeal joint. Although clinical history and presentation are important in developing a reasonable differential diagnosis, there is often considerable overlap in the clinical presentation and physical findings between various pathologic entities. Imaging plays an important role in narrowing the differential diagnosis and in directing appropriate therapy. This article reviews the normal anatomy of the hallucal sesamoidal complex and the plantar capsular structures of the first metatarsophalangeal joint. Typical clinical presentations are discussed for various pathologic entities that involve this area of the hallux, followed by a summary of the various imaging findings that occur when using conventional radiography, nuclear medicine bone scan, CT and MR imaging. Finally, general treatment guidelines are discussed for each entity.

**Imaging of Soft Tissue Lesions of the Foot and Ankle**     1093

Laura W. Bancroft, Jeffrey J. Peterson, and Mark J. Kransdorf

Differential diagnosis of soft tissue lesions of the foot can be narrowed with imaging. The cystic nature of ganglia, synovial cysts, and bursitis can be confirmed with MR imaging or sonography. Location and signal characteristics of noncystic lesions can suggest Morton's neuroma, giant cell tumor of tendon sheath, and plantar fibromatosis. Synovial-based lesions of the foot and ankle can be differentiated based on presence or absence of mineralization, lesion density, signal intensity, and enhancement pattern. Knowledge of the incidence of specific neoplasms of the foot and ankle based on patient age aids in providing a limited differential diagnosis.

**Current Concepts in Imaging Diabetic Pedal Osteomyelitis**     1105

Andrea Donovan and Mark E. Schweitzer

Diabetic pedal osteomyelitis is primarily a manifestation of vascular insufficiency with resultant tissue ischemia, neuropathy, and infection. Nearly all cases of pedal osteomyelitis arise from a contiguous ulcer and soft tissue infection. MR imaging is the modality of choice to assess for the presence of osteomyelitis and associated soft tissue complications, to guide patient management, and to aid in limited limb resection.

**Index**     1125

## GOAL STATEMENT

The goal of the *Radiologic Clinics of North America* is to keep practicing radiologists and radiology residents up to date with current clinical practice in radiology by providing timely articles reviewing the state of the art in patient care.

## ACCREDITATION

The *Radiologic Clinics of North America* is planned and implemented in accordance with the Essential Areas and Policies of the Accreditation Council for Continuing Medical Education (ACCME) through the joint sponsorship of the University of Virginia School of Medicine and Elsevier. The University of Virginia School of Medicine is accredited by the ACCME to provide continuing medical education for physicians.

The University of Virginia School of Medicine designates this educational activity for a maximum of 15 *AMA PRA Category 1 Credits*™. Physicians should only claim credit commensurate with the extent of their participation in the activity.

The American Medical Association has determined that physicians not licensed in the US who participate in this CME activity are eligible for 15 *AMA PRA Category 1 Credits*™.

Credit can be earned by reading the text material, taking the CME examination online at http://www.theclinics.com/home/cme, and completing the evaluation. After taking the test, you will be required to review any and all incorrect answers. Following completion of the test and evaluation, your credit will be awarded and you may print your certificate.

## FACULTY DISCLOSURE/CONFLICT OF INTEREST

The University of Virginia School of Medicine, as an ACCME accredited provider, endorses and strives to comply with the Accreditation Council for Continuing Medical Education (ACCME) Standards of Commercial Support, Commonwealth of Virginia statutes, University of Virginia policies and procedures, and associated federal and private regulations and guidelines on the need for disclosure and monitoring of proprietary and financial interests that may affect the scientific integrity and balance of content delivered in continuing medical education activities under our auspices.

The University of Virginia School of Medicine requires that all CME activities accredited through this institution be developed independently and be scientifically rigorous, balanced and objective in the presentation/discussion of its content, theories and practices.

All authors/editors participating in an accredited CME activity are expected to disclose to the readers relevant financial relationships with commercial entities occurring within the past 12 months (such as grants or research support, employee, consultant, stock holder, member of speakers bureau, etc.). The University of Virginia School of Medicine will employ appropriate mechanisms to resolve potential conflicts of interest to maintain the standards of fair and balanced education to the reader. Questions about specific strategies can be directed to the Office of Continuing Medical Education, University of Virginia School of Medicine, Charlottesville, Virginia.

The faculty and staff of the University of Virginia Office of Continuing Medical Education have no financial affiliations to disclose.

**The authors/editors listed below have identified no financial or professional relationships for themselves or their spouse/partner:**

Joseph M. Bestic, MD; Ana Canga, MD; Luis Cerezal, MD; Julia R. Crim, MD; Andrea Donovan, MD; Barton Dudlick (Acquisitions Editor); Julie M. Gregg, GDU, PhD; Stephen F. Hatem, MD; Melanie Hopper, MD, MBChB, MRCS, FRCR; Theodore E. Keats, MD (Test Author); Mark J. Kransdorf, MD; Eva Llopis, MD; Paul Marks, MD; Ketan N. Naran, MD; Jeffrey J. Peterson, MD; Sharik Kabir Rathur, MD; Alejandro Rolón, MD; Philip Robinson, MD, MBChB, MRCP, FRCR; Timothy G. Sanders, MD; Timothy E. Schneider, MD; Mark E. Schweitzer, MD; and Hilary Umans, MD (Guest Editor).

**The authors/editors listed below have identified the following financial or professional relationships for themselves or their spouse/partner:**

**Laura W. Bancroft, MD** serves on the Speakers Bureau for Ryals Meeting Planner.
**David P. Fessell, MD** is a consultant for Bioimaging.
**Jon A. Jacobson, MD** receives an honorarium from Elsevier Saunders and is a consultant for Sonosite, Hitachi, and Bio!maging Technologies.
**Adam C. Zoga, MD** serves on the Speakers Bureau for Bayer Healthcare North America.

*Disclosure of Discussion of Non-FDA Approved Uses for Pharmaceutical and/or Medical Devices*

**The University of Virginia School of Medicine, as an ACCME provider, requires that all faculty presenters identify and disclose any off-label uses for pharmaceutical and medical device products. The University of Virginia School of Medicine recommends that each physician fully review all the available data on new products or procedures prior to clinical use.**

## TO ENROLL

To enroll in the Radiologic Clinics of North America Continuing Medical Education program, call customer service at 1-800-654-2452 or sign up online at http://www.theclinics.com/home/cme. The CME program is available to subscribers for an additional annual fee USD 205.

# Radiologic Clinics of North America

## FORTHCOMING ISSUES

*January 2009*

**New Imaging Technologies**
Dushyant Sahani, MD and
Vahid Yaghmai, MD, *Guest Editors*

*March 2009*

**Imaging of Airway Diseases**
Philippe Grenier, MD, *Guest Editor*

## RECENT ISSUES

*September 2008*

**Imaging of Intestinal Ischemia and Infarction**
Stefania Romano, MD, *Guest Editor*

*July 2008*

**Imaging of the Geriatric Patient**
Giuseppe Guglielmi, MD, *Guest Editor*

## RELATED INTEREST

*November 2008*
Magnetic Resonance Imaging Clinics of North America
**Foot and Ankle**
Douglas P. Beall, MD and Scot E. Campbell, MD, *Guest Editors*

**THE CLINICS ARE NOW AVAILABLE ONLINE!**

Access your subscription at:
**www.theclinics.com**

# Preface

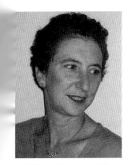

Hilary Umans, MD
*Guest Editor*

I confess I have always been a musculoskeletal radiologist with a bit of a foot fetish. It has frustrated me that many texts and articles entitled "Foot and Ankle Imaging" tend to give the foot short shrift, although it usually commands first billing. Having been disappointed with available texts on the subject, I have relied on original research articles to find the answers to the many questions I have had. So you can imagine my enthusiasm when I was presented with the opportunity to fashion my own custom-ordered text on foot and ankle imaging. That is the deal I was offered when I was invited to guest edit this issue. I had the unique opportunity to invite review articles on topics of my choice from foremost experts in the field from around the country and around the world.

I have chosen to include the mid- and forefoot in the mix with articles on sesamoiditis and metatarsalgia, in addition to midfoot sprain and tarsal coalition. I have tried to focus on conditions that present a diagnostic challenge, including ankle impingement syndromes, osteochondral lesions, and soft tissue lesions. I sought to extend the scope of ankle imaging beyond conventional radiography, CT, and MR imaging by including a comprehensive review of magnetic resonance arthrography, which is commonly used in the evaluation of shoulder instability but may provide critical information in assessment of refractory painful ankle syndromes. For that matter, sonography is ideally suited for evaluation of foot and ankle pathologic conditions, permitting high resolution and real-time assessment and combining dynamic maneuvers with direct physical examination and communication with the patient. It is my goal to bring these modalities out of the closet of subspecialty journals and take the discussion to a wider audience.

Inasmuch as diabetic pedal osteomyelitis remains a major public health problem and drives much of the inpatient foot and ankle imaging, no monograph on foot and ankle imaging would be complete without a comprehensive review of the current concepts of imaging foot infection and neuropathic arthropathy. Finally, ankle arthroplasty represents one of the final frontiers in joint replacement and is unfamiliar to most of us. There are a variety of prostheses with a range of normal postoperative appearances and unique complications that have been expertly illustrated and thoroughly reviewed in this issue.

It is my sincere hope that these excellent comprehensive articles inspire the readers to venture south of the knee and discover what I find so challenging and alluring in imaging the foot and ankle.

Hilary Umans, MD
Department of Radiology
Jacobi Medical Center
Albert Einstein College of Medicine
1400 Pelham Parkway
Bronx, NY 10461

E-mail address:
hilary.umans@gmail.com (H. Umans)

Radiol Clin N Am 46 (2008) xi
doi:10.1016/j.rcl.2008.10.002

# Ankle Impingement Syndromes

Melanie A. Hopper, MBChB, MRCS, FRCR,
Philip Robinson, MBChB, MRCP, FRCR*

**KEYWORDS**

- Ankle impingement • MR imaging • Ultrasound
- Athletic injury

The ankle impingement syndromes are defined as pathologic conditions causing painful restriction of movement at the tibiotalar joint caused by osseous or soft tissue overgrowth or by the presence of accessory ossification centers. First described by Morris[1] in 1943 and then by McMurray[2] in 1950, who termed the condition "footballer's ankle," ankle impingement is now an established cause of ongoing ankle dysfunction, often following seemingly trivial trauma. Originally studied in athletes, impingement is now also acknowledged as a cause of persisting symptoms in the general population. Ankle sprains are common, and although in most no significant sequelae develop, 15% to 20% of sports injuries result in continuing symptoms caused by a range of chronic and subacute pathologies including osteochondral defects, tendon injuries, mechanical instability, and impingement.[3]

Classification of the ankle impingement syndromes is anatomic according to their relationship to the tibiotalar joint. Each anatomic site may have similar injury etiology, but presents with differing clinical signs and symptoms and imaging findings.

## ANTERIOR IMPINGEMENT SYNDROME

Anterior impingement is a relatively common cause of chronic ankle pain seen particularly in such athletes as ballet dancers and soccer players.[4–6] Symptoms are generally progressive and are caused by impingement of hypertrophied soft tissue and bony spurs within the anterior ankle joint.

### Anatomy and Pathophysiology

Characteristically, there is formation of bony prominences at the anterior rim of the tibial plafond and at the opposing aspect of the talus. Originally, these bony spurs were thought to represent a response to capsular traction during plantar flexion.[1,2] Anatomic studies have demonstrated, however, that these anterior tibiotalar spurs are formed within the anterior ankle joint capsule (**Figs. 1** and **2**), rather than at the site of capsular insertion, making repetitive capsular traction an unlikely etiology.[4,7]

These bony spurs are thought to develop in response to repetitive trauma to the anterior articular cartilage rim either from repeated dorsiflexion when there is impaction between the anterior tibia and talus,[4,7] or from external direct trauma to the anterior ankle joint as is seen during ball strike in soccer players. Evaluation of ankle biomechanics during ball strike has revealed that spurs typically form at the location of ball impact, suggesting that the spurs develop in response to the direct trauma rather than capsular traction.[6] Microfractures of trabecular bone and periosteal hemorrhage resulting from the repetitive trauma heal to form new bone that develops into the characteristic bony spurs. In addition to injury to the bony articular rim, trauma to the anterior chondral margin of the ankle joint may lead to reparative formation of fibrous tissue and subsequent ossification.[8]

In addition to the osseous element of anterior impingement there is an important associated soft tissue component.[7] Bony spurs have been noted to be present in both athletes and

Leeds Teaching Hospitals, Chapel Allerton Hospital, Leeds, UK LS7 4SA
* Corresponding author. Musculoskeletal Centre X-Ray Department, Chapel Allerton Hospital, Leeds, UK LS7 4SA.
*E-mail address:* p.robinson@leedsth.nhs.uk (P. Robinson).

Radiol Clin N Am 46 (2008) 957–971
doi:10.1016/j.rcl.2008.08.001

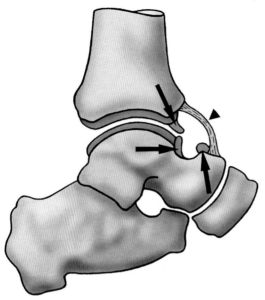

Fig. 1. Diagrammatic representation of the ankle shows the most common sites for anterior tibiotalar spur development (*arrows*) within the joint capsule (*arrowhead*).

nonathletes who have no symptoms of anterior ankle impingement.[4,7,9] In addition, postexcision recurrence of the bony spurs is not accompanied by recurrence of symptoms indicating the

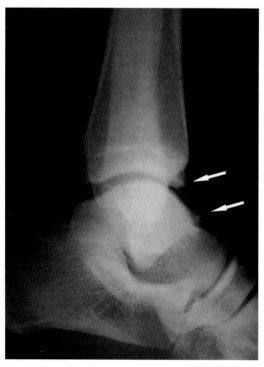

Fig. 2. Lateral radiograph shows anterior tibiotalar spurs (*arrows*) in a soccer player with clinical anterior impingement.

significance of the associated soft tissue abnormality in precipitating the clinical syndrome.[8,10]

## Clinical Features

Typically, anterior impingement syndrome presents with anterior ankle pain exacerbated by dorsiflexion. Clinical examination may reveal soft tissue swelling over the anterior aspect of the ankle joint with reduced range of dorsiflexion. Movement limitation can sometimes be overcome by excessive ankle pronation, but this additional abnormality in ankle biomechanics may have further consequences.[5] In some instances the anterior bony spurs may be palpable.

## Imaging

The diagnosis of anterior impingement is primarily a clinical one. Imaging can exclude other causes of ankle pain, such as osteochondral defects or fracture, and conventional radiography can confirm the presence of anterior tibiotalar spurs, although anteromedial spurs may be more difficult to identify. Combining a lateral radiograph with an oblique anteromedial impingement radiograph has been shown to increase the sensitivity of plain radiography, but there is a concomitant decrease in specificity.[11] Although there is a grading system for anterior impingement based on clinical findings and the size of spurs on conventional radiography,[12] these features have not been shown to correlate well with outcome. The absence of preoperative degenerative changes within the ankle joint is a more consistent indicator of likely treatment success. Several studies have demonstrated that patients with associated ankle joint degenerative changes are significantly more likely to have poor long-term outcome following surgical treatment.[8,10] Further imaging is often unnecessary but, particularly if coexistent ankle pathology is suspected, MR imaging may be useful.[13] As in anterolateral impingement demonstration of extensive bone marrow edema is uncommon, but the extent of synovitis and joint capsule thickening may be evident (**Fig. 3**).[14]

## Treatment

Conservative management including limitation of symptom-provoking activity combined with physiotherapy is successful in most patients. Particularly in ballet dancers this should be performed in conjunction with correction of technique to correct overpronation where appropriate.

Surgical intervention is generally reserved for those cases where conservative therapies have failed to provide adequate relief. Long-term follow-up studies have shown open and arthroscopic

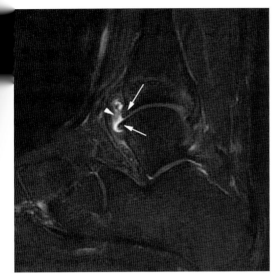

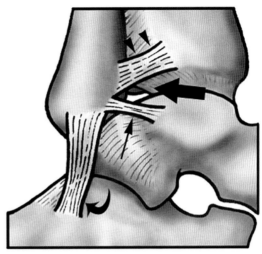

**Fig. 3.** Sagittal T2-weighted fat-suppressed MR image shows anterior tibial and talar spurs (*arrows*), anterior effusion, and irregular capsular thickening (*arrowhead*).

**Fig. 4.** Illustration of anterolateral anatomy of the ankle. Anterolateral recess (*thick arrow*) sited between anterior tibiofibular ligament (*arrowheads*) and anterior talofibular ligament (*thin arrow*). Note calcaneofibular ligament (*curved arrow*).

excision of the bony spurs, hypertrophic synovium, and scar tissue to be effective treatments for anterior impingement providing there is no evidence of preoperative joint space narrowing.[8,10,15,16] With either technique a return to full activity is expected, even in elite athletes.

## ANTEROLATERAL IMPINGEMENT

Anterolateral impingement is a relatively uncommon cause of anterolateral ankle pain caused by entrapment of hypertrophied soft tissues within the anterolateral recess of the ankle.

### Anatomy and Pathophysiology

The anterolateral recess is triangular in cross-section and is limited posteriorly by the anterolateral tibia and talus, anteromedial fibula, and anteriorly by the joint capsule, the anterior inferior tibiofibular, anterior talofibular, and calcaneofibular ligaments (**Fig. 4**).[17] Classically anterolateral impingement syndrome is described in young athletic patients who have experienced a relatively minor injury to the anterolateral ankle ligaments or the joint capsule, either as a single inversion injury or because of repetitive plantar flexion and inversion.[18,19] The initial sprain may be minor and not recalled. Despite no initial apparent sequelae, recurrent subclinical instability and associated microtrauma may cause intra-articular and soft tissue hemorrhage, localized reactive synovial hyperplasia, and scarring. Compression of the abnormal anterolateral soft tissue during

eversion or dorsiflexion causes symptoms of impingement. In advanced cases the soft tissue can become molded within the anterolateral recess to form a reactive hyalinzed connective tissue mass termed the "meniscoid lesion" by Wolin and colleagues.[20]

Anterolateral impingement has also been described in a subset of individuals with a distal or accessory fascicle of the anterior inferior tibiofibular ligament.[17,21] This ligament is multifascicular and may be present as two or three separate bands extending from the anterior aspect of the lateral malleolus to the anterolateral tubercle of the tibia. An accessory fascicle has been identified in 21% to 97% of patients as a band oriented in parallel to the main ligament but separated from it by a fibrofatty septum.[22] The apparent disparity in incidence is likely to be caused by lack of consensus as to the definition of a separate fascicle but its presence is thought to represent a normal anatomic variant. Contact between the anterolateral corner of the talus and the anteroinferior tibiofibular ligament may be normal in some cases, but if the anterolateral ankle is lax this allows increased pressure because of anterior extrusion of the talar dome in dorsiflexion. This potentially initiates inflammatory changes within the ligament with resultant hypertrophy and injury, predisposing it to impingement. Chondral injury of the anterolateral corner of the talus caused by abrasion from the impinging anteroinferior tibiofibular ligament can be identified at arthroscopy and on imaging.[17,21]

## Clinical Features

Clinical assessment is reasonably accurate in the diagnosis of anterolateral impingement.[23] Antero-lateral ankle pain with tenderness and swelling are suggestive of the diagnosis but can be present in other entities, such as peroneal tendon pathology, sinus tarsi syndrome, stress fractures, chronic ankle instability, and intra-articular loose bodies, many of which may also develop subsequent to ankle trauma.

Several clinical tests have been described but symptoms exacerbated by single leg squatting and ankle eversion or dorsiflexion have been shown retrospectively to correlate best with positive findings of impingement at arthroscopy.[24] Molloy and colleagues[25] have described a clinical sign elicited by impinging abnormal hypertrophic synovium within the tibiotalar joint causing pain. They report a 94.8% sensitivity and 88% specificity in a prospective study of this lateral impingement test. The subset of individuals with impingement secondary to an accessory anteroinferior tibiofibular ligament may describe a popping sensation or an audible pop on ankle dorsiflexion and eversion.

## Imaging

A study of ultrasound assessment in patients with clinical anterolateral impingement identified a nodular, mixed echogenic, synovitic mass within the anterolateral recess of 100% of eight patients (**Fig. 5A**).[26] The mass could be extruded anteriorly with manual compression and in the study group measured greater than 1 cm diameter. Power Doppler interrogation was found to be unhelpful. Importantly, findings were not dependent on the presence of an ankle joint effusion, unlike MR imaging.[27] Ultrasound also identified bony spurs and injury to the anterior talofibular ligament (**Fig. 5B**). Similar findings were seen in two of the control group, however, where anterolateral masses were identified in patients without accompanying symptoms.[26] A similar study of 14 sportsmen, however, concluded that ultrasound evaluation was nonspecific with changes demonstrated within the anterior talofibular ligaments of all subjects.[28]

The predominating soft tissue changes and lack of a bony component to anterolateral impingement makes plain radiography and conventional CT assessment unhelpful. A study of CT arthrography showed nodular fraying or thickening, seen best on coronal images that correlated well with soft tissue impingement at arthroscopy.[29]

The use of conventional MR imaging in anterolateral impingement remains controversial. Some authors have found it to be beneficial, but several studies have found conventional MR imaging to be unhelpful.[30–33] Thickening of the anterior talofibular ligament and lateral gutter fullness is suggestive of the diagnosis and is most reliably demonstrated on T1 axial imaging (**Fig. 5; Fig. 6**).[18,34] Confirmation of axial findings using a sagittal T1 sequence has been suggested, because displacement of the normal fat anterior to the fibula by synovitis or scar tissue can be evaluated (**Fig. 5D**).[34] Most groups, however, believe that conventional MR imaging is only reliably diagnostic in the presence of an ankle effusion.[14,27]

MR arthrography has proved to be an accurate method of evaluation of the anterolateral recess. Positive findings of anterolateral scarring and synovitis can be identified as capsular adherence to the fibula and tibia, presumably because of adhesion formation (**Fig. 6C**). As in ultrasound assessment, clinical correlation is essential because these features can also be seen without symptoms of anterolateral impingement. MR arthrography also demonstrates additional pathology, such as abnormalities of the anterior talofibular ligament, chondral damage, and bony spurs.[23]

## Management

As in other impingement syndromes, initial treatment is conservative with immobilization, physiotherapy, and nonsteroidal anti-inflammatory medication, reserving surgery for resistant cases.[24,35] Dry needling with injection of steroid and local anesthetic can be performed under ultrasound guidance allowing a return to previous levels of activity even in elite athletes, but this technique has not been evaluated in the literature. Arthroscopic resection of hypertrophic synovium and scar tissue gives symptomatic and functional improvement and allows resection of a distal fascicle of the anterior talofibular ligament when that is the underlying etiology (**Fig. 6B**).

## ANTEROMEDIAL IMPINGEMENT

An uncommon cause of chronic ankle pain, anteromedial impingement rarely occurs as an isolated finding.[36,37]

## Anatomy and Pathophysiology

First described in a case report of an anteromedial meniscoid lesion similar to that seen in anterolateral impingement, the initial proposed mechanism of injury was eversion of the ankle joint with resultant traction of the anterior tibiotalar ligament.[38] Subsequent surgical and radiologic series, although

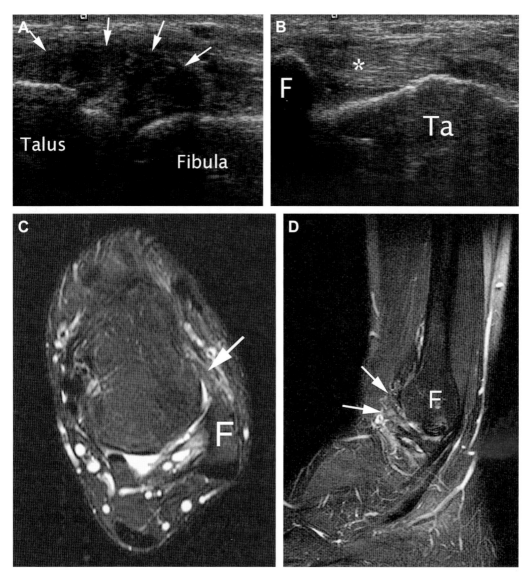

**Fig. 5.** Patients with clinical anterolateral impingement. Axial ultrasounds show (*A*) hypoechoic nodule (*arrows*) in anterolateral recess and (*B*) thickening of anterior talofibular ligament (*) F, fibula; Ta, talus axial (*C*) and sagittal (*D*) T2-weighted fat-suppressed MR images show anterolateral synovitis (*arrows*) anterior to the fibula (F).

not large, have suggested that anteromedial impingement instead represents a rare complication of inversion trauma at the tibiotalar joint, perhaps with a rotational component.[36,37] As in anterolateral impingement it is thought that subsequent microtrauma and healing following the original inversion injury initiates synovial, ligamentous, and capsular thickening within the anteromedial compartment that can become compressed during dorsiflexion and inversion.

### Clinical Features

Patients describe focal anteromedial tenderness and pain that is exacerbated by dorsiflexion and inversion, clinical examination shows restriction of these movements. There may be associated soft tissue thickening.

### Imaging

Although in some patients bony spurs have been shown to be a feature of anteromedial impingement,[36] they are not the dominant feature and so plain radiography and conventional CT assessment are usually not of use.

There have been no imaging studies assessing the use of ultrasound or conventional MR imaging in anteromedial impingement. In the largest clinical series 2 of 11 patients underwent MR imaging that

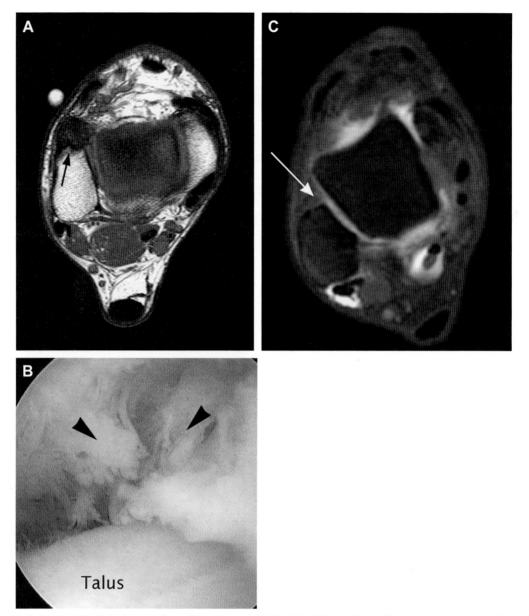

Fig. 6. Patients with clinical anterolateral impingement. (*A*) Axial T1-weighted MR image shows irregular soft tissue thickening (*arrow*) in anterolateral recess. (*B*) Corresponding arthroscopic image shows synovitis and nodularity (*arrowheads*) within anterolateral recess. (*Courtesy of* Steve Bollen, MD, Bradford, UK.) (*C*) Axial T1-weighted fat-suppressed MR arthrogram image shows capsular adherence with no recess of fluid anterior to the fibula (*arrow*).

was thought to be inconclusive. Perhaps unsurprisingly given the proposed mechanism of injury, five cases were found at surgery to have lateral ligamentous injury.[36] A prospective evaluation of MR arthrography in two patients with clinical anteromedial impingement demonstrated irregular soft tissue thickening anterior to the anterior tibiotalar ligament in both patients, which was shown to represent synovitis at subsequent arthroscopy (**Fig. 7**). One patient also had an anteromedial joint capsule tear diagnosed at MR imaging arthrography and confirmed surgically.[37] In some patients, bony spurs have been shown to be a feature of anteromedial impingement and have been described on imaging and at surgery.

## Management

There are currently no cases describing nonsurgical treatment of anteromedial impingement in the

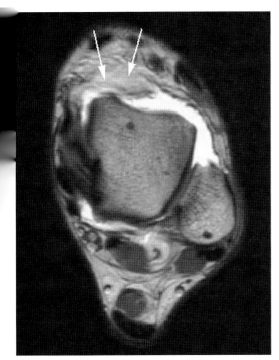

Fig. 7. Axial T1-weighted MR arthrogram image from patient with anteromedial impingement shows irregular soft tissue thickening within anteromedial ankle joint (*arrows*).

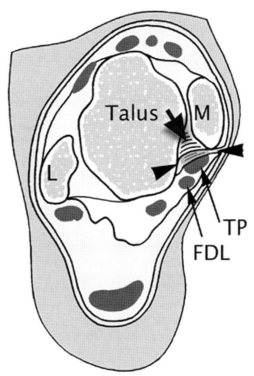

Fig. 8. Axial illustration shows structures involved in posteromedial impingement (see text). M, medial malleolus; TP, tibialis posterior tendon; FDL, flexor digitorum longus tendon; L, lateral malleolus. Arrowheads denote posterior fibers of tibiotalar ligament; short arrow indicates deep fibers of tibiotalar ligament.

literature. Surgical excision of abnormal synovial tissue and bony spurs gives symptomatic relief and functional improvement.[35,36,38]

## POSTEROMEDIAL IMPINGEMENT

Until recently posteromedial impingement was one of the least described ankle impingement syndromes and accordingly its etiology was less well understood. Although there are few reported series they have identified relatively characteristic imaging findings.

### Anatomy and Pathophysiology

Surgical and radiologic studies have identified posteromedial impingement following severe inversion injury at the ankle joint.[39,40] Injury of the anterior talofibular ligament during inversion allows compression of posteromedial structures including the posteromedial joint capsule, posterior tibiotalar ligament, and posteromedial flexor tendons between the medial wall of the talus and the medial malleolus (**Fig. 8**). In some cases inadequate healing of posteromedial soft tissues forms thickened and disorganized fibrous tissue within the posteromedial ankle joint, which impinges

between the posterior aspect of the medial malleolus and the medial talus.[39]

### Clinical Features

Following the initial injury lateral symptoms predominate; as these settle there is insidious onset of posteromedial and medial activity-related pain, typically after 4 to 6 weeks.[39] There is focal posteromedial tenderness on examination and pain can be elicited by posteromedial palpation during plantar flexion and inversion. Similar symptoms may also be found in early tibialis posterior dysfunction, although patients have no history of trauma. Distinction between posteromedial impingement and tibialis posterior dysfunction is clinical; in the latter patients describe progressive pes planus and are restricted in their ability to stand on tiptoe with loss of normal heel inversion during this maneuver.

### Imaging

Because soft tissue abnormality is the basis of posteromedial impingement, plain radiography and CT are usually unhelpful but very rarely accessory medial talar tubercle ossification can contribute to soft tissue thickening (**Fig. 9**).

A single study identified increased radionuclide uptake in the region of the posteromedial ankle on isotope bone scanning; however, bone scanning was unable to define further associated injuries subsequently identified and treated at arthroscopy.[41]

Ultrasound and MR imaging have been jointly assessed in radiologic studies of patients with clinically diagnosed posteromedial impingement. Messiou and colleagues[40] imaged nine elite athletes 4 to 6 weeks following injury using both modalities as did Koulouris and colleagues[41] who assessed 25 patients greater than 1 year following initial trauma. Despite small numbers of subjects, these studies revealed relatively consistent findings on MR imaging and on ultrasound. MR imaging demonstrated loss of the normal fat striations within the posterior tibiotalar ligament, posteromedial synovitis, and abnormal signal and thickening within the posteromedial joint capsule that in some cases displaced or surrounded the adjacent tendons (**Fig. 9B; Fig. 10A**).[40,41] Posteromedial capsulitis, however, was also identified in the control group of one study. These patients clinically had posterolateral impingement and no symptoms or signs of posteromedial impingement.[40] A total of 100% of patients in both studies were shown to have posteromedial abnormalities on ultrasound either thickening of the posteromedial capsule or posteromedial synovial hypertrophy and, as on MR imaging, displacement or entrapment of adjacent tendons was also elicited (**Fig. 10B**).[40,41] It is possible that the apparent differences in scarring around the tendons between the two studies are related to differences in timing of imaging following the initial trauma and reflect the natural history and development of posteromedial impingement syndrome.

## Management

In addition to identifying posteromedial impingement, MR imaging helps to exclude or confirm other pathologies particularly within the anterolateral ankle.[40,41] Clinical correlation is essential, because imaging findings do not always reflect symptomatic impingement.[40] Ultrasound-guided dry needling of the capsular abnormality with injection of steroid and local anesthetic, in most cases, allows a return to previous levels of activity even in elite athletes (**Fig. 10**).[40] Successful outcome has also been demonstrated following surgical resection of abnormal posteromedial soft

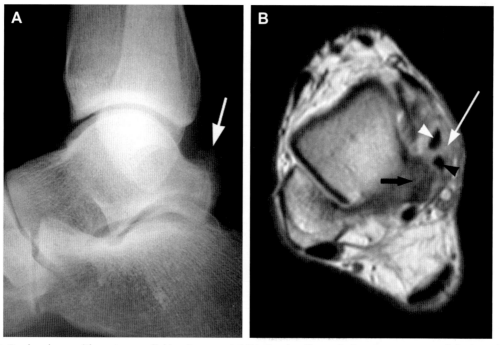

**Fig. 9.** Rugby player with posteromedial impingement. (*A*) Lateral radiograph shows accessory medial talar tubercle (*arrow*). (*B*) Axial proton-density weighted MR image shows accessory medial talar tubercle (*black arrow*). Posteromedial soft tissue thickening (*white arrow*) encases tendons of tibialis posterior (*white arrowhead*) and flexor digitorum longus (*black arrowhead*).

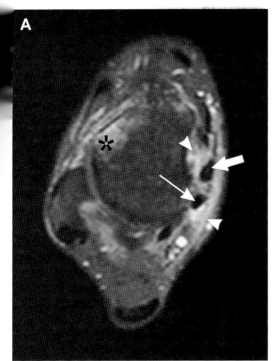

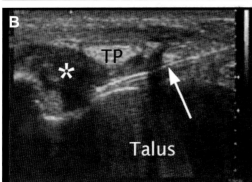

Fig. 10. Soccer player with clinical posteromedial impingement. (A) Axial T1 fat-suppressed image following IV gadolinium shows posteromedial synovitis (*arrowheads*) displacing tibialis posterior (*thick arrow*) and flexor digitorum longus (*thin arrow*) tendons. Note resolving anterolateral talar injury (*). (B) Axial ultrasound image of posteromedial recess during guided injection (*arrow*) shows displacement of tibialis posterior (TP) by hypoechoic synovitis (*).

tissue without ligamentous repair,[39,41] but should be reserved for cases resistant to ultrasound-guided therapy.

## POSTERIOR IMPINGEMENT

Posterior impingement syndrome encompasses a group of pathologies that are characterized by posterior ankle pain in plantar flexion. Symptoms result from compression of the talus and soft tissues between the posterior tibia and calcaneum. Other terms, such as "os trigonum syndrome," "talar compression syndrome," and "posterior block," have also been used to describe the same collection of signs and symptoms. Posterior ankle pain is a common symptom and may be caused by a range of soft tissue and osseous abnormalities. Overall, pathology of the Achilles tendon is the most common cause of posterior ankle pain but similar symptoms are also experienced with flexor hallucis longus tendonopathy, osteochondritis dissecans, retrocalcaneal bursitis, and tarsal tunnel syndrome.

### Anatomy and Pathophysiology

Pathology related to the os-trigonum-talar process is the most common cause of posterior impingement and has been extensively studied. The posterior talar process extends posteromedial to the tibiotalar joint and has two projections. The smaller medial process is separated from the larger lateral tubercle by a shallow groove that contains the flexor hallucis longus tendon. Ossification of the talar body is evident from 6 months of fetal development. The posterior talus ossifies from a secondary ossification center, mineralization starts between 7 and 13 years, and generally fusion with the talar body occurs within 12 months to form the lateral tubercle. In some individuals the lateral tubercle is particularly elongated and is termed the "Steida process." Failure of fusion between the talar body and the lateral tubercle occurs in 14% to 25% of the normal population[42] and is bilateral in 1.4%. The ossicle formed is known as the "os trigonum" and articulates with the main body of the talus at a cartilaginous synchondrosis (**Fig. 11**). Although the os trigonum appears round or oval on radiographs it is, as its name suggests, triangular in shape having three articular surfaces.[42] The anterior articular surface articulates with the talar body, the posterior facet gives attachment for the posterior talofibular and posterior talocalcaneal ligaments,[43] and the inferior aspect may articulate with the superior surface of the calcaneum.

Although the presence or absence of a Steida process or os trigonum is important in posterior impingement, the articular surface of the posterior tibia and the calcaneal tuberosity are also involved in the impingement mechanism. The posterior tibial articular surface, or posterior malleolus, may have a more or less downward sloping configuration and in some individuals the posterior process of the calcaneum may be prominent.

Soft tissue impingement may involve the posterior capsule, the posterior talofibular, and posterior

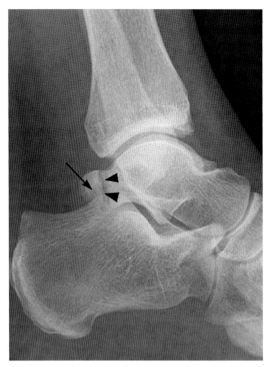

Fig. 11. Lateral radiograph shows os trigonum (*arrow*) separated from talus by cartilaginous synchondrosis (*arrowheads*).

intermalleolar and tibiofibular ligaments, any of which can become compressed between the posterior tibial plafond and the superior aspect of the calcaneum. The flexor hallucis longus tendon runs between the medial and lateral talar tubercles where it is held in a fibro-osseous tunnel by the overlying extensor retinaculum. Injury to the tendon as part of posterior impingement is typically, but not exclusively, seen in ballet dancers and can result in tenosynovitis; in extreme cases the tendon can become tethered.[44,45]

The posterior intermalleolar ligament is an anatomic variant of the posterior ligaments of the ankle. The ligament extends obliquely from the posterior margin of the medial malleolus to the superior margin of the fibular malleolar fossa between the inferior transverse ligament and the posterior talofibular ligament (**Fig. 12**A). Cadaveric studies suggest it is present in 56% of individuals, although it was identified in only 19% of MR images of asymptomatic patients (**Fig. 12**B).[46] During its course the posterior intermalleolar ligament can herniate into the posterior ankle joint and bucket handle tears and entrapment of the ligament have been described as a cause of posterior impingement in ballet dancers.[47]

Whatever the underlying anatomy, the typical etiology for the development of posterior ankle impingement is chronic repetitive stress in plantar flexion. This is commonly encountered in ballet dancers because of the forced plantar flexion position required en pointe, and in this group posterior impingement has been extensively described.[43–45,47,48] Other athletes, such as soccer players and downhill runners, are also prone to posterior impingement because of stresses placed on the ankle joint during sporting activity. Soccer players experience forced plantar flexion during ball strike; the impact of the ball on the anterior ankle is a cause of anterior impingement but the compression of posterior structures also means this group of athletes is also at risk of posterior impingement.[49] Although posterior impingement is generally diagnosed because of repetitive stresses on the posterior ankle, the syndrome is also encountered following acute trauma. Forced plantar flexion can cause fracture of the lateral talar tubercle or separation of the cartilaginous synchondrosis if an os trigonum is present. Soccer players are prone to inversion injury with the ankle in a neutral position that places strain on the calcaneofibular and posterior talofibular ligaments and can result in posterior impingement subacutely.[49]

## Clinical Features

The predominant symptom is progressive posterior ankle pain. Patients may also complain of mild posterior swelling. Tenderness can be elicited on palpation of the posterolateral ankle between the Achilles and peroneal tendons.[48,49] On examination, pain is reproduced by plantar flexion or by dorsiflexion of the great toe. Associated tethering of the flexor hallucis longus tendon within the fibro-osseous tunnel behind the talus causes restricted plantar and dorsiflexion movement of the great toe itself.[48]

## Imaging

Plain radiography may demonstrate a Steida process or an os trigonum (see **Fig. 11**) that may or may not be the source of symptoms; however, it is not always possible to differentiate between a fractured lateral tubercle and an os trigonum even using more complex imaging.[48,50] Lateral radiographs taken in plantar flexion may reveal impingement of the lateral tubercle–os trigonum between the posterior tibia and the calcaneal tuberosity, although the size of the os trigonum is not a good predictor of symptoms.[51] Improved bony detail may be displayed using CT that more accurately demonstrates fractures of the lateral tubercle or separation at the cartilaginous synchondrosis.[50,52] More recently ultrasound has been used to interrogate the ankle in soccer players with

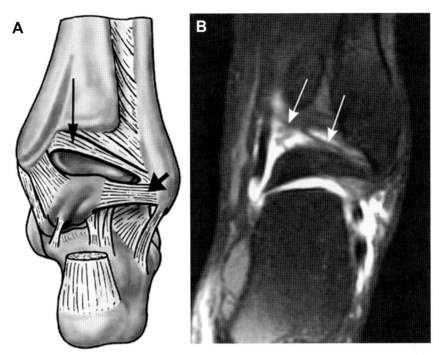

Fig. 12. (A) Illustration of posterior ankle shows posterior intermalleolar (*long arrow*) and posterior talofibular ligaments (*short arrow*). (B) Coronal T2-weighted MR image shows normal posterior intermalleolar ligament (*arrows*).

posterior impingement. This revealed nodular, hypoechoic thickening of the posterolateral joint capsule in 100% of 10 patients (**Fig. 13**).[49]

Posterolateral capsule thickening and synovitis within the posterior ankle is seen on MR imaging, which may also demonstrate osseous abnormalities, such as bone marrow edema, fragmentation of the lateral tubercle–os trigonum, and the presence of a pseudoarthrosis (**Figs. 14–16**).[50] Fluid within the flexor hallucis tendon sheath can also be identified (**Fig. 14B**);[50] however, care must be taken in interpretation of this finding because in 20% of normal individuals the tendon sheath communicates with the ankle joint and, not infrequently, a sizeable volume of fluid is seen in asymptomatic individuals.[53] A differential quantity of fluid above and below the level of the posterior talus has been suggested as the most likely finding consistent with entrapment of the flexor hallucis tendon.[51] Conventional MR imaging may also detect thickening of the posterior intermalleolar ligament, but this requires separate identification of the adjacent posterior talofibular and inferior tibiofibular ligaments and this is not always possible.[54]

*Management*

Initial management of posterior impingement is conservative. Confirmation of the os trigonum

synchondrosis as the site of pain can be achieved by injection of local anesthetic under fluoroscopic guidance if there is clinical uncertainty as to the diagnosis (**Fig. 17**).[55] Ultrasound-guided dry needling combined with local anesthetic and corticosteroid has been shown to be successful in the treatment of posterior impingement syndrome in soccer players, particularly in the absence of an os trigonum (see **Fig. 13**).[49] Surgical excision of

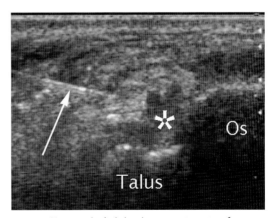

Fig. 13. Nonsurgical injection treatment of soccer player with clinical posterior impingement. Axial ultrasound shows nodular hypoechoic synovitis (*), os trigonum (Os), talus, and needle placement (*arrow*).

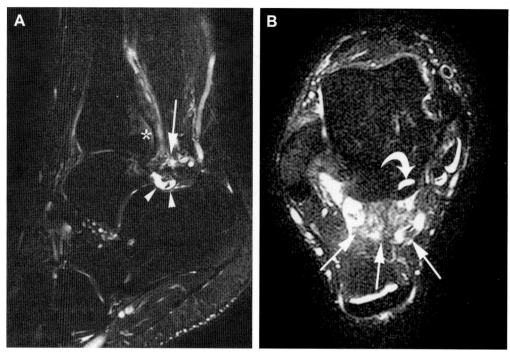

**Fig.14.** Ballet dancer with clinical posterior impingement. (*A*) Sagittal T2-weighted fat-suppressed MR image with the ankle in dorsiflexion to simulate en pointe position shows bone marrow edema in posterior tibia (*), joint effusion (*arrowheads*), posterior recess nodularity, and thickening (*arrow*). (*B*) Axial T2-weighted fat-suppressed MR image shows marked nodular synovitis (*arrows*) and minor fluid around flexor hallucis longus tendon (*curved arrow*).

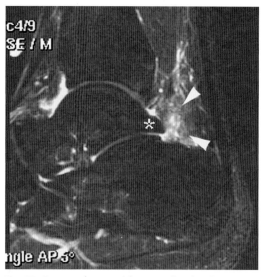

**Fig. 15.** Soccer player with posterior impingement. Sagittal T2-weighted fat-suppressed MR image shows steida process (*) and posterior capsular synovitis (*arrowheads*).

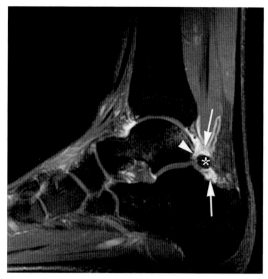

**Fig. 16.** Soccer player with posterior impingement. Sagittal T1-weighted fat-suppressed MR image following IV gadolinium shows os trigonum (*), cartilaginous synchondrosis (*arrowhead*), and posterior capsule enhancement (*arrows*).

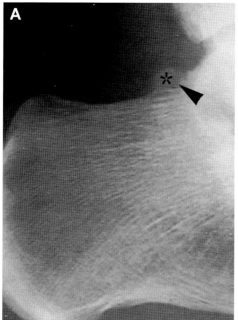
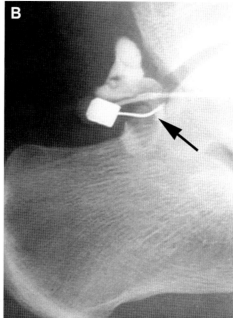

**Fig. 17.** Fluoroscopic-guided injection into os trigonum synchondrosis. (*A*) Os trigonum (*) and synchondrosis (*arrowhead*). (*B*) Contrast within synchondrosis (*arrow*).

osseous elements and any soft tissue component has a good prognosis in patients who fail to respond satisfactorily to conservative measures and can be combined with release of the flexor hallucis tendon if involved.[43,48]

## SUMMARY

The ankle impingement syndromes are an established cause of ankle dysfunction within the general population and within the athletic community. In many cases the diagnosis is clinical, although imaging has a significant role to play particularly in the exclusion of alternative or concomitant pathology or when the diagnosis is in doubt. For most patients conservative management or nonsurgical intervention allows resumption of their previous level of activity, even in elite athletes. Surgical treatment for more resistant cases has a low complication rate and a high level of success.

## REFERENCES

1. Morris LH. Athlete's ankle. J Bone Joint Surg 1943; 25:220.
2. McMurray TP. Footballer's ankle. J Bone Joint Surg Br 1950;32B:68–9.
3. Ogilvie-Harris DJ, Gilbart MK, Chorney K. Chronic pain following ankle sprains in athletes the role of arthroscopic surgery. Arthroscopy 1997;13:564–74.
4. O'Donoghue DH. Impingement exostoses of the talus and tibia. J Bone Joint Surg Am 1957;39:835–920.
5. O'Kane JW, Kadel N. Anterior impingement syndrome in dancers. Journal of Current Reviews in Musculoskeletal Medicine 2008;1:12–6.
6. Tol JL, Slim E, van Soest AJ, et al. The relationship of the kicking action in soccer and anterior ankle impingement syndrome: a biomechanical analysis. Am J Sports Med 2002;30:45–50.
7. Tol JL, van Dijk CN. Aetiology of the anterior ankle impingement syndrome: a descriptive anatomical study. Foot Ankle Int 2004;25(6):382–6.
8. Tol JL, Verheyen CP, van Dijk CN. Arthroscopic treatment of anterior impingement in the ankle. J Bone Joint Surg Br 2001;83:9–13.
9. Stoller SM, Hekmat F, Kleiger B. A comparative study of the frequency of anterior impingement exostoses in dancers and non-dancers. Foot Ankle 1984;4(4):201–3.
10. Coull R, Raffiq T, James LE, et al. Open treatment of anterior impingement of the ankle. J Bone Joint Surg Br 2003;85:550–3.
11. Tol JL, Verhagen RA, Krips R, et al. The anterior ankle impingement syndrome: diagnostic value of oblique radiographs. Foot Ankle Int 2004;25:63–8.
12. Van Dijk CN, Tol JL, Verheyen C. A prospective study of prognostic factors concerning the outcome of arthroscopic surgery for anterior ankle impingement. Am J Sports Med 1997;25:737–45.
13. Haller J, Bernt R, Seeger T, et al. MR-imaging of anterior tibiotalar impingement syndrome: agreement,

sensitivity and specificity of MR-imaging and indirect MR-arthrography. Eur J Radiol 2006;58:450–60.

14. Robinson P, White LM. Soft-tissue and osseous impingement syndromes of the ankle: role of imaging in diagnosis and management. Radiographics 2002;22:1457–69.

15. Scranton PE, McDermott JE. Anterior tibiotalar spurs: a comparison of open versus arthroscopic debridement. Foot Ankle 1992;13:125–9.

16. Nihal A, Rose DJ, Trepman E. Arthroscopic treatment of anterior impingement syndrome in dancers. Foot Ankle Int 2003;26(11):908–12.

17. Bassett FH III, Gates HS III, Billys JB, et al. Talar impingement by the anteroinferior tibiofibular ligament: a cause of chronic pain in the ankle after inversion sprain. J Bone Joint Surg Am 1990;72:55–9.

18. Ferkel RD, Karzel RP, Del Pizzo W, et al. Arthroscopic treatment of anterolateral impingement of the ankle. Am J Sports Med 1991;19:440–6.

19. Kim SH, Ha KI. Arthroscopic treatment for impingement of the anterolateral soft tissues of the ankle. J Bone Joint Surg Br 2000;82:1019–21.

20. Wolin I, Glassman F, Sideman S, et al. Internal derangement of the talofibular component of the ankle. Surg Gynecol Obstet 1950;91:193–200.

21. van den Bekerom MP, Raven EP. The distal fascicle of the anterior inferior tibiofibular ligament as a cause of tibiotalar impingement syndrome: a current concepts review. Knee Surg Sports Traumatol Arthrosc 2007;15:465–71.

22. Nikolopoulos CE, Tsirikos AI, Sourmelis S, et al. The accessory anteroinferior tibiofibular ligament as a cause of talar impingement: a cadaveric study. Am J Sports Med 2004;32:389–95.

23. Robinson P, White LM, Salonen DC, et al. Anterolateral ankle impingement: MR arthrographic assessment of the anterolateral recess. Radiology 2001; 221:186–90.

24. Lui HI, Raskin A, Osti I, et al. Arthroscopic treatment of anterolateral ankle impingement. Arthroscopy 1994;10:215–8.

25. Molloy S, Solan MC, Bendall SP. Synovial impingement in the ankle: a physical sign. J Bone Joint Surg Br 2003;85:330–3.

26. McCarthy CL, Wilson DJ, Coltman TP. Anterolateral ankle impingement: findings and diagnostic accuracy with ultrasound imaging. Skeletal Radiol 2008; 37(3):209–16.

27. Rubin DA, Tishkoff NW, Britton CA, et al. Anterolateral soft-tissue impingement in the ankle: diagnosis using MR imaging. AJR Am J Roentgenol 1997; 169:829–35.

28. Bagnolesi P, Zampa V, Carafoli D, et al. Anterolateral fibrous impingement of the ankle: report of 14 cases. Radiol Med (Torino) 1998;95(4):293–7.

29. Hauger O, Moinard M, Lasalarie JC, et al. Anterolateral compartment of the ankle in the lateral

impingement syndrome: appearance on CT arthrography. AJR Am J Roentgenol 1999;173:685–90.

30. Liu ST, Nuccion SL, Finerman G. Diagnosis of anterolateral ankle impingement: comparison between magnetic resonance imaging and clinical examination. Am J Sports Med 1997;25:389–93.

31. Farooki S, Yao L, Seeger LL. Anterolateral impingement of the ankle: effectiveness of MR imaging. Radiology 1998;207:357–60.

32. Jordan LK, Helms CA, Cooperman AE, et al. Magnetic resonance imaging findings in anterolateral impingement of the ankle. Skeletal Radiol 2000;29:34–9.

33. Cerezal L, Abascal F, Canga A, et al. MR imaging of ankle impingement syndromes. AJR Am J Roentgenol 2003;181:551–9.

34. Duncan D, Mologne T, Hildebrand H, et al. The usefulness of magnetic resonance imaging in the diagnosis of anterolateral impingement of the ankle. J Foot Ankle Surg 2006;45(5):304–7.

35. Meislin RJ. Arthroscopic treatment of synovial impingement of the ankle. Am J Sports Med 1993;21: 186–9.

36. Mosier-La Clair SM, Monroe MT, Manoli A. Medial impingement syndrome of the anterior tibiotalar fascicle of the deltoid ligament on the talus. Foot Ankle Int 2000;21:385–91.

37. Robinson P, White LM, Salonen D, et al. Anteromedial impingement of the ankle: using MR arthrography to assess the anteromedial recess. AJR Am J Roentgenol 2002;178:601–4.

38. Egol KA, Parisien JS. Impingement syndrome of the ankle caused by a medial meniscoid lesion. Arthroscopy 1997;13:522–5.

39. Paterson RS, Brown JN. The posteromedial impingement lesion of the ankle: a series of six cases. Am J Sports Med 2001;29:550–7.

40. Messiou C, Robinson P, O'Connor PJ, et al. Subacute posteromedial impingement of the ankle in athletes: MR imaging evaluation and ultrasound guided therapy. Skeletal Radiol 2006;35:88–94.

41. Koulouris G, Connell D, Schneider T, et al. Posterior tibitotalar ligament injury resulting in posteromedial impingement. Foot Ankle Int 2003;24(8):575–83.

42. Lawson JP. Clinically significant radiological anatomic variants of the skeleton. AJR Am J Roentgenol 1994;163:249–55.

43. Marotta JJ, Micheli LJ. Os trigonum impingement in dancers. Am J Sports Med 1992;20:533–6.

44. Hamilton WG, Geppert MJ, Thompson FM. Pain in the posterior aspect of the ankle in dancers: differential diagnosis and operative treatment. J Bone Joint Surg 1996;78:1491–500.

45. Hillier JC, Peace K, Hulme A, et al. MRI features of foot and ankle injuries in ballet dancers. Br J Radiol 2004;77:532–7.

46. Rosenburg ZS, Cheung YY, Beltran J, et al. Posterior intermalleolar ligament of the ankle: normal anatomy

and MR imaging features. AJR Am J Roentgenol 1995;165:387–90.

47. Hamilton WG. Foot and ankle injuries in dancers. Clin Sports Med 1988;143–73.

48. Brodsky AE, Momtaz AK. Talar compression syndrome. Am J Sports Med 1986;14:472–6.

49. Robinson P, Bollen SR. Posterior ankle impingement in professional soccer players: effectiveness of sonographically guided therapy. AJR Am J Roentgenol 2006;187:W53–8.

50. Bureau NJ, Cardinale E, Hobden R, et al. Posterior ankle impingement syndrome: MR imaging in seven patients. Radiology 2000;215:497–503.

51. Lo LD, Schweitzer ME, Fan JF, et al. MR imaging findings of entrapment of the flexor hallucis longus tendon. AJR Am J Roentgenol 2001;176:1145–8.

52. Karasick D, Schweitzer ME. The os trigonum syndrome: imaging features. AJR Am J Roentgenol 1996;166:125–9.

53. Schweitzer ME, van Leersum M, Ehrlich SS, et al. Fluid in normal and abnormal ankle joints: amount and distribution as seen on MR images. AJR Am J Roentgenol 1994;162:111–4.

54. Fiorella D, Helms CA, Nunley JA. The MR imaging features of the posterior intermalleolar ligament in patients with posterior impingement syndrome of the ankle. Skeletal Radiol 1999;28:573–6.

55. Mitchell MJ, Bielecki D, Bergman AG, et al. Localization of specific joint causing hindfoot pain: value of injecting local anesthetics into individual joints during arthrography. AJR Am J Roentgenol 1995;64: 1473–6.

# MR Arthrography of the Ankle: Indications and Technique

Luis Cerezal, MD[a],*, Eva Llopis, MD[b], Ana Canga, MD[c], Alejandro Rolón, MD[d]

**KEYWORDS**
- Ankle joint • Arthrography • Magnetic resonance imaging
- Ankle injuries • Ligaments • Articular • Athletic injuries

MR imaging has become established as the most effective imaging technique in the diagnosis of articular pathology. MR arthrography is a minimally invasive procedure that extends the capabilities of conventional MR imaging. Intra-articular contrast permits capsular distention and delineates articular structures as it separates adjacent anatomic structures and fills potential spaces that communicate with the joint.

In recent years there has been rapid development and improvement of arthroscopic treatments in multiple joints such as the shoulder, hip, and wrist. As a result, musculoskeletal radiologists have been required to provide more accurate detection and characterization of articular pathology. MR arthrography has emerged as the imaging technique of choice for precise preoperative diagnosis in a spectrum of conditions, such as biceps pulley and biceps-labral complex injuries in the shoulder and femoroacetabular impingement syndrome in the hip. Despite the widespread use of MR arthrography for evaluation of intra-articular pathology at the shoulder, hip, and wrist, ankle MR arthrography is performed less frequently and its indications still seem to be limited. It should be recognized that MR arthrography can improve diagnostic accuracy in the context of certain ankle injuries and can greatly enhance the diagnostic utility of conventional MR imaging for a range of clinically suspected intra-articular pathologies. It is likely that future improvements in ankle arthroscopy will expand the indications for ankle MR arthrography.

Indirect MR arthrography with intravenous administration of gadolinium permits articular enhancement without capsular distention. For joints with less capacity for distention, such as the ankle, it is considered an alternative to direct MR arthrography in some cases.

This article reviews the role of ankle MR arthrography focusing on technique, pitfalls, complications, pertinent anatomy, and clinical applications.

## DIRECT MR ARTHROGRAPHY TECHNIQUE

MR arthrography of the ankle is a two-step procedure involving intra-articular injection of contrast solution before MR imaging. The skin puncture can be performed in two main sites (**Fig. 1**A) at the anterior aspect of the ankle: immediately medial to the anterior tibial tendon or medial to the tendon of the extensor hallucis longus.[1–5] The arthrogram is usually performed under fluoroscopic control; however sonographic, CT, or MR guidance may be used.[6–11] Blind joint puncture can be performed in the MR imaging suite, using

[a] Radiology Department, Instituto Radiologico Cantabro, Clínica Mompía, Avenida de los Condes sn, Mompía 39108, Cantabria, Spain
[b] Radiology Department, Hospital de la Ribera, Carretera de Corbera km1, Alzira 46600, Valencia, Spain
[c] Radiology Department, Hospital Universitario Marqués de Valdecilla, Avenida de Valdecilla sn, Santander 39008, Cantabria, Spain
[d] Radiology Department, Centro de Diagnóstico Dr. Enrique Rossi, Arenales 2777 - CP: C1425BEE, Buenos Aires, Argentina
* Corresponding author.
*E-mail address:* lcerezal@gmail.com (L. Cerezal).

Radiol Clin N Am 46 (2008) 973–994
doi:10.1016/j.rcl.2008.09.002

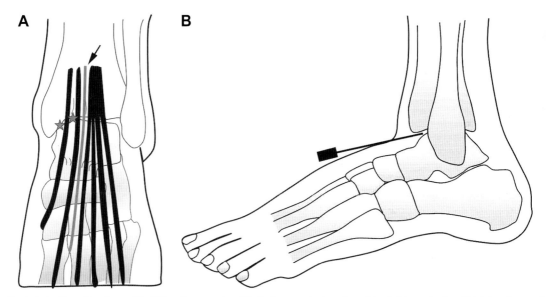

**Fig. 1.** Injection sites for ankle MR arthrography. (*A*) Anteroposterior view: Medial to anterior tibial tendon and medial to extensor hallucis longus tendon (*stars*). The course of dorsalis pedis artery (*arrow*) should be avoided, skin can be marked. (*B*) The needle is placed slightly cranial beneath the anterior lip of the tibia and advanced until its tip is seen between the distal tibia and the talus.

anatomic landmarks, thereby avoiding the need for iodinated contrast agents and ionizing radiation. Having achieved successful ankle arthrography under fluoroscopic guidance, blind ankle injection is easily performed.[1] The preferred puncture site is located at the level of the anteromedial ankle joint, just medial to the tibialis anterior tendon, approximately 5 mm proximal to the medial malleolus.

The authors recommend the following technique:[1,2] the patient is placed in lateral decubitus position with the ankle in the lateral position and the dorsal ankle facing the examiner. The course of the dorsalis pedis artery is palpated and marked to avoid arterial puncture. Using fluoroscopic guidance, a 22-23 gauge needle is inserted under sterile conditions into the tibiotalar joint medial to the anterior tibial tendon with a slight cranial tilt to avoid the overhanging anterior margin of the tibia (**Fig. 1**B). Before the injection of contrast material, any fluid within the joint is aspirated to avoid diluting the contrast material. Intra-articular needle placement is confirmed with an injection of 1 to 2 mL of iodinated contrast material. If the needle is intra-articular, the contrast medium flows away from the needle tip toward the capsular recesses. Subsequently, a mixture of 0.1 to 0.2 mL of gadolinium, 10 mL of saline solution, 5 mL of iodinated contrast material, and 5 mL of lidocaine 1% is injected until the joint capsule is properly distended (approximately 6–10 mL). The presence of iodinated contrast material in the mixture ensures

correct needle position and adequate capsular distention.[12] To prevent capsular disruption, the contrast injection is stopped if the patient expresses discomfort or if high resistance is felt during the instillation of the solution. In the normal ankle, the injected contrast material forms an umbrella shape over the articular surface of the talus with prominence of the anterior and posterior capsular recesses. Cranial extension of contrast material is seen between the distal tibia and fibula into the syndesmotic recess. In up to 25% of cases the contrast solution enters the flexor hallucis longus and flexor digitorum longus tendon sheaths as well as the subtalar joint.[5] There should be no tendon sheath filling on the lateral side of a normal ankle. Following the injection, the needle is removed and the ankle is manipulated briefly to distribute the contrast medium uniformly.

Although saline solution may be used as MR arthrographic contrast material, saline is not an ideal contrast medium as it has the same signal characteristics as preexisting joint effusion and periarticular fluid.[6–11]

MR arthrography is a safe procedure without significant side effects. Studies have shown that patients who have undergone MR arthrography considered the discomfort less than expected.[13,14] The main complications of MR arthrography are joint pain, which may persist one to three days after joint puncture, and vasovagal reaction. Articular distention in arthrography produces a feeling of pressure in the joint and pain of variable intensity on joint motion, which progressively decreases in the days following the procedure.[13] Vasovagal reactions may occur, particularly in young athletic patients with low resting heart rates; coexisting anxiety, apprehension, and pain increase the risk. Vasovagal reactions are easily managed in the radiology suite with prompt recovery. The routine administration of prophylactic atropine before ankle arthrography to block vasovagal reactions is unnecessary given the low incidence of these reactions (about 1% in the authors' experience). We believe that vasovagal reactions decrease when the patient is not allowed to see the needle or observe the procedure. Joint infection is an extremely rare major complication of arthrography that is independent of the type of substance injected into the joint.[13]

MR images is ideally performed within 20 to 30 minutes of injection, to minimize absorption of contrast and guarantee the desired capsular distention, although imaging delays of up to 1.5 to 2 hours are tolerated in the lower limbs joints.[5,15]

Imaging protocol sequences are oriented in axial, sagittal, and coronal planes with dedicated extremity coil and using small field of view to optimize the visualization of intra-articular structures. Several authors have used forced projections to stress ankle ligaments and improve its visualization, axial plane with dorsiflexion for anterior talofibular ligament (ATFL), or oblique coronal with plantar flexion for calcaneofibular ligament (CFL).[16] The choice of sequence depends on radiologist preference and MR device, but T1-weighted spin echo with and without fat saturation should be included. Three-dimensional gradient-echo images allow reconstruction in any plane making forced projections unnecessary and are also helpful detecting cartilage lesions and loose bodies. To rule out subtle bone marrow edema and extra-articular fluid collections, one sequence on T2-weighted fat suppression or short tau inversion recovery (STIR) is necessary.[1,2,4–11]

The most common pitfalls of MR arthrography of the ankle are extra-articular injection or reflux of contrast material through the capsular puncture site that can be confused with capsular disruption.[17] Accumulation of contrast material in the anterior and posterior recesses of the tibiotalar joint, which manifests as smooth, encapsulated fluid outside the ligaments, can be misinterpreted as a ligamentous tear. The bulbous appearance of the posterior talofibular ligament (PTFL) and posterior tibiofibular ligament (PITF) on sagittal images can simulate loose bodies. This pitfall is easily avoided by the evaluation of consecutive sagittal images and knowledge of the ligamentous anatomy. A pseudodefect of the talar dome is a normal

groove at the posterior aspect of the talus. This defect should not be misinterpreted as an articular erosion or osteochondral defect.

Inadvertent use of undiluted gadolinium or higher gadolinium concentration dilution decreases signal-to-noise ratio and decreases signal intensity on T1-weighted imaging. This effect decreases with time; therefore, delay images could be helpful. The instillation of air bubbles during injection may mimic loose bodies; although air bubbles tend to rise to nondependent regions of the joint (Fig. 2), whereas loose bodies fall dependently.[1,5,11]

## INDIRECT MR ARTHROGRAPHY

Indirect MR arthrography has been proposed as an alternative to direct MR arthrography. Intravenous administration of a standard dose of gadolinium followed by 5 to 10 minutes of light exercise can provide arthrogram-like images of the ankle joint.[18–22] Imaging delay is essential, as time is required for the contrast agent to transfer from the blood pool into the joint. The degree of articular enhancement is dependent on the blood concentration of contrast, joint volume, intra-articular pressure, synovial area, inflammation and permeability, and the time delay following contrast injection. These variables are difficult to control and result in the heterogeneous quality of indirect MR arthrography.[19]

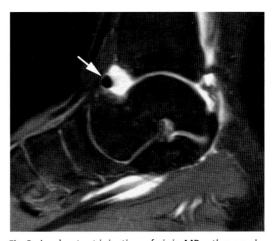

Fig. 2. Inadvertent injection of air in MR arthrography mimicking a loose body. Sagittal fat suppressed T1-weighted MR arthrogram image of the right ankle shows a gas bubble located in the upper part of the joint (arrow). Most air bubbles can be easily distinguished from loose bodies by their nondependent position and typical appearance caused by susceptibility artifact.

The main drawback of indirect MR arthrography is the lack of capsular distention. Another limitation is that juxta-articular structures, such as vessels, and the synovial membranes of bursae and tendon sheaths also demonstrate enhancement, which can lead to confusion with capsular disruption or the presence of abnormal joint recesses.

Indirect MR arthrography may be useful in detection of subtle cartilaginous defects with enhancement of the cartilaginous defect and the subchondral bone due to trabecular disruption and hyperemia.[18–22]

In the assessment of osteochondral lesions of the talus with indirect MR arthrography, high signal intensity on T1-weighted imaging surrounding the bone fragment interface is a sign of a loose osteochondral fragment, which might be secondary to synovial fluid entering the defect indicating partial or complete detachment of the fragment or granulation tissue enhancement, correlation with signal intensity on T2-weighted sequence helps to differentiate detachment fragment which has higher T2-weighted signal intensity following fluid signal than granulation that is slightly lower signal intensity on T2-weighted (**Fig. 3**).[18–22]

Partial ligament tears may be identified by focal enhancement indicating hyperemia. Complete tears may be seen as enhanced joint fluid extending into the ligament defect.

Indirect MR arthrography may also be useful in the evaluation of anterolateral impingement outlining the impinging lesion in the anterolateral gutter of the ankle.[18–22]

Indirect MR arthrography provides further assessment of extra-articular soft tissues of the ankle. Enhancement of extra-articular structures can highlight focal pathology while lack of abnormal enhancement invariably indicates absence of disease in the region of interest. For instance enhancement around the plantar fascia is observed in patients with plantar fasciitis. Enhancement of fluid within the tendon sheath indicates tenosynovitis. Synovitis in the region of the tarsal tunnel with enhancement around the posterior tibial nerve may suggest tarsal tunnel syndrome. Focal enhancement in the region of the sinus tarsi suggests sinus tarsi pathology.[18–22]

## INDICATIONS

Indications for the use of MR arthroscopy include: ligamentous injuries, ankle impingement syndromes, osteochondral and cartilage lesions, intra-articular loose bodies, and adhesive capsulitis. The anatomy, pathophysiology, imaging, and treatment of each is discussed below.

### Ligamentous Injuries

The ankle joint is stabilized by three ligamentous groups: the distal tibiofibular ligamentous or syndesmotic complex, the lateral collateral ligament (LCL) complex, and the deltoid ligament.[22–24]

Ankle sprains are common and account for up to 10% of emergency department visits and are the most common sports-related injury, accounting for 16% to 21% of all sports-related injuries.[25,26] Athletic activities requiring frequent pivoting and jumping are particularly susceptible to ankle injuries, so the highest incidences of ankle sprains are found in sports such as football, soccer, and basketball.[25]

Approximately 85% of all ankle sprains are due to inversion forces involving the LCL complex.[22–25] Syndesmotic sprains are the second most prevalent (10%), followed by isolated medial sprains. Multiligamentous injuries are frequent: an inversion

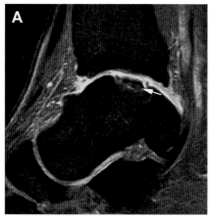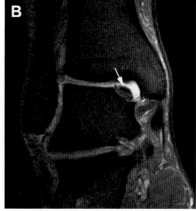

**Fig. 3.** Stage III osteochondral lesion of the talus. (*A, B*) Sagittal and coronal fat-suppressed T1-weighted indirect MR ankle arthrogram of the right ankle show contrast-enhanced fluid around osteochondral lesion of the talar dome (*arrows*) which indicates complete loosening of the osteochondral fragment.

mechanism often involves both lateral and syndesmotic ligaments, whereas an eversion mechanism may affect both deltoid and syndesmotic ligaments.

Regardless of the pattern of injury, the outcome of ankle sprain is similar. As such, clinical evaluation with or without conventional radiography is sufficient. However, chronic pain or instability can limit activity and affect up to 20% to 40% of patients following ankle sprain.[27]

MR arthrography improves visualization of the ankle ligaments. The role of MR arthrography is in preoperative planning for chronic ankle pain, to determine the extent and severity of ligamentous injuries, and to identify associated intra-articular pathology; especially to determine causes of ankle impingement syndromes.

### Lateral collateral ligament complex

**Anatomy** The LCL complex includes three ligaments: ATFL, CFL, and PTFL.[23,24,26] The ATFL is located within the anterolateral joint capsule extending from the anteroinferior aspect of the lateral malleolus to the lateral talar neck. The CFL is a cord-like structure that arises from the tip of the lateral malleolus and passes obliquely downward and posterior to insert at the posterolateral aspect of the calcaneus. It is an extra-articular structure and forms the floor of the peroneal tendon sheath. The CFL controls two joints, talocrural and subtalar; unlike the other two elements of LCL, which only support the talocrural joint. The PTFL is an intra-articular ligament that arises from the medial aspect of the distal fibula and passes almost horizontally to insert along the posterolateral tubercle of the talus. On MR imaging the ATFL is better visualized in the axial plane, CFL in the axial or coronal plane, and PTFL in the axial or coronal plane.

**Pathophysiology** Plantar flexion with inversion and internal rotation of the foot is the most common mechanism of ankle injury and follows a predictable sequence: ATFL is torn first, followed by CFL and, only under extreme inversion, the PTFL is torn usually with an avulsion fracture. Isolated tear of CFL is unusual.[24–26]

Chronic pain secondary to lateral ankle sprains presents a diagnostic and therapeutic challenge, as it can be due to a variety of pathology, including: instability, soft-tissue impingement, posttraumatic arthritis, syndesmotic injuries, sinus tarsi syndrome, subtalar instability, peroneal tendon lesions, or osteochondral lesions of the talar dome.[27–29]

Patients describe ankle instability as recurrent, intermittent episodes of a feeling of "giving way"

with asymptomatic periods in between.[30–32] It can be divided into mechanical or functional. Instability without evidence of anatomic ligamentous injury is referred as "functional instability" whereas when specific ligament incompetency (mobility beyond the physiologic range of motion) is termed "mechanical instability." The reported prevalence of functional instability ranges from 15 to 60% following ankle sprain, and appears to be independent of the severity of the initial injury. Mechanical instability is less prevalent.[29–32]

### Imaging

*MR imaging* Indications for MR imaging to evaluate ligamentous injury and instability are limited to: the evaluation of acute ankle injuries with instability, stable acute injuries suffered by athletes or in cases of litigation, and patients with repeated injuries or chronic ankle instability in whom surgery is contemplated. MR imaging may depict lesions commonly associated with ligament injuries, such as impingement syndromes, sinus tarsi syndrome, osteochondral lesions, and tendon tears.[23,24]

Ankle ligaments are readily identified on MR images as low-signal intensity structures joining adjacent bones usually delimited by contiguous high signal intensity fat. Heterogeneity and striation may be noted in some ligaments, such as the PTFL or deep component of the deltoid ligament, owing to the presence of interposed fat between their fascicles.[33]

MR imaging criteria for the diagnosis of acute tears of the ankle ligaments include morphologic and signal intensity alterations within the ligament (primary signs) or surrounding the ligament (secondary signs). Primary signs of ligament tear include: discontinuity, detachment, nonvisualization, or thickening of the ligament associated with increased intrasubstance signal intensity on T2-weighted images indicative of edema or hemorrhage. Secondary signs of acute ligament injury include: extravasation of joint fluid into the adjacent soft tissues, joint effusion, and bone bruises. Fluid within the peroneal tendon sheath is an important secondary sign of acute CFL injury. In chronic tears secondary signs disappear and the ligament can appear thickened, thinned, elongated, with an irregular or wavy contour.[23,24,33] Avulsion injuries are easily diagnosed in either the acute and chronic setting as a bone fragment adjacent to an irregular lateral or medial malleolus.

*MR arthrography* Normal ankle ligaments of the LCL complex are better depicted by MR arthrography as compared with conventional MR imaging.[1–5,16] Intra-articular joint distention with diluted contrast lifts the ligaments away from the adjacent bones, outlining the ligaments and improving their visualization. MR arthrography allows precise assessment of the thickness of the ligaments and their integrity at insertion sites.

Nonvisualization of the ligament or extravasation of contrast material anterior to the ATFL indicates tear of the ligament (**Figs. 4** and **5**). A capacious anterior recess of the ankle joint which may permit the contrast agent to outline the anterior border of the capsular ligament due to capsular distention beyond the ligament should not be confused with a tear. Disruption of the CFL often results in pathologic communication of contrast material lateral to the ligament from the ankle joint into the peroneal tendon sheath (see **Fig. 5**), which is attached to the superficial surface of the ligament. Therefore, contrast material in the peroneal tendons sheath at MR arthrography is an indirect but specific sign of CFL injury. Extravasation of contrast material into the soft tissues posterior to the PTFL indicates a tear of this ligament.[1–5,16]

**Treatment** Treatment of injuries to lateral ankle ligaments is conservative. Surgical management of ankle sprains is rarely indicated, and is limited to ankle instability refractory to conservative treatment. Numerous surgical techniques have been described to correct ankle instability with an 80% to 90% success rate.[31,34] Current methods of direct repair of the ATFL and CFL offers better functional results than reconstructive techniques using tendon transfer.[29–32,34]

## Syndesmosis

Syndesmotic ligament injuries, also known as high ankle sprains, are the second most prevalent ankle ligament injury (10%).[23,24,27,35] The incidence of syndesmotic sprains is probably higher than reported,[23,24,35,36] and occurs as an isolated injury or in association with lateral and medial collateral ligament injuries. Syndesmotic disruption is commonly associated with Lauge-Hansen fractures (Weber B and C). The injury is common in young athletic individuals, especially those involved in contact sports, such as soccer and football.[26]

Syndesmotic injuries are more debilitating than lateral collateral ligament sprains and require a longer recovery time. Isolated syndesmotic injuries often do not present with appreciable diastasis and can be difficult to diagnose, leading to underestimation of injury, incomplete rehabilitation, and prolonged pain and disability.[27,35]

**Anatomy** Three ligaments join the distal tibial and fibular epiphyses: the anterior or anteroinferior tibiofibular ligament (AITF), the PITF, and the interosseous tibiofibular ligament.[37] The AITF has a multifascicular morphology and is the weakest of the three. The most distal fascicle of the AITF seems to be an independent structure, situated slightly deeper and separated by a fibroadipose septum from the rest of the ligament. The AITF normally contacts the dorsolateral border of the talus during ankle dorsiflexion and eversion.[37] Nikolopoulous[38] considered the accessory AITF to be a separate structure from the AITF with

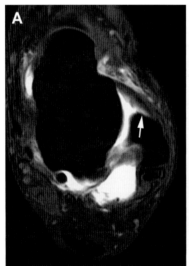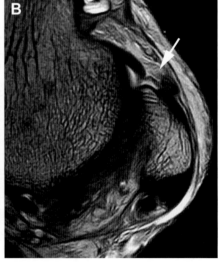

Fig. 4. Chronic tear of the ATFL. (*A*) Axial fat-suppressed T1-weighted MR arthrogram image shows diffuse irregular thickening and partial detachment at peroneal insertion of the ATFL (*arrow*). (*B*) Axial T1-weighted MR arthrogram image demonstrates focal disruption of the peroneal insertion of the ATFL (*arrow*).

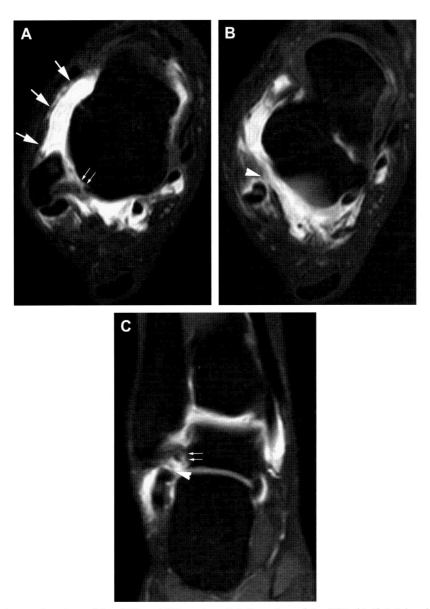

Fig. 5. Chronic complete tear of the ATFL and CFL, and partial disruption of the PTFL. (*A–C*) Axial and coronal fat suppressed T1-weighted MR arthrogram images of the right ankle show complete absence of the ATFL (*arrows in A*), complete rupture of the CFL with contrast communication with the peroneal tendon sheath (*arrowheads in B and C*), and partial disruption of the PTFL at the insertion on posterolateral tubercle of the talus (*small arrows in A and C*).

a reported incidence of 21% to 92%.[38] This theory was refuted by Bassett and colleagues,[39] whose anatomic cadaveric study designated the distal fascicle of the AITF as a constant structure (also known as Bassett's ligament).

The PITF is formed by two components: one superficial and one deep or transverse ligament. The interosseous tibiofibular ligament is simply the continuation of the interosseous membrane at this level.[24,37]

There is a synovial-lined interosseous recess or diverticulum that extends from the ankle joint, between the distal tibia and fibula, and ends close to the base of the interosseous ligament. The recess is formed by a posteriorly located V-shaped synovial plica that blends laterally with the fibula.[37] The medial aspect of the plica lies loosely on the tibia, creating the diverticulum. The normal tibiofibular recess measures approximately 1 cm in height in anatomic studies and averages 0.5 cm on MR imaging.[36]

**Pathophysiology** Syndesmotic ligaments stabilize the distal tibiofibular articulation and prevent diastasis of the tibia and fibula at the ankle. The most common mechanism of injury is pronation and eversion of the foot combined with internal rotation of the tibia on a fixed foot. Syndesmotic injuries are frequently associated with eversion-type ankle fractures, particularly high fibular fractures (Weber B and C), and rupture of the deltoid ligament.[27–29] Syndesmotic sprains requires a longer recovery period than isolated LCL sprains. Incomplete reduction of syndesmotic injury may produce chronic syndesmotic widening, persistent pain, and ankle arthrosis.

### Imaging

**MR imaging** MR imaging is sensitive and specific for identification of tibiofibular syndesmotic injuries. Findings indicative of a syndesmotic interruption include ligament discontinuity, contour alteration (wavy or curved ligaments), or ligament nonvisualization.[36,40] Using these criteria, the reported sensitivity and specificity of MR imaging compared with arthroscopy are 100% and 83% to 92%, respectively.[40] Common findings associated with syndesmotic injury include an increase in the height of the tibiofibular recess, osteochondral lesions of the talus (28%), and tibiofibular joint incongruity (33%).

**MR arthrography** MR arthrography permits better assessment of syndesmotic injury, which appears as thickening, nonvisualization, or irregularity of the syndesmotic ligaments (Fig. 6), and is helpful for detection of associated lesions.[1,16] The oblique course of the syndesmotic ligaments must be kept in mind when assessing syndesmotic tears, because they may appear falsely torn on routine axial images. In addition, the normal fascicular pattern especially of the AITFL, should not be misinterpreted as a tear.[1]

A common indirect finding in syndesmotic ligament complex injury on MR arthrography is an increase in the height of the tibiofibular recess, averaging 1.2 cm in acute tears and 1.4 cm in chronic tears.

**Treatment** Treatment of isolated syndesmotic ligament injury without diastasis is conservative. Indications for surgery are: symptoms refractory to conservative management, presence of diastasis on routine or stress radiographs, and delayed presentation of more than three months. A complete tear is managed by suture of the ligament and temporary fixation of the tibia and fibula with a syndesmosis screw, cerclage or Kirschner wires.[29–34]

### Deltoid ligament

Deltoid ligament sprains without other ligamentous injuries are rare (5% of all ankle ligament injuries).[23,24,27,41] Deltoid or medial collateral ligament (MCL) sprain is often more painful than lateral ankle sprain and can be a significant source of chronic medial ankle pain.[42] Sequelae of deltoid ligament tear include: ankle instability, chondral injuries, ankle joint arthritis, and medial impingement.[41]

**Anatomy** Deltoid ligament anatomy is confusing since the division of its components is difficult

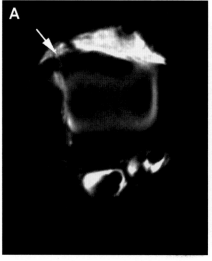
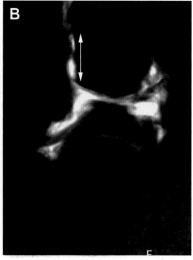

Fig. 6. Chronic syndesmosis sprain. (*A, B*) Axial and coronal fat suppressed T1-weighted images of right ankle show thickening and complete disruption of the AITF (*arrow*), and increase in the height of the tibiofibular recess (*double-headed arrow*).

during dissection, and its origins and insertions are complex.[37] Most investigators agree that the MCL has a superficial and deep layer.[37,43] Milner and Soames[43] describe the deltoid ligament as being composed of four superficial (tibionavicular, tibiospring, tibiocalcaneal, and superficial posterior tibiotalar) and two deep (anterior and posterior tibiotalar) bands or components.[24,37] The deltoid ligament blends with the tendon sheaths of the posterior tibial tendon, flexor hallucis longus, and flexor digitorum longus tendons. The superficial layer of the ligament crosses both the ankle and subtalar joints, whereas the deep layer only crosses the ankle joint.[43]

**Pathophysiology** Traumatic deltoid ligament injury is most commonly associated with concomitant malleolar fracture, lateral ankle sprain, and syndesmotic injury; whereas nontraumatic injuries occur frequently in patients with posterior tibial tendon dysfunction.[23,24,41,43] Isolated ruptures of the deltoid ligament are rare but can occur as a consequence of an eversion-lateral rotation mechanism. Contusions and partial tears of the deltoid ligament, particularly of its posterior tibiotalar component, are frequently associated with inversion sprains, in which the deep posterior fibers of the medial deltoid ligament are crushed between the medial wall of the talus and the medial malleolus.[42]

### Imaging
*MR imaging* The normal uninjured bands of the MCL can usually be easily distinguished from one other, optimally seen in the coronal and axial plane.[23,24,33] Deltoid ligament injury is clearly demonstrated by MRI as morphologic and signal alterations of the ligament. Loss of the normal striated appearance and increased interstitial signal of the deep tibiotalar component are common findings. Interstitial edema signal is not infrequently seen on MR imaging in stable ankles and likely reflects contusion rather than a tear of the tibiotalar component of the deltoid ligament. Thickening or attenuation of the deltoid ligament may be seen with healing.[23,24,33] Osseous abnormalities that are associated with deltoid ligament injury include fibular and medial malleolar fractures, bone bruises at the medial malleolar/tibial plafond junction, and talar displacement. Concomitant LCL and syndesmotic ligament injuries are also common.

*MR arthrography* MR arthrography with optimal articular distention outlines the deep deltoid ligament and improves evaluation of partial tears (**Fig. 7**).[1] Detection of associated lesions, such as chondral and osteochondral defects, and medial impingement is also improved with MR arthrography.[1]

**Treatment** Management of deltoid ligament injury focuses on associated bone or ligamentous injuries. Partial deltoid ligament tears are managed conservatively. Isolated complete acute deltoid tear, avulsion of the medial malleolus, and chronic deltoid sprains are surgically repaired using arthroscopy or open reduction.[41]

## Ankle Impingement Syndromes

Ankle impingement syndromes are chronic, painful conditions due to repetitive friction of joint tissues, precipitated and exacerbated by altered ankle joint biomechanics.[44,45] The main cause of impingement lesions is posttraumatic ankle injury, usually ankle sprain. Ankle impingement syndrome is a clinical exclusion diagnosis; its symptoms

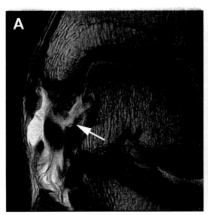
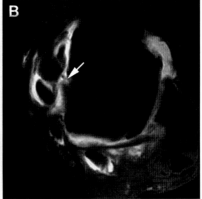

**Fig. 7.** Chronic complete tear of the deltoid ligament. (*A*) Coronal T1-weighted and (*B*) axial fat suppressed T1-weighted MR arthrogram images of left ankle demonstrate complete tear of the deltoid ligament involving both superficial and deep components (*arrows*).

mimic a wide variety of common disorders such as osteochondral fracture, mechanical instability, peroneal tendon rupture, subluxation or tenosynovitis, and sinus tarsi syndrome.

These syndromes are classified in anatomic and clinical terms as anterolateral, anterior, anteromedial, posteromedial, and posterior.[44,46–48]

Careful analysis of patient history, and signs and symptoms at physical examination can suggest a specific diagnosis in most patients. MR imaging and MR arthrography are the most useful imaging methods for detecting the osseous and soft-tissue abnormalities present in these syndromes and for ruling out other potential causes of chronic ankle pain.[44,46]

The initial treatment of all ankle impingement syndromes is conservative, but when this fails, arthroscopic examination is indicated to identify and resect the impinging lesion.[1,2]

### Anterolateral impingement syndrome

**Prevalence, epidemiology, and definitions** Anterolateral impingement is a relatively uncommon cause of chronic ankle pain produced by entrapment of abnormal soft tissue in the anterolateral gutter of the ankle after single or multiple ankle inversion injuries (**Fig. 8**). The anterolateral recess of the ankle is defined by the talus and tibia posteromedially, the fibula laterally, and the anterior ankle joint capsule along with the AITF, ATFL, and CFL anteriorly. The space extends inferiorly to the CFL and superiorly to the tibial plafond and distal tibiofibular syndesmosis.[49,50] Approximately 3% of ankle sprains may lead to anterolateral impingement. This type of ankle impingement is most common in athletic young males.[49,50]

**Pathophysiology** Anterolateral impingement is thought to occur subsequent to relatively minor trauma involving forced ankle plantarflexion and supination. Repeated microtrauma produce synovial scarring, inflammation, and hypertrophy in the anterolateral gutter of the ankle, and may cause impingement. Wolin and colleagues[51] coined the term "meniscoid lesion" owing to its resemblance at surgery to meniscal tissue.

Other contributing factors are osseous spurs and hypertrophy of the inferior fascicle of the AITF.[44,46] A chronic ATFL tear results in anterolateral joint laxity, permitting anterior talar extrusion in dorsiflexion and increasing contact between the talus and the inferior fascicle of the AITF or Bassett ligament. Constant rubbing of the fascicle against the talus thickens the fascicle, developing an impinging lesion in the anterolateral gutter. This condition has also been referred to as "syndesmotic impingement." There may be associated chondral abrasion at the apposed anterosuperior lateral margin of the talus.[37,44,46]

### Imaging

**MR imaging** There is controversy about the accuracy of the MR imaging for the diagnosis of anterolateral impingement, but most of the authors believe that assessment of the anterolateral recess with conventional MR imaging is only accurate when a substantial joint effusion is present.[48]

**MR arthrography** MR arthrography has proved to be an accurate technique for assessing the presence of soft tissue scarring in the anterolateral recess of the ankle and determining its extent in patients with anterolateral impingement before arthroscopy, seen as a nodular or irregular deep contour of the anterolateral joint capsule (**Fig. 9**).[1,52] Robinson and colleagues[52] found that MR arthrography was 100% accurate for evaluation of soft tissue abnormality in 13 patients with suspected clinical anterolateral impingement that had scarring and synovitis in the anterolateral recess. A highly specific but insensitive MR arthrographic finding is the absence of a normal fluid-filled recess between the anterolateral soft tissues and the anterior surface of the fibula. This may be due to the presence of adhesions and scar tissue that impairs the entrance of fluid into the normal recess between the fibula and joint capsule.

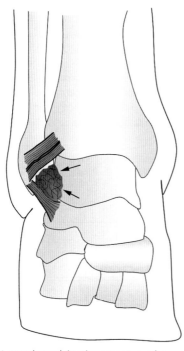

Fig. 8. Anterolateral impingement syndrome: typical location of anterolateral ankle impingement, with irregular fibrosis and synovitis in the anterolateral capsular recess of tibiotalar joint (*arrows*).

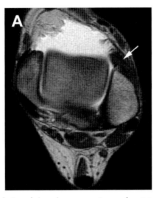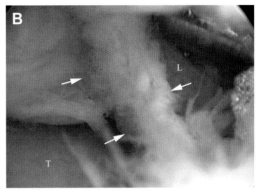

Fig. 9. Anterolateral impingement syndrome. (A) Axial T1-weighted spin echo MR arthrography of left ankle shows irregular soft tissue thickening in the anterolateral gutter (arrows). (B) Arthroscopic image demonstrating scarring and synovitis in the anterolateral gutter (arrows). L, lateral malleolus; T, talus.

Clinical correlation is essential because abnormal soft tissue scarring with or without synovitis can be seen in asymptomatic patients.[46,52]

Articular distention by MR arthrography allows more precise diagnosis of anterolateral impingement caused by thickening of the inferior fascicle of the AITF ligament (syndesmotic impingement) (Fig. 10). Fibrosis and focal synovitis often are observed surrounding the AITF ligament in syndesmotic impingement.[1,45]

### Anterior impingement syndrome

Prevalence, epidemiology, and definitions Anterior impingement is a relatively common cause of chronic anterior ankle pain, especially in young athletes subjected to repeated stress in dorsiflexion of the ankle, such as soccer players and dancers.[44,46,47,53]

Pathophysiology The origin of anterior impingement is uncertain, and many mechanical factors are probably involved.[46,53] Three different hypotheses have been proposed to explain the formation of talotibial osteophytes in the anterior ankle impingement syndrome.[53] Forced dorsiflexion results in repeated microtrauma on the tibia and talus, leading to microfractures of trabecular bone or periosteal hemorrhage, healing with new bone formation. Another mechanism suggested is forced plantarflexion trauma, with capsular avulsion injury. However, the majority of the talotibial osteophytes are not located at the capsular attachment but are found in arthroscopy to be intra-articular at the anterior tibiotalar articular margin, approximately 5 to 8 mm distant from the capsular attachments.[53] Thus this hyperplantarflexion mechanism has been largely discredited. A recent hypothesis has suggested that formation of osteophytes in the ankle is related to direct damage to the rim of the anterior ankle cartilage combined with recurrent microtrauma, such as by direct impact of a soccer ball on the anterior ankle region.

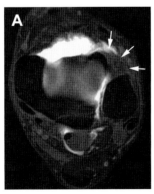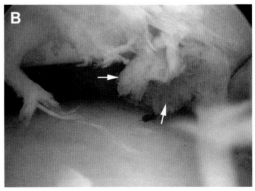

Fig. 10. Anterolateral impingement syndrome. (A) Axial fat-suppressed T1-weighted spin echo MR arthrogram of left ankle demonstrates nodular irregular lesion surrounding inferior fascicle of AITF (Bassett's ligament) in the superior aspect of the anterolateral gutter (arrows). (B) Corresponding arthroscopic image showing focal fibrosis and synovitis (arrows) surrounding inferior fascicle of AITF.

Once formed, forced dorsiflexion of the ankle causes impingement between reciprocating talotibial "kissing" lesions (**Fig. 11**).[44–47,53]

*Imaging* Conventional radiography is the only imaging study required in most cases, allowing evaluation of osseous spurs and the tibiotalar joint space. An oblique ankle radiograph, anteromedial impingement view, is a useful adjunct to routine views to detect tibial and anteromedial talar osteophytes.[53]

*MR imaging* MR imaging is useful to confirm the diagnosis, to depict associated findings and to rule out other causes of chronic ankle pain. The presence of anterior tibiotalar joint effusion and bone marrow edema in the anterior talar neck or distal anterior tibia are the findings most consistent with symptomatic anterior impingement.[44]

*MR arthrography* MR arthrography is useful in assessing the degree of cartilage damage, in delineating loose bodies, and in the detection of capsular thickening and synovitis in the anterior capsular recess (**Fig. 12**).[44,46]

### Medial impingement syndrome

**Prevalence, epidemiology, and definitions** Medial impingement is an uncommon cause of chronic ankle pain after an ankle trauma. Medial impingement is commonly associated with lateral and medial ligament injury. Depending on its anatomic location it is referred to as anteromedial or posteromedial impingement.[44,46,54,55]

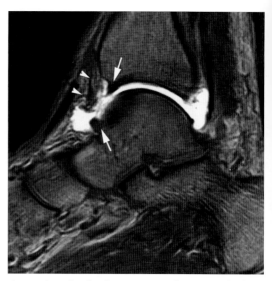

Fig. 12. Anterior impingement syndrome. Sagittal T1-weighted spin echo MR arthrogram of right ankle shows anterior tibial and talar osteophytes ("kissing lesion") (*arrows*), and irregular soft tissue mass in the anterior capsular recess (*arrowheads*).

**Pathophysiology** Medial impingement is rarely an isolated condition; it is most commonly associated with an inversion mechanism resulting in lateral ligament injury. It can occur after a severe ankle-inversion injury with the deep anterior or posterior fibers of the deltoid ligament becoming crushed between the talus and the medial malleolus. Inadequate healing of the contused deep deltoid ligament fibers may lead to chronic inflammation and fibrosis. In these cases, the anomalous soft tissue may impinge between the medial wall of the talus and the medial malleolus (**Fig. 13**).[44,46,54,55]

**Imaging** Conventional MR imaging has not been proved useful for diagnosis of anteromedial ankle impingement.

*MR arthrography* MR arthrography is the imaging method of choice, clearly defining a medial meniscoid lesion (**Fig. 14**), thickened and irregular tibiotalar ligaments, capsular abnormalities, and chondral or osteochondral associated lesions.[44–46,55] Occasionally, MR arthrography reveals the existence of fibrosis encasing the sheaths of the internal retromalleolar tendons that can interfere with the proper sliding of the medial posterior tendons and contribute to medial ankle pain in patients with medial impingement (see **Fig. 14**).

### Posterior impingement syndrome

**Prevalence, epidemiology, and definitions** Posterior ankle impingement syndrome is a clinical disorder characterized by posterior ankle pain, including

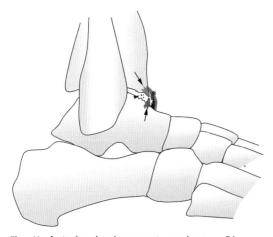

Fig. 11. Anterior impingement syndrome. Diagram shows typical features of anterior ankle impingement including chondral fraying, anterior tibial and talar osteophytes (*arrows*), synovitis in anterior capsular recess (*asterisk*), reduction of joint space, and osteochondral loose bodies (*arrowhead*).

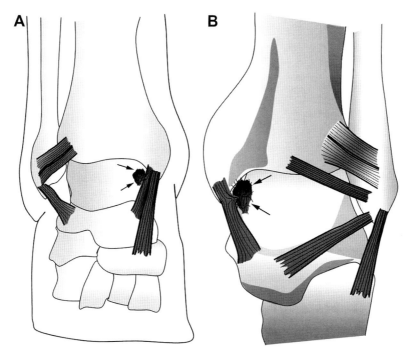

**Fig. 13.** Anteromedial and posteromedial ankle impingement. Diagrams illustrating findings of anteromedial (*A*) and posteromedial (*B*) ankle impingement including meniscoid lesions (*arrows*), and thickened anterior or posterior tibiotalar ligaments.

a group of pathologic conditions secondary to repetitive or acute forced plantarflexion of the foot, which produce compression of the talus and surrounding soft tissue between the tibia and the calcaneus.[44,46,56]

**Pathophysiology** Posterior impingement has been described as a "nut in a nutcracker"

mechanism. The posterior talus and surrounding soft tissues are compressed between the tibia and the calcaneus during plantarflexion of the foot.[44,46,56]

Posterior ankle impingement syndrome may manifest as an inflammation of the posterior ankle soft tissues, as an osseous injury, or as a combination of both. The most common

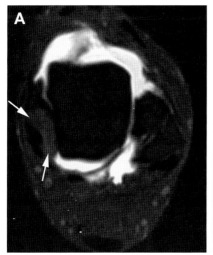
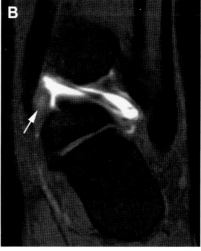

**Fig. 14.** Posteromedial impingement syndrome. (*A, B*) Axial and coronal fat-suppressed T1-weighted MR arthrograms of the left ankle show hypertrophic fibrotic tissue in the posteromedial aspect of the ankle (*arrows*) behind the posterior tibiotalar ligament and deep to the posterior tibial tendon.

causes are osseous (**Fig. 15**), such as the os trigonum, an elongated lateral tubercle termed a "Stieda process," a downward sloping posterior lip of the tibia, the prominent posterior process of the calcaneus, and loose bodies. Injuries include fracture, fragmentation, and pseudarthrosis of the os trigonum or lateral talar tubercle.[44,46]

Soft tissue causes of impingement include synovitis of the flexor hallucis longus tendon sheath, the posterior synovial recess of the subtalar and tibiotalar joints, ganglia, low-lying flexor hallucis longus muscle belly, anomalous muscles, and the intermalleolar ligament (IML).[44,46,56]

The IML is a normal variant of the posterior ankle ligaments of the ankle that courses obliquely from lateral to medial and from downward to upward, connecting the malleolar fossa of the fibula to the medial posterior tibial cortex.[37,57,58] Repeated intra-articular entrapment of the IML during plantar flexion can produce thickening of the ligament, focal synovitis, and fibrosis.[57,58]

**Imaging** The diagnosis of posterior ankle impingement syndrome is based primarily on the patient's clinical history and physical examination, and is supported by radiographic and MR imaging findings.[44,46,56]

*MR imaging* MR imaging can specifically identify the wide range of pathology that may contribute to posterior ankle impingement and to rule out other causes of posterior ankle pain.

*MR arthrography* MR arthrography offers few advantages over conventional MR imaging in the assessment of posterior ankle impingement syndrome (**Figs. 16** and **17**).[1] MR arthrography is primarily useful for the diagnosis of uncommon cases of posterior impingement caused by the IML. The IML is often not well visualized on conventional MR imaging. MR arthrography improves the visualization of this ligament, which can readily be separated from the surrounding PTFL and the deeper fibers of the PITF or transverse ligament. Irregular focal or diffuse thickening of the intermalleolar ligament (see **Fig. 17**), and focal fibrosis or synovitis are the MR arthrographic findings frequently observed.[1]

### Osteochondral and cartilage lesions of the talus

**Prevalence, epidemiology, and definitions** Chondral injuries are common in the ankle and predispose

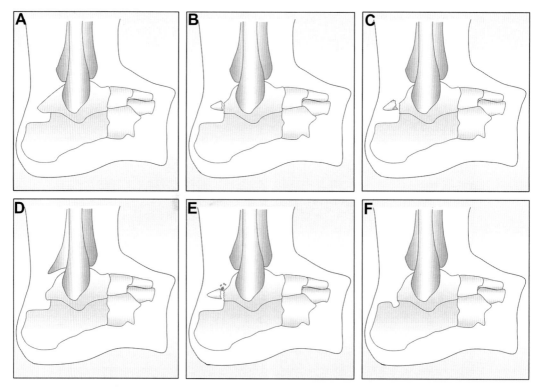

**Fig. 15.** Osseous anatomic structures involved in posterior impingement. (*A*) Stieda process. (*B*) Os trigonum. (*C*) Fractured lateral tubercle of the talus. (*D*) Prominent downslope of the posterior tibial articular surface. (*E*) Calcified inflammatory tissue. (*F*) Prominent superior surface of the calcaneal tuberosity.

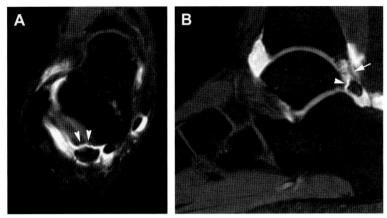

**Fig. 16.** Posterior impingement syndrome. (*A, B*) Axial and sagittal fat-suppressed MR arthrograms of the right ankle demonstrate irregularity of the os trigonum synchondrosis (*arrowheads*) and irregular fibrosis in the posterior recesses (*arrow in B*).

to development of degenerative arthritis. Osteo-chondral injuries reflect injury not only to the articular cartilage, but also the subchondral bone. "Osteo-chondral lesion of the talus" (OLT) is the accepted term for a variety of disorders including: osteochondritis dissecans, osteochondral fracture, transchondral fracture, and talar dome fracture.[59,60] OLT are more common in men than women and represent

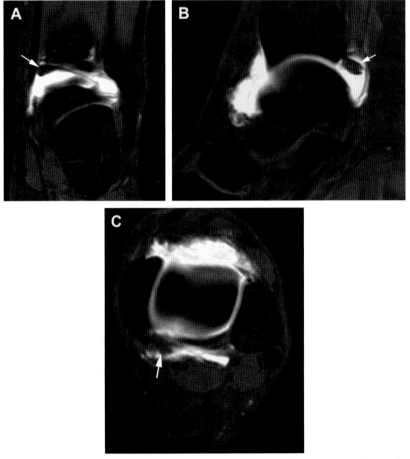

**Fig. 17.** Posterior impingement syndrome. (*A–C*) Coronal, sagittal, and axial fat-suppressed MR arthrograms of the left ankle show focal nodular thickening of the medial aspect of IML (*arrows*).

4% of all osteochondral lesions in the body. After the knee and elbow, the talus is the third most common location of osteochondral lesions.[59,60]

Medial and lateral aspects of the talar dome are involved in approximately 55% and 45% of the cases, respectively (**Fig. 18**). Lateral OLT are typically located over the anterolateral portion of the talar dome. Medial lesions are most commonly located over the posteromedial portion.[59,60]

**Clinical symptoms and physical findings** Osteochondral and chondral lesions of the talus usually manifest as persistent ankle pain ipsilateral to the lesion, accompanied by intermittent joint swelling, catching, and limitation of motion of the joint in the context of prior ankle inversion injury.[59,60]

**Pathophysiology** Lateral OLT are almost always associated with an acute traumatic episode and most probably represent true osteochondral or transchondral fractures, whereas patients with medial OLT usually do not have a clear recent trauma. Although trauma is the most common cause of OLT, ischemic necrosis, endocrine disorders, and genetic factors may have etiologic significance. In 10% to 25% of affected individuals, OLT is bilateral.[59,60]

The primary mechanism of injury is talar dome impaction due to ankle inversion. Lateral OLT results from inversion and dorsiflexion with impaction of the anterolateral aspect of the talar dome against the fibula. Traumatic medial OLT results from a combination of inversion, plantarflexion, and external rotation with impaction of the posteromedial tibia and medial talar margin.[59,60]

**Imaging** The Berndt and Harty classification schema[61] is the most widely accepted staging system for OLT (**Fig. 18B**). Stage I represents subchondral compression fracture. Stage II consists of a partially detached osteochondral fragment. In stage III, the osteochondral fragment is completely detached but not displaced from its donor site. In stage IV, the osteochondral fragment is detached and displaced.

Bilateral radiographs, including anteroposterior, lateral, and mortise views, should be the initial imaging method when OLT is suspected. Morphologically, lateral lesions tend to be shallower and more wafer shaped than medial lesions, which appear as deeper, cup-shaped defects.[60] It should be noted that radiographs are insensitive for detection of chondral injuries and relatively insensitive for detection of stage I and stage II OLT.

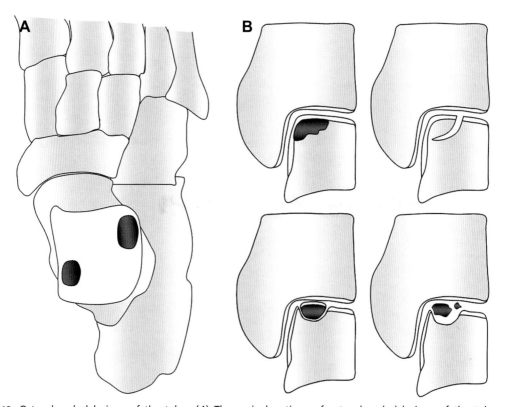

**Fig. 18.** Osteochondral lesions of the talus. (*A*) The main locations of osteochondral lesions of the talus and (*B*) diagram of Berndt and Harty classification system.

*MR imaging* MR imaging is sensitive for detecting and characterizing radiographically occult OLT, and permits assessment of the integrity of the overlying cartilage. MR imaging can also determine the viability of the osteochondral fragment. Necrotic fragments appear dark on both T1- and T2-weighted images and do not enhance after gadolinium administration.[23,33]

Multiple-pulse sequences are used for cartilage assessment with extremely variable reported sensitivity and specificity. For cartilage evaluation the following MR imaging, grading is most commonly used: grade I lesions MR images show abnormal intrachondral signal with smooth chondral surface and without alterations of the chondral thickness. Grade II lesions show mild surface irregularity with or without focal loss of less than 50% of the cartilage thickness. Severe surface irregularities with thinning of the cartilage thickness by more than 50% are present in grade III lesions and grade IV lesions consist of complete loss of articular cartilage with denuded subchondral bone.[5]

There is some controversy concerning the accuracy of MR imaging for assessing the stability of the osteochondral fragment.[62,63] Although arthroscopy remains the gold standard, MR imaging is an excellent predictor of fragment stability. MR imaging diagnosis of instability of osteochondral lesions of the talus has relied on the interface between the osteochondral fragment and the parent bone on T2-weighted images. A stable or healed osteochondral fragment is characterized by lack of high signal intensity at the interface between the lesion and the parent bone. The presence of a high signal line on T2-weighted images at the talar interface with the osteochondral fragment is the most reliable sign of instability.[63] It may represent granulation tissue or fluid. Usually, a moderately hyperintense interface, not as hyperintense as fluid, indicates the presence of fibrovascular granulation tissue or developing fibrocartilage. At this stage, the lesion is unstable but can heal after a period of non–weight bearing or internal fixation. If the interface is isointense with fluid or associated with cystic-appearing areas at the base of a non-displaced lesion, surgery is indicated.

*MR arthrography* MR arthrography is more accurate than conventional MR imaging in the evaluation of articular cartilage, the assessment of stability of osteochondral lesions (**Fig. 19**), and the detection of intra-articular bodies.[1,2,64]

MR arthrography aids in prearthroscopic assessment, differentiating between stage II and stage III OLT by documenting intra-articular communication of fluid around the lesion.[1,5]

MR arthrography allows excellent delineation of the chondral surface and provides good discrimination of higher grade cartilaginous lesions (**Fig. 20**).[64] MR arthrography is superior to unenhanced MR imaging because fluid is forced into the chondral defects at the interface between the OLT and its donor site. MR arthrography can detect chondral lesions as small as 2 mm. It should be noted that grade I chondral lesions have no surface contour defect or irregularity and may not be detected with MR arthrography.[5,64]

### Treatment
*Treatment of osteochondral injuries* Lesion stability determines treatment. In stable OLT (stage

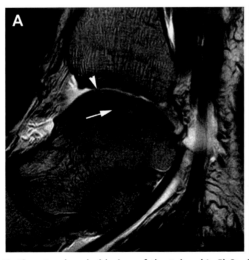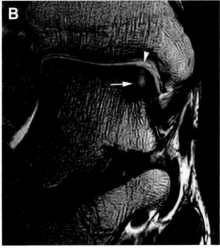

**Fig. 19.** Cystic osteochondral lesion of the talus. (*A, B*) Sagittal and coronal T1-weighted MR arthrograms of the right ankle demonstrate cystic medial osteochondral lesion of the talus (*arrows*). Note existence of cartilage detached flap (*arrowheads*).

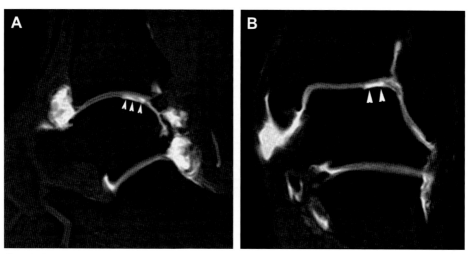

**Fig. 20.** Chondral grade IV lesion of the talar dome. (*A, B*) Sagittal and coronal fat-suppressed MR arthrograms of the left ankle show large cartilage defect (grade IV lesion) in the posterolateral aspect of the talar dome (*arrowheads*).

I and most stage II lesions) conservative treatment is recommended. Surgical treatment is advocated for unstable lesions, including stage IV and the majority of stage III lesions.[59,60,62]

Current principles of surgical treatment[65] fall into one of three categories: (1) loose body removal with or without stimulation of fibrocartilage growth (microfracture, curettage, abrasion, or transarticular drilling), (2) securing the OLT to the talar dome through retrograde drilling, bone grafting, or internal fixation, and (3) stimulating development of hyaline cartilage through osteochondral autografts, allografts, or cell culture.

*Treatment of cartilage injuries* As no stem cells are found within hyaline cartilage, the intrinsic repair capabilities of cartilage are limited. Many surgical repair techniques have been developed, with new cartilage-dedicated therapeutic strategies targeted at therapy for early stages of osteoarthritis. These strategies include: palliative (debridement or stabilization of loose articular cartilage), reparative (stimulation of repair from the subchondral bone, such as microfracturing), and restorative procedures (replacement of damaged cartilage; the most promising technique being cell transplantation–based repair).[62]

*Imaging cartilage repair* The advent of new procedures for repairing cartilage has increased the need for accurate noninvasive methods to objectively evaluate the success of repair. MR imaging is less invasive than arthroscopy, and allows a more comprehensive evaluation of repair tissue, from the articular surface of the joint to the bone–cartilage interface.[62] Despite the higher spatial

resolution of new pulse sequences, higher field strength MR imaging, and promising new techniques that evaluate cartilage matrix characteristics, many authors[62,64] suggest that MR arthrography is superior to MR imaging because it allows a more accurate characterization of the overlying repair tissue (**Fig. 21**). MR arthrography is helpful in evaluating detachment of the graft, facilitated differentiation between delamination of the base of the graft, and normal high-signal-intensity repair tissue in the immediate postoperative period.[62]

### Intra-articular loose bodies

Intra-articular loose bodies in the ankle joint may produce impingement symptoms. Loose bodies may be bone, cartilage, or bone and cartilage.[66]

Imaging is usually required to confirm the clinical diagnosis and localize the intra-articular loose bodies before surgery. Radiographs are useful only when calcified intra-articular bodies are present.

MR arthrography is the optimal imaging technique for detecting osseous and cartilaginous loose bodies with an accuracy of 92%, which is significantly better than MR imaging (57%–70%).[66] Air bubbles can mimic loose bodies on MR arthrography, but the distinction can usually be made by their nondependent position and typical appearance (see **Fig. 2**).[7–11]

### Adhesive capsulitis

**Prevalence, epidemiology, and definitions** Adhesive capsulitis, also known as a frozen ankle, is post-traumatic stiffness of the ankle joint that can severely affect the patient's movement and ability

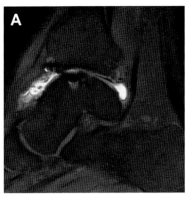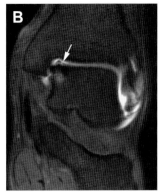

Fig. 21. Autologous osteochondral plug transfer in the medial talar dome. (*A, B*) Sagittal and coronal fat-suppressed MR arthrograms of the left ankle show good integration of osteochondral plug into the medial talar dome. The subchondral plate is flush, and there is only a slight cartilage fissure at the lateral margin of the graft (*arrow in B*).

to carry out activities of daily life. It can be caused by intra-articular or extra-articular pathology. It is a diagnostic and therapeutic challenge. Limited information concerning diagnosis and treatment is available in the musculoskeletal literature. Although the incidence of ankle adhesive capsulitis is unknown, some reports suggest that it may be more frequent than recognized.[67,68]

**Clinical symptoms and physical findings** Clinically, patients present with ankle pain, stiffness, and swelling. Calf muscle atrophy also may be present. Symptoms may start immediately after immobilization or several months after a traumatic ankle injury. Physical examination reveals decreased range of motion of the ankle joint, with limitation of both dorsi and plantar flexion because the entire capsule is involved.[67,68]

**Pathophysiology** The exact pathophysiology of posttraumatic adhesive capsulitis is unknown.[67,68]

Although all reported patients had traumatic ankle joint injury, a specific etiology has not been yet identified. Trauma may occur in the form of a single catastrophic event or repetitive minor injuries. Immobilization after trauma also may play a role in promoting fibrosis and subsequent progression to adhesive capsulitis. Although it has only been reported as a consequence of trauma, it is possible that nontraumatic ankle pain may be caused by adhesive capsulitis and may be secondary to other etiologies such as inflammatory synovitis or degenerative joint disease.[67,68]

Shoulder adhesive capsulitis is more common than in the ankle or other joints and has been extensively studied, demonstrating association with other conditions including diabetes, hypothyroidism, and hyperthyroidism. Pathologic studies indicate that the entire shoulder joint capsule is involved (**Fig. 22**), not just the site of the initial injury. The primary lesion occurs in the fibrous layer

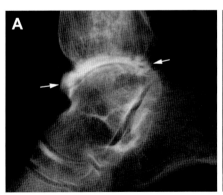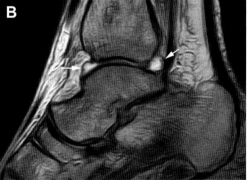

Fig. 22. Adhesive capsulitis of tibiotalar joint. (*A*) Lateral ankle arthrogram and (*B*) sagittal T1-weighted MR arthrogram of the right ankle in a patient previously surgically treated for bimalleolar fracture show restricted filling of the anterior and posterior capsular recesses (*arrows*). A decreased joint volume (4 mL) was encountered during arthrography as well.

of the capsule that becomes thickened by dense compact bundles of connective tissue containing new fibrocytes.

### Imaging

Classically, conventional arthrography was used for diagnosis of adhesive capsulitis of the ankle. Three arthrographic criteria were described: (1) reduction of joint volume from the normal 10 to 25 mL, to 3 to 5 mL (**Fig. 22**A), (2) high intra-articular pressure with back-flow of the contrast material, and (3) obliteration of the anterior, posterior, and syndesmotic recesses of the ankle.[67,68] Standard three-view ankle radiographs were usually non-specific. The value of CT and MR imaging has not been described.

The diagnostic value of MR imaging for ankle adhesive capsulitis is not clear, but remains an important tool for ruling out other causes of ankle pain and stiffness.

MR arthrography is currently the best method of diagnosis. It combines the advantages of MR imaging with conventional ankle arthrography criteria. MR arthrographic findings include: decrease in joint capacity, obliteration of normal joint recesses, and capsular thickening (**Fig. 22**B).[1]

### Treatment

Treatment of ankle adhesive capsulitis has not been reported in a significant number of patients, and there are no long-term outcome data. Range-of-motion ankle exercise programs and adjunctive therapies with or without intra-articular injection of steroids usually improve symptoms, but the long-term benefits are not documented. Arthroscopic synovectomy is potentially an effective treatment for posttraumatic ankle adhesive capsulitis.[67,68] Therapeutic effects may result from excision of the major intra-articular adhesions by partial synovectomy and removal of scar tissue. This is supported by improved range of ankle movement after ankle arthroscopy.

### SUMMARY

MR arthrography has become an important tool for the assessment of a wide variety of joint disorders. MR arthrography may facilitate the evaluation of patients with suspected intra-articular pathology in whom conventional MR imaging is not sufficient for obtaining an adequate diagnosis, and is thus useful for planning therapy. MR arthrography is an easy and safe procedure with a very low rate of complications. Indirect MR arthrography is a useful adjunct to conventional MR imaging and may be preferable to direct MR arthrography in cases where an invasive procedure is contraindicated or when fluoroscopy is not available.

In patients with a history of ankle sprains, chronic pain or instability can limit activity and affects up to 20% to 40% of patients. When conservative treatment has failed in these patients and surgical treatment is contemplated, MR arthrography of the ankle permits accurate diagnosis of ligament injuries, and other frequently associated pathology such as impingement syndromes, chondral and osteochondral injuries, and intra-articular loose bodies with greater reliability as compared with conventional MR imaging.

MR arthrography plays an important role in the diagnosis and staging of chondral and osteochondral injuries of the talar dome, and in monitoring the evolution of the different treatments available today.

Adhesive capsulitis or frozen ankle is a related posttraumatic disorder that severely limits ankle motion and may occur more frequently than recognized. MR arthrography of the ankle is a reliable way to diagnose this condition.

### REFERENCES

1. Cerezal L, Abascal F, Garcia-Valtuille R, et al. Ankle MR arthrography: how, why, when. Radiol Clin North Am 2005;43(4):693–707.
2. Cerezal L, Abascal F, Canga A, et al. Magnetic resonance arthrography indications and technique (II). Lower limb. Radiologia 2006;48(6):357–68.
3. Chandnani VP, Harper MT, Ficke JR, et al. Chronic ankle instability: evaluation with MR arthrography, MR imaging, and stress radiography. Radiology 1994;192(1):189–94.
4. Helgason JW, Chandnani VP. MR arthrography of the ankle. Radiol Clin North Am 1998;36(4):729–38.
5. Kramer J, Recht MP. MR arthrography of the lower extremity. Radiol Clin North Am 2002;40(5):1121–32.
6. Elentuck D, Palmer WE. Direct magnetic resonance arthrography. Eur Radiol 2004;14(11):1956–67.
7. Grainger AJ, Elliott JM, Campbell RS, et al. Direct MR arthrography: a review of current use. Clin Radiol 2000;55(3):163–76.
8. Osinski T, Malfair D, Steinbach L. Magnetic resonance arthrography. Orthop Clin North Am 2006;37(3):299–319.
9. Peh WC, Cassar-Pullicino VN. Magnetic resonance arthrography: current status. Clin Radiol 1999;54(9):575–87.
10. Sahin G, Demirtas M. An overview of MR arthrography with emphasis on the current technique and application hints and tips. Eur J Radiol 2006;58(3):416–30.
11. Steinbach LS, Palmer WE, Schweitzer ME. Special focus session. MR arthrography. Radiographics 2002;22(5):1223–46.

12. Brown RR, Clarke DW, Daffner RH. Is a mixture of gadolinium and iodinated contrast material safe during MR arthrography? AJR Am J Roentgenol 2000; 175(4):1087–90.

13. Schulte-Altedorneburg G, Gebhard M, Wohlgemuth WA, et al. MR arthrography: pharmacology, efficacy and safety in clinical trials. Skeletal Radiol 2003;32(1):1–12.

14. Robbins MI, Anzilotti KF Jr, Katz LD, et al. Patient perception of magnetic resonance arthrography. Skeletal Radiol 2000;29(5):265–9.

15. Wagner SC, Schweitzer ME, Weishaupt D. Temporal behavior of intra-articular gadolinium. J Comput Assist Tomogr 2001;25(5):661–70.

16. Lee SH, Jacobson J, Trudell D, et al. Ligaments of the ankle: normal anatomy with MR arthrography. J Comput Assist Tomogr 1998;22(5):807–13.

17. Hodler J. Technical errors in MR arthrography. Skeletal Radiol 2008;37(1):9–18.

18. Bergin D, Schweitzer ME. Indirect magnetic resonance arthrography. Skeletal Radiol 2003;32(10): 551–8.

19. Morrison WB. Indirect MR arthrography: concepts and controversies. Semin Musculoskelet Radiol 2005;9(2):125–34.

20. Schweitzer ME, Natale P, Winalski CS, et al. Indirect wrist MR arthrography: the effects of passive motion versus active exercise. Skeletal Radiol 2000; 29(1):10–4.

21. Vahlensieck M, Peterfy CG, Wischer T, et al. Indirect MR arthrography: optimization and clinical applications. Radiology 1996;200(1):249–54.

22. Zoga AC, Schweitzer ME. Indirect magnetic resonance arthrography: applications in sports imaging. Top Magn Reson Imaging 2003;14(1):25–33.

23. Bencardino J, Rosenberg ZS, Delfaut E. MR imaging in sports injuries of the foot and ankle. Magn Reson Imaging Clin N Am 1999;7(1):131–49.

24. Cheung Y, Rosenberg ZS. MR imaging of ligamentous abnormalities of the ankle and foot. Magn Reson Imaging Clin N Am 2001;9(3):507–31.

25. Garrick JG, Requa RK. The epidemiology of foot and ankle injuries in sports. Clin Sports Med 1988;7(1): 29–36.

26. Linklater J. Ligamentous, chondral, and osteochondral ankle injuries in athletes. Semin Musculoskelet Radiol 2004;8(1):81–98.

27. Gerber JP, Williams GN, Scoville CR, et al. Persistent disability associated with ankle sprains: a prospective examination of an athletic population. Foot Ankle Int 1998;19(10):653–60.

28. DiGiovanni BF, Fraga CJ, Cohen BE, et al. Associated injuries found in chronic lateral ankle instability. Foot Ankle Int 2000;21(10):809–15.

29. Renstrom PA. Persistently painful sprained ankle. J Am Acad Orthop Surg 1994;2(5):270–80.

30. Krips R, de Vries J, van Dijk CN. Ankle instability. Foot Ankle Clin 2006;11(2):311–29.

31. Colville MR. Surgical treatment of the unstable ankle. J Am Acad Orthop Surg 1998;6(6):368–77.

32. Peters JW, Trevino SG, Renstrom PA. Chronic lateral ankle instability. Foot Ankle 1991;12(3):182–91.

33. Rosenberg ZS, Beltran J, Bencardino JT. From the RSNA Refresher Courses. Radiological Society of North America. MR imaging of the ankle and foot. Radiographics 2000;20(Suppl):153–79.

34. Espinosa N, Smerek J, Kadakia AR, et al. Operative management of ankle instability: reconstruction with open and percutaneous methods. Foot Ankle Clin 2006;11(3):547–65.

35. Espinosa N, Smerek JP, Myerson MS. Acute and chronic syndesmosis injuries: pathomechanisms, diagnosis and management. Foot Ankle Clin 2006; 11(3):639–57.

36. Brown KW, Morrison WB, Schweitzer ME, et al. MRI findings associated with distal tibiofibular syndesmosis injury. AJR Am J Roentgenol 2004;182(1): 131–6.

37. Golano P, Vega J, Perez-Carro L, et al. Ankle anatomy for the arthroscopist. Part II: role of the ankle ligaments in soft tissue impingement. Foot Ankle Clin 2006;11(2):275–96.

38. Nikolopoulos CE, Tsirikos AI, Sourmelis S, et al. The accessory anteroinferior tibiofibular ligament as a cause of talar impingement: a cadaveric study. Am J Sports Med 2004;32(2):389–95.

39. Bassett FH III, Gates HS III, Billys JB, et al. Talar impingement by the anteroinferior tibiofibular ligament. A cause of chronic pain in the ankle after inversion sprain. J Bone Joint Surg Am 1990;72(1):55–9.

40. Oae K, Takao M, Naito K, et al. Injury of the tibiofibular syndesmosis: value of MR imaging for diagnosis. Radiology 2003;227(1):155–61.

41. Hintermann B, Knupp M, Pagenstert GI. Deltoid ligament injuries: diagnosis and management. Foot Ankle Clin 2006;11(3):625–37.

42. van Dijk CN, Bossuyt PM, Marti RK. Medial ankle pain after lateral ligament rupture. J Bone Joint Surg Br 1996;78(4):562–7.

43. Milner CE, Soames RW. The medial collateral ligaments of the human ankle joint: anatomical variations. Foot Ankle Int 1998;19(5):289–92.

44. Cerezal L, Abascal F, Canga A, et al. MR imaging of ankle impingement syndromes. AJR Am J Roentgenol 2003;181(2):551–9.

45. Umans HR, Cerezal L. Anterior ankle impingement syndromes. Semin Musculoskelet Radiol 2008; 12(2):146–53.

46. Robinson P, White LM. Soft-tissue and osseous impingement syndromes of the ankle: role of imaging in diagnosis and management. Radiographics 2002;22(6):1457–69.

47. Umans H. Ankle impingement syndromes. Semin Musculoskelet Radiol 2002;6(2):133–9.

48. Sanders TG, Rathur SK. Impingement syndromes of the ankle. Magn Reson Imaging Clin N Am 2008; 16(1):29–38.

49. Hauger O, Moinard M, Lasalarie JC, et al. Anterolateral compartment of the ankle in the lateral impingement syndrome: appearance on CT arthrography. AJR Am J Roentgenol 1999;173(3):685–90.

50. Rubin DA, Tishkoff NW, Britton CA, et al. Anterolateral soft-tissue impingement in the ankle: diagnosis using MR imaging. AJR Am J Roentgenol 1997; 169(3):829–35.

51. Wolin I, Glassman F, Sideman S, et al. Internal derangement of the talofibular component of the ankle. Surg Gynecol Obstet 1950;91(2):193–200.

52. Robinson P, White LM, Salonen DC, et al. Anterolateral ankle impingement: MR arthrographic assessment of the anterolateral recess. Radiology 2001; 221(1):186–90.

53. Tol JL, van Dijk CN. Anterior ankle impingement. Foot Ankle Clin 2006;11(2):297–310.

54. Paterson RS, Brown JN. The posteromedial impingement lesion of the ankle. A series of six cases. Am J Sports Med 2001;29(5):550–7.

55. Robinson P, White LM, Salonen D, et al. Anteromedial impingement of the ankle: using MR arthrography to assess the anteromedial recess. AJR Am J Roentgenol 2002;178(3):601–4.

56. Bureau NJ, Cardinal E, Hobden R, et al. Posterior ankle impingement syndrome: MR imaging findings in seven patients. Radiology 2000;215(2):497–503.

57. Fiorella D, Helms CA, Nunley JA. The MR imaging features of the posterior intermalleolar ligament in patients with posterior impingement syndrome of the ankle. Skeletal Radiol 1999;28(10):573–6.

58. Rosenberg ZS, Cheung YY, Beltran J, et al. Posterior intermalleolar ligament of the ankle: normal anatomy and MR imaging features. AJR Am J Roentgenol 1995;165(2):387–90.

59. Stone JW. Osteochondral lesions of the talar dome. Am J Orthop 2007;36(12):643–6.

60. Schachter AK, Chen AL, Reddy PD, et al. Osteochondral lesions of the talus. J Am Acad Orthop Surg 2005;13(3):152–8.

61. Berndt AL, Harty M. Transchondral fractures (osteochondritis dissecans) of the talus. Am J Orthop 1959;41-A:988–1020.

62. Choi YS, Potter HG, Chun TJ. MR imaging of cartilage repair in the knee and ankle. Radiographics 2008;28(4):1043–59.

63. De Smet AA, Fisher DR, Burnstein MI, et al. Value of MR imaging in staging osteochondral lesions of the talus (osteochondritis dissecans): results in 14 patients. AJR Am J Roentgenol 1990;154(3):555–8.

64. Schmid MR, Pfirrmann CW, Hodler J, et al. Cartilage lesions in the ankle joint: comparison of MR arthrography and CT arthrography. Skeletal Radiol 2003; 32(5):259–65.

65. Zengerink M, Szerb I, Hangody L, et al. Current concepts: treatment of osteochondral ankle defects. Foot Ankle Clin 2006;11(2):331–59.

66. Brossmann J, Preidler KW, Daenen B, et al. Imaging of osseous and cartilaginous intra-articular bodies in the knee: comparison of MR imaging and MR arthrography with CT and CT arthrography in cadavers. Radiology 1996;200(2):509–17.

67. Cui Q, Milbrandt T, Millington S, et al. Treatment of posttraumatic adhesive capsulitis of the ankle: a case series. Foot Ankle Int 2005;26(8):602–6.

68. Lui TH, Chan WK, Chan KB. The arthroscopic management of frozen ankle. Arthroscopy 2006;22(3):283–6.

# Osteochondral Lesions About the Ankle

Ketan N. Naran, MD, Adam C. Zoga, MD*

**KEYWORDS**

- Osteochondral lesions of the talus
- Ankle injury • Transchondral fracture

The term "osteochondral lesion" (OCL) indicates a posttraumatic or developmental injury simultaneously involving a region of hyaline cartilage at an articular surface and its underlying subchondral bone. Common locations for OCLs include, in order of published frequency, the femoral condyles, capitellum of the elbow, talar dome, and patella.[1,2] The OCL involves articular cartilage and the subjacent bone and can lead to loss of integrity or stability at an articular surface, with resultant decreased range of motion of the involved joint and, ultimately, premature osteoarthritis. OCLs are often a source of pain and dysfunction in the acute phase after injury and in the chronic phase owing to degenerative joint disease. Early diagnosis of OCLs is essential for development of an appropriate treatment plan to optimize pain relief in the acute phase of injury and to maintain and preserve long-term joint function.

In 1888, König[3] described osteochondritis dissecans in the knee, the first report of one of the many entities now documented in this spectrum of musculoskeletal injury. A similar pattern was subsequently described at the talar dome in 1922 by Kappis and colleagues.[3,4] The etiology of these lesions remains controversial today with numerous proposed biomechanical explanations and causes in the orthopaedic, pediatric, radiology, and sports medicine literature. Proposed etiologic factors for the development of OCLs include trauma, ischemia, genetics, abnormal vasculature, and metabolic disorders. Early on, the pathoetiology for osteochondritis dissecans was believed to be ischemic necrosis of subchondral bone with subsequent fragmentation of the articular surface and formation of free or loose osseous and cartilaginous bodies after detachment from the overlying articular cartilage. The current general consensus is that most, if not all, OCLs are posttraumatic in origin. Numerous series have shown that these lesions increase in prevalence in individuals who have a history of prior injury at the joint, and that OCL location can be predicted by knowledge of the injury mechanism.[1,4,5,6,7] Many OCLs, such as osteochondritis dissecans of the lateral aspect of the medial femoral condyle, continue to afflict young patients in reproducible locations that defy a weightbearing axis or easily explained biomechanical mechanism. Today, terms such as OCL and osteochondral defect are commonly used almost interchangeably to describe a spectrum of pathologic conditions that range from small, posttraumatic defects of articular cartilage to detached osteochondral fragments, including unstable lesions and even chronic, focal breaches at the articular surface with or without a history of antecedent trauma.[4,6]

## OSTEOCHONDRAL LESIONS OF THE ANKLE AND FOOT

OCLs about the ankle are particularly important to diagnose, because the tibiotalar joint is exposed to more compressive load per unit area than any other joint in the body. Failure of diagnosis can lead to evolution of a small, stable lesion into a larger lesion or an unstable fragment, which can result in chronic pain, joint instability, and premature osteoarthritis.[8,9] Most authors agree that tibiotalar OCLs are generally posttraumatic, and radiographs often are negative in the immediate period after injury. In the setting of a conservatively

Department of Radiology, Thomas Jefferson University Hospital, 132 South 10th Street, 10 Main, Philadelphia, PA 19107, USA
* Corresponding author.
*E-mail address:* adam.zoga@jefferson.edu (A.C. Zoga).

Radiol Clin N Am 46 (2008) 995–1002
doi:10.1016/j.rcl.2008.10.001
0033-8389/08/$ – see front matter © 2008 published by Elsevier Inc.

treated ankle sprain with normal radiographs and atypically prolonged pain refractory to treatment, an MR imaging study is often obtained to determine whether there is a radiographically occult nondisplaced fracture or an OCL.[2]

The most common OCLs about the ankle involve the talar dome. Elias and colleagues[5] described the exact locations of talar dome OCLs in 424 patients using a nine-zone anatomic grid. The grid is designed to promote consistency and reproducibility in OCL localization between radiologists and orthopaedic surgeons for preoperative planning (**Fig. 1**). Their study determined that medial talar dome lesions are more common than lateral lesions (62% versus 34%) and are both deeper and involve a greater surface area as compared with lateral lesions. Medial lesions were predominately located near the equator (midline of the talus in the anteroposterior dimension), and posteromedial/anterolateral lesions were rarely seen. Elias and colleagues[5] theorized that medial OCLs occur as a result of a combined inversion, plantar flexion, and external rotation injury causing impaction of the medial dome against the tibial articular surface.

Although the talar dome is the most frequent site of OCLs about the ankle, numerous other locations affected about the ankle and foot include

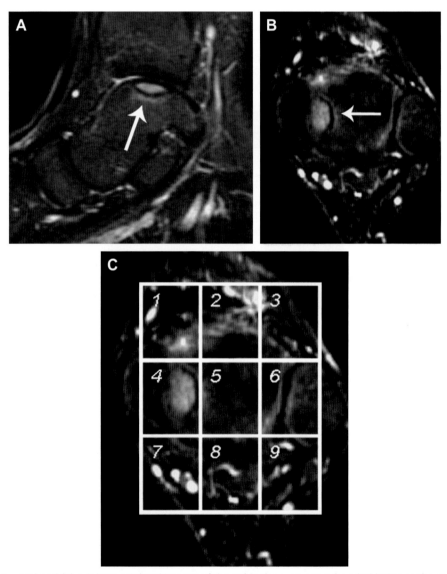

**Fig. 1.** (*A*) Sagittal and (*B*) axial T2-weighted images of the ankle show an osteochondral lesion at the medial talar dome at the equator (midline) of the anteroposterior (AP) dimension. (*C*) This corresponds to Zone 4 in the grid proposed by Elias and colleagues,[5] which was found to be the most common location for talar dome lesions and the location of the largest and deepest lesions.

he talar head, tibial plafond, cuboid, navicular, subtalar joint, and various metatarsal heads (Figs. 2–5). At the smaller joints of the mid and forefoot, MR imaging resolution suffers and more subtle findings may be relied on to diagnose an OCL. These include small chondral surface inhomogeneities and reactive subchondral marrow edema, often with a flame-shaped configuration but without reciprocal changes on the opposite side of the joint (see Fig. 4).

Common characteristics that exist among all of these posttraumatic OCLs in the foot and ankle are locations at reproducible sites of articular impaction with various ankle sprain mechanisms and a propensity for evolution to osteoarthritis and subsequent long-term disability if not treated effectively. With a history of inversion ankle sprain, the imager should take care to assess the middle subtalar facet and the talonavicular joint along with the more commonly involved tibiotalar surfaces. With an eversion injury, the calcaneocuboid joint should be carefully scrutinized along with the cuneiform bases and distal navicular. Dorsiflexion trauma can lead to OCLs in numerous locations from the anterior tibial plafond to the Lisfranc articulation. Regardless of location, every effort should be made to report any potential unstable osteochondral fragment or any articular surface collapse and to direct the managing physician toward a potentially more specific imaging modality if findings for such lesions are equivocal.

## IMAGING OF OSTEOCHONDRAL LESIONS

Berndt and Harty[1] developed a classification system in 1959 to characterize OCLs of the talus based on film/screen radiographic findings as follows: stage I, small focus of subchondral trabecular compression; stage II, partially detached fragment; stage III, fragment completely detached but nondisplaced; and stage IV, fragment detached and displaced. In the past 25 years, CT and MR imaging have come to play a greater role in the diagnosis and grading of OCLs, and conventional radiographs are now generally considered to be insensitive for the evaluation of suspected chondral injury, unless there is a significant subjacent osseous component.[10] As a result, standard of care for diagnosis of OCLs has shifted away from radiographs and toward either CT or, more frequently, MR imaging.

With the development of slip ring technology and numerous sequential detector rows in CT or multidetector CT (MDCT), the ability to evaluate subtle osseous injuries with multiplanar reconstructions has improved dramatically, although the authors know of no series pitting MDCT against MR imaging in the assessment of OCLs. Although current MDCT protocols clearly offer greater specificity than radiography for detection of many articular lesions, CT lacks the ability to demonstrate bone marrow edema and thus may be insensitive for early stage osteochondral lesions, particularly those that are nondisplaced or predominately involve articular cartilage. For these lesions, MR imaging remains the preferred imaging modality for detection of OCLs over CT.[7] Nevertheless, we believe that high-resolution MDCT plays a valuable role in the delineation of subchondral lesions that may present with instability of osteochondral fragments at the articular surface by detecting the presence of subchondral cysts, detachment, fragmentation, and displacement; we recommend MDCT in the setting of such lesions visible on MR imaging but equivocal for instability (Fig. 6).

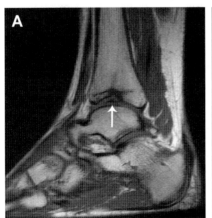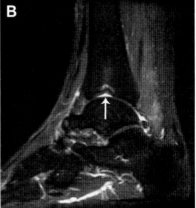

Fig. 2. (A) T1-weighted and (B) fat-saturated T2-weighted sagittal images of the ankle show an osteochondral lesion involving the lateral tibial plafond with impaction of the articular surface and subjacent reactive marrow edema in this patient status post an eversion injury.

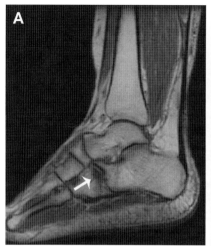
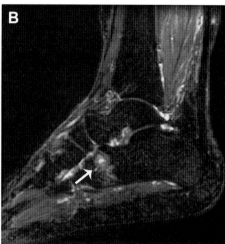

Fig. 3. (A) T1-weighted and (B) fat-saturated T2-weighted sagittal imaging of the ankle show an osteochondral lesion in the proximal cuboid in a patient who has refractory lateral ankle pain, failing conservative therapy after a severe sprain.

Although the resolution of noncontrast MR imaging does not begin to approach that of MDCT or conventional radiography, the superior contrast resolution between fluid and fat permits exquisite sensitivity for detection of bone marrow edema, whether related to acute trauma or chronic instability. Using MR imaging, in 1989 Anderson and colleagues[7] revised the original classification

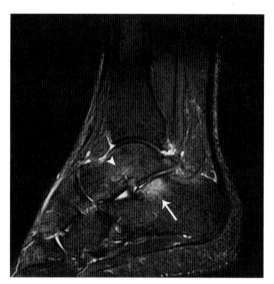

Fig. 4. Sagittal T2-weighted image with fat saturation demonstrates flame-shaped subchondral marrow edema involving the calcaneus at the posterior facet of the subtalar joint (arrow), consistent with an osteochondral lesion. Note the marrow edema in the body of the talus, not in a reciprocal subchondral location, likely reflecting altered biomechanics (arrowhead).

schema developed by Berndt and Harty, noting that there was no mention of subchondral cyst formation during the evolution of osteochondral lesions, for which stage IIA was added (Table 1). In 1993 Loomer and colleagues[11,12] noted that there was a high incidence of these "radiolucent lesions" or subchondral cysts on CT, with 77% of the patients in their series noted to have these findings, for which they subsequently added a stage V to the original Berndt and Harty classification to accommodate this finding. Numerous staging modifications have been proposed since, with MR imaging now evolving as the gold standard for diagnosing and classifying osteochondral lesions throughout the body (Fig. 7).

It is important to differentiate stable from unstable or potentially unstable OCL, because treatment varies accordingly. Unstable lesions are classically characterized on MR imaging as showing T2 hyperintense signal equal to joint fluid interposed between the detached osteochondral fragment and the parent bone. Using these strict criteria for determining OCL instability may lead to false negative assessments. Other relative indicators of instability on MR imaging include cystic change at the donor site undercutting the lesion, extensive bone marrow edema out of proportion to any recent trauma extending into the parent bone, or interval collapse of the articular surface at the site of the lesion since the inciting trauma. Absence of intervening fluid signal undercutting the OCL or other indirect MR imaging signs of fragment instability suggests a stable lesion that possesses vascular continuity with the parent bone (Figs. 8 and 9).

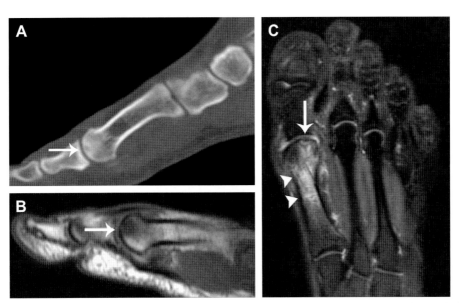

Fig. 5. (A) Sagittal MDCT reformatted image from a ballerina with chronic toe pain shows a subchondral lucency with surrounding sclerosis (arrow) involving the subchondral first metatarsal head. Corresponding (B) sagittal T1-weighted and (C) fat-saturated coronal T2-weighted images confirm an osteochondral lesion in the first metatarsal head (arrow) with associated reactive marrow edema extending far into the first metatarsal shaft (arrowheads). This lesion was treated successfully with microfracture.

At our institution, the noncontrast MR imaging ankle protocol includes an articular cartilage-sensitive sequence (T2-weighted fast spin echo with fat suppression) in a coronal plane prescribed by bisecting both malleoli on an axial localizer, for improved detection and localization of osteochondral lesions at the tibiotalar articular surfaces. The tibiotalar joint should, however, be routinely imaged in three orthogonal planes, particularly in patients who have a history of trauma or refractory ankle pain.[13]

Occasionally, differentiation between a stable and unstable OCL can be difficult using noncontrast MR imaging. In these cases, MR arthrography or MDCT may provide additional information. MR arthrography with distention of the joint can often help to determine whether the OCL is

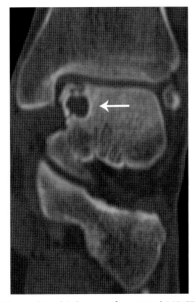

Fig. 6. Coronal multiplanar reformatted MDCT image of the ankle shows a large medial talar dome osteochondral lesion with subjacent cyst formation (arrow) and fragmentation indicating instability.

| Table 1 | |
|---|---|
| **Modified staging system for osteochondral lesions of the talus proposed by Anderson and colleagues** | |
| Stage I | Subchondral trabecular compression (radiographically occult but seen on MR imaging) |
| Stage II | Incomplete separation of the fragment |
| Stage IIA | Formation of a subchondral cyst |
| Stage III | Unattached, undisplaced fragment |
| Stage IV | Displaced fragment |

Data from Anderson IF, Crichton KJ, Grattan-Smith T, et al. Osteochondral fractures of the dome of the talus. J Bone Joint Surg Am 71:1989;1143–52.

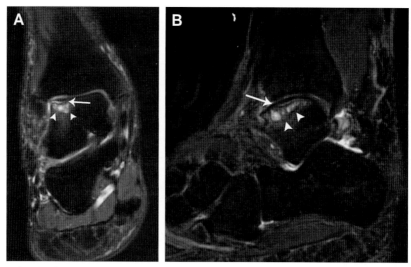

Fig. 7. (*A*) Coronal and (*B*) sagittal T2-weighed FSE MR images with fat saturation demonstrate an osteochondral lesion of the lateral talar dome, which is undercut by subchondral cystic changes (*arrowheads*), implying instability.

detached and deemed unstable by demonstrating contrast material insinuating between the fragment and the parent bone. In addition, direct MR arthrography can be more sensitive for detection of small, focal articular cartilage defects and intra-articular bodies because of capsular distension and excellent contrast resolution.[2]

Indirect MR arthrography, using high-resolution arthrographic sequences acquired at some interval after an intravenous contrast injection, has been proposed as another useful tool for establishing the stability of OCLs at the talar dome. In our experience, however, the potential for enhancement of granulation tissue undercutting a healing osteochondral lesion and the lack of direct joint distention compromise the specificity of indirect as compared with direct MR arthrography. Nevertheless, in an outpatient MR imaging setting

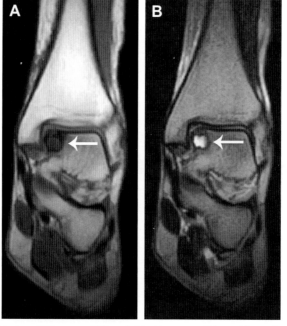

Fig. 8. (*A*) Coronal T1-weighted and (*B*) coronal T2-weighted images of the ankle performed on a 0.3-T open magnet show a medial talar dome osteochondral lesion with cystic change (*arrow*), suggesting instability. This patient went on to MDCT, which confirmed instability of the lesion. (See Fig. 6; same patient.)

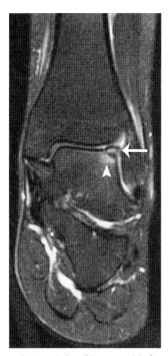

Fig. 9. Coronal T2-weighted image with fat saturation shows a lateral talar dome osteochondral lesion (*arrow*), which is displaced and thus characterized as unstable. Extensive subjacent reactive bone marrow edema is also seen (*arrowhead*). This patient went on to operative débridement of the unstable fragment and microfracture.

without the availability of either MDCT or direct MR arthrography, indirect MR arthrography may improve confidence or specificity in the assessment of OCL stability.

## OSTEOCHONDRAL LESIONS VERSUS AVASCULAR NECROSIS AND OSTEOARTHRITIS

The MR imaging pattern of OCLs we have discussed should be distinguished from that of subchondral avascular necrosis (AVN), which is more common in larger joints, such as the hip, but can occur in the talus, navicular, and metatarsal heads. AVN causes large regions of significant marrow signal abnormality similar to osteochondral lesions, but spares the articular surface and thus is isolated to the osseous structures themselves (**Fig. 10**). Both end-stage OCL and AVN can result in collapse of the articular surface isolated to one side of a joint, which connotes a poor prognosis.[14] In addition, OCLs should be distinguished from osteoarthritis, whether because of trauma or chronic biomechanical alterations. Although a single articular surface in an osteoarthritic joint can resemble an osteochondral lesion at MR imaging, the reciprocal changes spanning both sides of the joint reliably indicate the presence of osteoarthritis, along with hallmark findings of eburnation and osteophytes. Once these reciprocal findings are present at both sides of a joint, osteoarthritis exists, even if the predisposing injury was a posttraumatic OCL.

## TREATMENT OF OSTEOCHONDRAL LESIONS

Stable lesions are generally treated conservatively with nonweightbearing cast immobilization followed by progressive weightbearing over 3 to 4 months, a period that typically allows for adequate healing.[1,8] Unstable lesions are more likely to be managed surgically with arthroscopic or open approaches. Surgical techniques are aimed at removal of the subchondral fragment with curettage

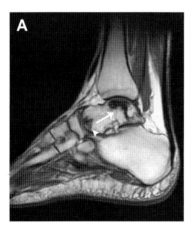
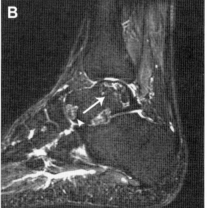

Fig. 10. (A) T1- and (B) T2-weighted FSE sagittal images show marked marrow signal abnormality involving the talar dome (*arrow*) with sparing of the articular surface, typical of avascular necrosis. Note the distinct pattern, not extending through the articular surface, in contrast to the osteochondral lesion of the talus demonstrated in Fig. 7. Ironically, this patient does have an osteochondral lesion at the talar head (*arrowhead*).

of the residual surface and removal of damaged cartilage and debris. Using microfracture technique, the remnant subchondral bone is then drilled to incite vascular recruitment and growth to promote new fibrocartilage to cover the original lesion. Alternatively, internal fixation can be performed with screws, wires, or bioabsorbable devices for larger unstable lesions measuring 7.5 mm or more in diameter.[8,15,16] A newer surgical approach involves using osteochondral allografts or autografts, which have been shown to heal with type II collagen instead of fibrocartilage. Type II collagen is similar in morphology to hyaline cartilage and should theoretically restore better physiologic function to the ankle joint.[4,8]

## SUMMARY

OCLs about the foot and ankle often manifest clinically as prolonged joint pain after trauma, often an ankle sprain, which is refractory to conventional, conservative therapeutic treatment. Noncontrast MR imaging is the standard of care imaging modality for diagnosing and classifying osteochondral lesions, but equivocal or difficult lesions can be assessed more specifically with direct MR arthrography or in conjunction with MDCT. Once an OCL has been identified, the imager should make every effort to determine whether it is stable or potentially unstable. At the talar dome, the most frequent site of OCL in the foot and ankle, the most common location is the mid anteroposterior equator of the medial dome articular surface. OCLs at the medial talar dome are larger and deeper than those at the lateral talar dome. Other typical locations for posttraumatic OCLs of the ankle and foot include the talar head, the calcaneocuboid joint, the tibial plafond, and the metatarsal heads. Using MR imaging, osteochondral lesions can be reliably distinguished from avascular necrosis and osteoarthritis.

## REFERENCES

1. Berndt AL, Harty M. Transchondral fractures (osteochondritis dissecans) of the talus. J Bone Joint Surg Am 1959;41-A:988–1020.
2. Loredo R, Sanders TG. Imaging of osteochondra injuries. Clin Sports Med 2001;20:249–78.
3. König F. Über freie körpee in den gelenken. Deut schen eitschrift für Chirurgie 1888;27:90–10 [in German].
4. Assenmacher JA, Kelikian AS, Gottlob C, et al Arthroscopically assisted autologous osteochondra transplantation for osteochondral lesions of the talar dome: an MRI and clinical follow-up study. Foot Ankle Int 2001;22:544–51.
5. Elias I, Zoga AC, Morrison WB, et al. Osteochondral lesions of the talus: localization and morphologic data from 424 patients using a novel anatomical grid scheme. Foot & Ankle International 2007;28:154–61.
6. Mosher TJ. MRI of osteochondral injuries of the knee and ankle in the athlete. Clin Sports Med 2006;25: 843–66.
7. Anderson IF, Crichton KJ, Grattan-Smith T, et al. Osteochondral fractures of the dome of the talus. J Bone Joint Surg Am 1989;71:1143–52.
8. Schachter AK, Chen AL, Reddy PD, et al. Osteochondral lesions of the talus. J Am Acad Orthop Surg 2005;13:152–8.
9. Boyd HS, Knight RA. Fractures of the astralgus. Southampt Med J 1942;35:160–7.
10. Wright RW, Boyce RH, Michener T, et al. Radiographs are not useful in detecting arthroscopically confirmed mild chondral damage. Clin Orthop & Relat Res 2006;442:245–51.
11. Loomer R, Fisher C, Lloyd-Smith R, et al. Osteochondral lesions of the talus. Am J Sports Med 1993;21:13–9.
12. Hepple S, Winson IG, Glew D. Osteochondral lesions of the talus: a revised classification. Foot Ankle Int 1999;20:789–93.
13. Kavanagh EC, Zoga AC. MRI of trauma to the foot and ankle. Semin Musculoskeletal Radiol 2006;10: 308–27.
14. Zoga AC, Schweitzer ME. Imaging sports injuries of the foot and ankle. Magn Reson Imaging Clin N Am 2003;11:295–310.
15. Tol JL, Struijs PA, Bossuyt PM, et al. Treatment strategies in osteochondral defects of the talar dome: a systematic review. Foot Ankle Int 2000;21:119–26.
16. Stone JW. Osteochondral lesions of the talar dome. J Am Acad Orthop Surg 1996;4:63–73.

# Postoperative Imaging of the Total Ankle Arthroplasty

Joseph M. Bestic, MD[a],*, Laura W. Bancroft, MD[a,b], Jeffrey J. Peterson, MD[a], Mark J. Kransdorf, MD[a,c]

**KEYWORDS**

• Ankle • Arthroplasty • Musculoskeletal

Interest in total ankle arthroplasty continues to expand since its initial introduction more than 30 years ago. Continued improvements in implant design and surgical technique are aimed at mitigating unacceptably high complication rates associated with earlier devices. Several major modifications of earlier devices have resulted in improved implant survival and cautious enthusiasm for newer designs, referred to as *second-generation devices*. Promising intermediate-term (5- to 7-year) results reported with second-generation total ankle arthroplasties have led to increased use as an alternative to ankle arthrodesis and prompted the development of new devices and surgical techniques. As with knee and hip arthroplasties, postoperative evaluation of total ankle arthroplasties requires clinical and radiologic assessment. Familiarity with the commonly used total ankle arthroplasty devices and appropriate postoperative imaging techniques is imperative to confirm expected postoperative imaging findings and facilitate detection of potential postoperative complications. This article focuses on both normal and abnormal postoperative imaging findings associated with commonly used second-generation total ankle arthroplasties.

## INDICATIONS

The complex biomechanics of the ankle make appropriate patient selection a crucial component in optimizing survival of total ankle arthroplasties. The ideal candidate for total ankle arthroplasty is an older individual (preferably with limited physical demands) who has painful ankle arthritis secondary to trauma or an inflammatory arthropathy. Absolute contraindications for total ankle arthroplasty include inadequate peripheral perfusion, active infection, overlying soft tissue or skin disorders, and neuropathic arthropathy (Charcot's joint). History of prior infection, severe lower-extremity malalignment or ankle instability, advanced osteoporosis, and osteonecrosis (depending on extent of involvement) are considered relative contraindications to total ankle arthroplasty.[1,2]

## IMPLANT DESIGN

Second-generation total ankle arthroplasty devices have evolved in an attempt to rectify inherent technical and design flaws of earlier models. Despite continual modifications in component design, the ideal total ankle has not been developed. These second-generation arthroplasty designs differ in degrees of articular conformity and constraint. Conformity is a measure of the extent of articular contact between components. Fully conforming prostheses have matching articular geometry so that they remain in direct contact along the entire articular surface. This relationship results in lower stress at any point of contact along the articular surface, theoretically reducing wear on the components. Constraint is defined as the resistance of an implant to a particular direction

[a] Department of Radiology, Mayo Clinic, 4500 San Pablo Road, Jacksonville, FL 32224-3899, USA
[b] Department of Radiology, Florida Hospital, 601 East Rollins Street, Orlando, FL 32789, USA
[c] Department of Radiologic Pathology, Armed Forces Institute of Pathology, 6825 16th Street NW, Building 54, Room M-133A, Washington, DC 20306, USA
* Corresponding author.
*E-mail address:* bestic.joseph@mayo.edu (J.M. Bestic).

Radiol Clin N Am 46 (2008) 1003–1015
doi:10.1016/j.rcl.2008.08.002

or range of motion. Although increased constraint is associated with improved stability at the ankle joint, excessive constraint leads to transfer of significant shear and rotatory forces at the prosthesis–bone interface, predisposing components to early loosening.

Existing second-generation devices incorporate two basic design philosophies: three- and two-component designs (mobile- and fixed-bearing, respectively). Three-component (mobile-bearing) designs are characterized by individual tibial and talar devices separated by a fully conforming mobile polyethylene spacer. These devices have the potential benefit of less wear and loosening, attributable to improved component conformity with minimal constraint. Two-component (fixed-bearing) devices have only a single articulation between tibial and talar devices, with the polyethylene spacer fixed to the tibial component. To reduce constraint, two-component designs typically demonstrate only partial articular conformity, theoretically increasing polyethylene contact stress and component wear.[1]

A multitude of total ankle arthroplasty devices are currently available, with at least 20 different systems in use worldwide and new devices in continual development. In the United States, some of the more commonly used second-generation total ankle arthroplasty devices include the STAR (Scandinavian Total Ankle Replacement, Waldemar Link, Hamburg, Germany), the Buechel-Pappas Total Ankle Replacement (Endotec, South Orange, New Jersey), and the Agility Total Ankle System (DePuy, Warsaw, Indiana).

Of these devices, only the Agility Ankle was approved by the U.S. Food and Drug Administration (FDA) for use in the United States before 2006.

Since then, three new devices were approved by the FDA, including the INBONE (formerly Topez) Total Ankle (INBONE Orthopedics, Boulder, Colorado), the Salto Talaris Anatomic Ankle Prosthesis (Tornier, Stafford, Texas), and the Eclipse Total Ankle Implant (Kinetikos Medical Inc., Carlsbad, California). Although these devices are FDA-approved for use with cement, they are almost exclusively used off-label without cement and feature bone in-growth components. In early 2007, the STAR device (intended for use without cement) was the first three-component design to receive conditional FDA approval.[2]

The STAR prosthesis (**Fig. 1**) is a cementless, three-component (mobile-bearing) design developed by H. Kofoed in 1981. Two characteristic cylindric bars or barrels positioned on the superior aspect of a flat trapezoidal tibial component anchor the implant in the subchondral tibia. A mobile, ultra-high molecular weight polyethylene (UHMWPE) meniscus or spacer articulates superiorly with the tibial plate and inferiorly with a longitudinally ridged convex talar component. The talar component is stabilized with a small fin that projects inferiorly into the talus.

Similar to the STAR device, the Buechel-Pappas Total Ankle Replacement (**Fig. 2**) is made of three components. The tibial component consists of a flat platform stabilized by a stem that extends superiorly into the tibial metaphysis. Placement of the stem into the tibial metaphysis requires violation of the anterior tibial cortex. A UHMWPE meniscus glides along the convex metallic talar component stabilized by a ridge on its undersurface, which articulates with a corresponding longitudinal groove on the talar component. Design features allow for limited inversion and eversion

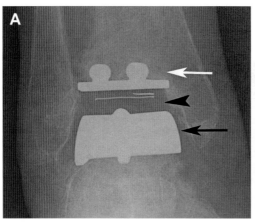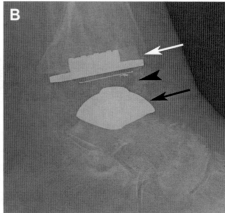

**Fig. 1.** STAR (Scandinavian Total Ankle Replacement, Waldemar Link, Hamburg, Germany). Anterior-posterior (*A*) and lateral (*B*) radiographs of the STAR device show implant components: tibial component (*white arrow*) with paired cylindric bars or barrels, polyethylene spacer (*arrowhead*) with internal wire marker, and talar component (*black arrow*).

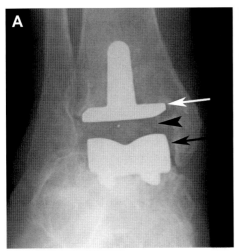
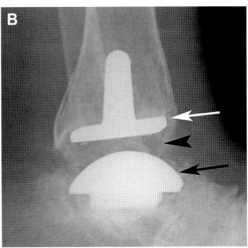

Fig. 2. Buechel-Pappas Total Ankle Replacement (Endotec, South Orange, New Jersey). Anterior-posterior (A) and lateral (B) radiographs of the Buechel-Pappas device show implant components: tibial component (*white arrow*) stabilized by a stem that extends superiorly into the tibial metaphysis, polyethylene spacer (*arrowhead*), and convex talar component (*black arrow*).

of the ankle joint without loss of conformity, and require minimal talar bone resection.

The Agility Total Ankle System (**Fig. 3**), which has been available since 1984, is the longest-used total ankle replacement system in the United States. The Agility Ankle is a two-component (fixed-bearing) implant with a partially conforming articulation. A characteristically broad-based tibial component abuts the tibial plafond and the medial and lateral malleoli. A concave polyethylene insert slides into the tibial component. In an attempt to mimic normal ankle anatomy, the superiorly convex talar component articulates with the tibial component in approximately 22° of external rotation. The tibial and talar components are stabilized with individual perpendicularly oriented fins. A syndesmotic fusion (unique to the Agility Ankle) provides a combined tibial and fibular support, while simultaneously increasing the surface area of the tibial component prosthesis–bone interface.

The INBONE (formerly Topez) Total Ankle (**Fig. 4**) is a two-component (fixed-bearing) device

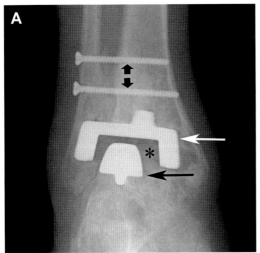
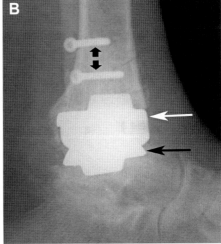

Fig. 3. Agility Total Ankle System (DePuy, Warsaw, Indiana). Anterior-posterior (A) and lateral (B) radiographs of the Agility device show implant components: broad-based tibial component (*white arrow*), polyethylene insert (*asterisk*), and convex talar component (*black arrow*). Also note the syndesmotic fusion (*double black arrows*), unique to the Agility Ankle.

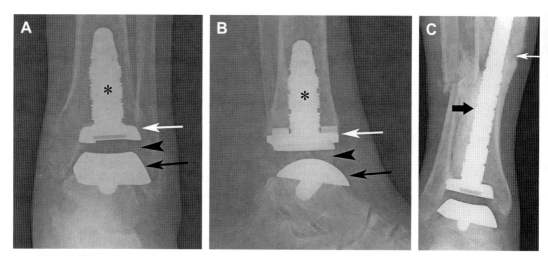

Fig. 4. INBONE (formerly Topez) Total Ankle (INBONE Orthopedics, Boulder, Colorado). Anterior-posterior (A) and lateral (B) radiographs of the INBONE device shows implant components: tibial component (*white arrow*) with modular anchoring stem (*asterisk*), polyethylene insert (*arrowhead*), and talar component (*black arrow*). (C) AP radiograph of the INBONE device with a long modular stem (*black arrow*) extending beyond the level of a tibial shaft fracture (*white arrow*) in an attempt to improve implant stability. Also note the slightly angulated fibular shaft fracture.

with modular anchoring stems extending from the tibial and anatomically designed talar components. The length of the modular stems can be adjusted to optimize component stability. Vertical fixation allows for less bone removal and leaves the fibula and most of the medial malleolus intact. As with other two-component devices, a polyethylene insert attaches to the tibial component. An innovative intraoperative guidance system has

been developed for use with the INBONE Total Ankle to facilitate proper alignment of the components.

The Salto Talaris Anatomic Ankle Prosthesis (**Fig. 5**) is a two-component (fixed-bearing) device with design features mimicking normal ankle anatomy. A tapered fixation plug on the superior aspect of the tibial component secures the implant against the bone surface. This fixation plug

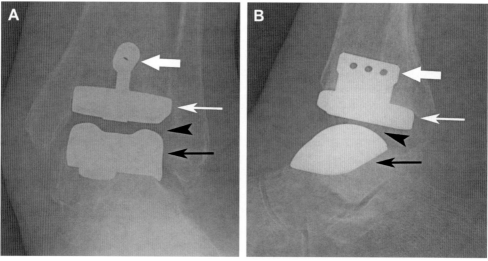

Fig. 5. Salto Talaris Anatomic Ankle Prosthesis (Tornier, Stafford, Texas). Anterior-posterior (A) and lateral (B) radiographs of the Salto Talaris device show implant components: tibial component (*thin white arrow*) with superiorly extending tapered fixation plug (*large white arrow*), polyethylene insert (*arrowhead*), and talar component (*black arrow*).

requires the formation of a keyhole-shaped anterior cortical window during component placement. A slide-on UHMWPE insert is attached to the tibial component and demonstrates matching articular geometry with the convex talar implant.

## POSTOPERATIVE IMAGING

Serial radiographs complement postoperative clinical assessment. Appropriate imaging techniques facilitate identification of early postoperative complications, which may not be apparent on clinical examination. CT can supplement evaluation of total ankle arthroplasty devices by providing a more detailed evaluation of implant components and surrounding osseous change.

Routine postoperative radiographs provide valuable information for orthopedic surgeons about the anatomic relationship between osseous structures and implant components and the presence and extent of bone loss or bony overgrowth. Anterior-posterior (AP) and lateral views of the ankle should ideally be obtained in the standing position to ensure physiologic positioning. Non-weight-bearing lateral radiographs obtained with the ankle in maximal dorsiflexion and plantar flexion can be obtained to evaluate for changes in range of motion at the ankle joint. Fluoroscopy is used to confirm component alignment intraoperatively and optimize radiographic alignment of the component–bone or bone–cement interfaces in the postoperative setting.[3]

The ability of radiography to detect progressive changes in component position, which may signify evidence of component loosening, is an integral component of the postoperative evaluation of total ankle arthroplasties. Changes in component position are often readily apparent. More subtle changes in component angulation or position relative to surrounding osseous structures can be detected when evaluating angular and linear measurements on serial radiographic examinations.

Several techniques have been proposed for establishing radiologic reference points used to monitor for evidence of component migration (**Fig. 6**).[4–7] Using the STAR device as an example, reference angular and linear values can be defined. On AP view of the ankle, the alpha angle ($\alpha$) is formed by the intersection of lines drawn parallel to the flat plate of the tibial component and the long axis of the tibial shaft (normal = 90°). On the lateral view of the ankle, the beta angle ($\beta$) is formed by the intersection of lines drawn parallel to the flat plate of the tibial component and the long axis of the tibial shaft (normal = 90°). The gamma angle ($\gamma$) is formed by the intersection of a line drawn through the long axis of the talar

component with a line drawn from the posterior talar component through the middle of the talar neck. The gamma angle in the postoperative setting has been shown to range from 11.1° to 33.4°, with an average measurement of 18.8°.[6]

Linear values are established by measuring position of components relative to surrounding osseous structures. Measurement "a" is the perpendicular distance between the tip of the lateral malleolus and a line drawn through the base of the tibial component on AP view. Measurement "b" is the perpendicular distance from the anterior aspect of the talar component to a line intersecting the calcaneal tubercle and dorsal aspect of the talonavicular joint on the lateral view. Measurement "c" is the perpendicular distance from the posterior aspect of the talar component to a line intersecting the calcaneal tubercle and dorsal aspect of the talonavicular joint.

Routine use of these measurements may not be practical, but when loosening is suspected based on history or physical examination, these measurements allow detection of subtle abnormalities and can provide surgeons with evidence of quantifiable change. An angular change of greater than 5° of either component has been suggested as a threshold for evidence of component migration or subsidence.[6] Greater than 5 mm subsidence of the talar component on lateral view is considered suggestive of loosening.[5]

In addition to changes in component position, lucent lines at the component–bone interface may suggest hardware loosening. Linear lucencies that increase in width or extent from baseline or measure greater than 2 mm are considered significant.[3] These lucencies must be differentiated from those related to surgical technique. Examples of lucencies seen after surgery include osseous defects attributable to a discrepancy between drill-hole size and cylindric barrel diameter with the STAR device or excessive medullary reaming with the INBONE device (**Fig. 7**). Lucencies related to surgical technique can be expected to become less well-defined over time, as they are replaced with physiologic bone production.[2]

To better localize abnormalities of the components, a zonal system (similar to Gruen's classification for hip arthroplasty) can be used for each device.[4,8–10] For example, for the STAR device, bone surrounding the tibial component can be divided into distinct zones.[7] Individual zones are demarcated by lines drawn perpendicular to the tibial plate on each side of the cylindrical bars, which are seen en face in the AP projection. Five zones (labeled 1–5, medial to lateral) are thus established, spanning the length of the tibial plate. In a similar fashion, the tibial component can be divided into

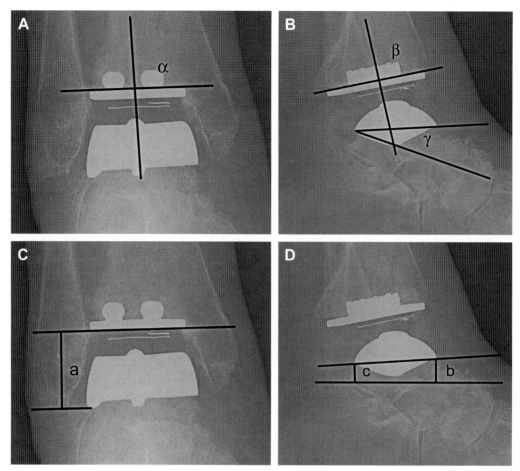

**Fig. 6.** Method of establishing angular and linear measurements to evaluate for component migration/subsidence (illustrated with the STAR device). AP (*A*) and lateral (*B*) views of the STAR device depict method of angular evaluation. The alpha angle (α) is formed by the intersection of lines drawn parallel to the flat plate of the tibial component and the long axis of the tibial shaft. The beta angle (β) is formed by the intersection of lines drawn parallel to the flat plate of the tibial component and the long axis of the tibial shaft. The gamma angle (γ) is formed by the intersection of a line drawn through the long axis of the talar component with a line drawn from the posterior talar component through the middle of the talar neck. AP (*C*) and lateral (*D*) views of the STAR device depict method of linear evaluation. (a) Perpendicular distance between the tip of the lateral malleolus and a line drawn through the base of the tibial component on AP view. (b) Perpendicular distance from the anterior aspect of the talar component to a line intersecting the calcaneal tubercle and dorsal aspect of the talonavicular joint on the lateral view. (c) Perpendicular distance from the posterior aspect of the talar component to a line intersecting the calcaneal tubercle and dorsal aspect of the talonavicular joint.

individual zones on the lateral radiograph. Using the cylindrical bars of the tibial plate as an internal reference, lines are drawn perpendicular to the tibial plate at the anterior and posterior aspect of the cylindrical bars now viewed in long axis. In the lateral projection, three zones are established (labeled A–C, anterior to posterior). Dividing the components into distinct zones allows for accurate serial assessment of questioned abnormalities and facilitates effective communication between the radiologist and orthopedic surgeon.

For a suspected radiographic abnormality, CT may be used to further evaluate or confirm postoperative complications. CT has been proven to be superior to conventional radiography for early detection and more accurate quantification of periprosthetic lucencies.[11] CT may permit evaluation of radiographically occult abnormalities specifically pertaining to the polyethylene component.

CT technique must be modified to reduce attenuation and streak artifact related to metal with high attenuation coefficient. The effective energy of the X-ray beam should be increased (140 kilovolt-peak [kVp], 200 milliampere-second [mAs]) to enhance penetration of dense metal and improve

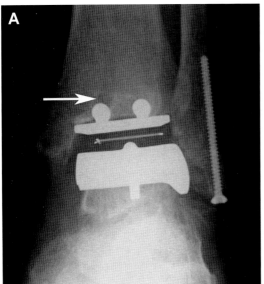
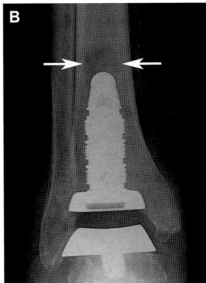

Fig. 7. Periprosthetic lucencies related to operative technique should not be misinterpreted as osteolysis. (*A*) Initial postoperative AP radiograph of a STAR total ankle shows discordance between the surgical drill hole (*arrow*) and medial cylindric bar of the tibial component. (*B*) AP radiograph of an INBONE device shows excessive medullary reaming (*arrows*).

accuracy of projection data. Aligning the axis of the implant so that the beam traverses the smallest possible cross-sectional area can reduce artifact, which can be further minimized by using narrow collimation settings and extended range postprocessing.[12] A standard or smooth reconstruction filter is often preferred, because metallic artifact is accentuated with the use of a sharp or bone algorithm. CT scale may be manually increased (up to 40,000 Hounsfield units) to accommodate the high linear attenuation coefficients of metal, which lie outside the normal range of reconstructed CT numbers.[12] Multiplanar reformatted imaging, which is often helpful in troublesome cases, requires thin-slice selection to achieve isotropic imaging.

## COMPLICATIONS

Second-generation total ankle arthroplasty devices have been reported to have promising intermediate-term results. The long-term outcome of total ankle arthroplasty is under continual scrutiny, with recent success tempered by the poor performance of cemented first-generation devices and the realization that complications occur with second-generation devices.[4–6,9,10,13–20] Published evidence concerning the safety and efficacy of total ankle arthroplasties consists largely of retrospective, uncontrolled case studies. Furthermore, existing data are often difficult to interpret secondary to heterogeneous patient populations and

poorly defined variables, such as differences in operator experience and individual surgical technique.[2]

In a systematic review of the literature addressing the intermediate- and long-term outcomes of total ankle arthroplasties, Haddad and colleagues[18] reported 5- and 10-year implant survival rates of 78% and 77%, respectively. The same review showed an overall revision rate of 7%, with loosening or subsidence the most common indication for revision. In a meta-analysis specifically reviewing the efficacy of three-component total ankle arthroplasties, Stengel and colleagues[19] found an overall 5-year implant survival rate of 90.6%. Weighted complication rates ranged from 1.6% (deep infections) to 14.7% (impingement). The same meta-analysis showed that secondary surgery was required in 12.5% of cases, with secondary arthrodesis performed in 6.3%.

Total ankle arthroplasties are predisposed to various complications because of the substantial shearing and axial loading forces transmitted through the small ankle joint. Complications associated with total ankle arthroplasties are categorized as intraoperative, early postoperative, or delayed. Intraoperative complications include injury to neurovascular and tendinous structures, malpositioning or improper sizing of prosthetic components, excessive bone resection, and periprosthetic fractures. Malleolar fractures constitute one of the most frequent complications observed with total ankle arthroplasties, with a reported incidence of approximately 20%.[19,21,22] Periprosthetic fractures may result from inappropriate excursion of the oscillating saw blade or drill, excessive levering with instrumentation, improper component sizing, or component malpositioning (**Fig. 8**).[2] Some authors have proposed prophylactic pinning of the malleoli.[22] Infection, impaired wound healing, stress fractures across the medial malleolus, and syndesmotic nonunions (Agility Ankle only) may be observed in the early postoperative period. Problems with wound healing have been reported in approximately 10% of cases.[5,16,21] Infection is considered a rare occurrence after total ankle arthroplasty, with a reported incidence of less than 4%.[4,6,9,16,19] Deep infections frequently require debridement with complete implant removal followed by placement of a temporary antibiotic impregnated spacer (**Fig. 9**).

Delayed postoperative complications include osteolysis and aseptic loosening, subsidence

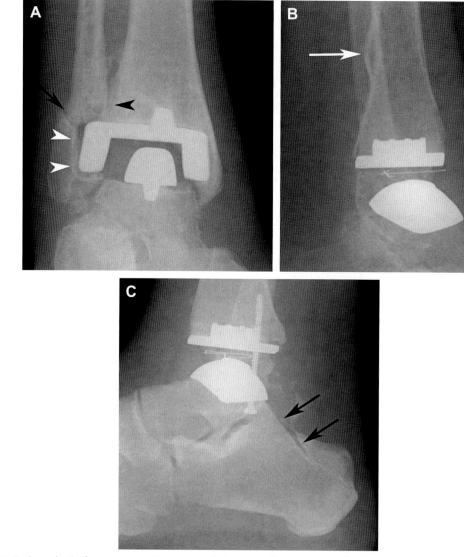

Fig. 8. Periprosthetic fractures constitute one of the most frequent complications observed with total ankle arthroplasties. (*A*) AP radiograph of an Agility Ankle shows a periprosthetic fracture through the distal fibula (*black arrow*) likely caused by altered stress distribution. Note lack of syndesmotic fusion (*black arrowhead*) and circumferential lucency (*white arrowheads*) about the lateral aspect of the tibial component, which is concerning for implant loosening. (*B*) Lateral radiograph of a STAR total ankle shows buckling of the posterior tibial cortex (*arrow*) related to protrusion of a drill bit used during placement of the tibial component saw guide. (*C*) Lateral radiograph of a STAR total ankle shows a linear defect (*arrows*) through the posterior calcaneus secondary to excessive excursion of the oscillating saw used during implant placement.

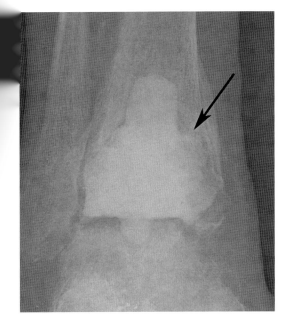

Fig. 9. Temporary antibiotic impregnated spacer (*arrow*) was placed after complete implant removal of an INBONE total ankle for deep infection.

and component migration, periprosthetic fractures (often related to altered stress distribution), polyethylene spacer migration or fracture, bony overgrowth with resultant impingement, syndesmotic

nonunion (Agility Ankle only), progressive ankle instability, and reflex sympathetic dystrophy. One of the most frequently encountered delayed complications leading to revision surgery involves the development of bony overgrowth and subsequent impingement, with a reported prevalence of up to 63% (**Fig. 10**).[6,13]

Failure secondary to osteolysis with subsequent aseptic loosening is generally considered the major delayed complication of total ankle arthroplasty.[20] Osteolysis results from a foreign body reaction to polyethylene particulate debris with resultant bony destruction (**Fig. 11**). Polyethylene osteolysis is primarily the result of poor component alignment with incongruent polyethylene articulation between the tibial and talar components.[2] Available data suggest the incidence of aseptic loosening is approximately 5% to 6%.[19,21] Revision total ankle arthroplasty or arthrodesis may be necessary if loosening is secondary to extensive osteolysis.[2]

Subsidence and component migration are believed to be caused by inadequate component support or poor in-growth of bone, with resultant failure of initial component stabilization (**Fig. 10**).[2] A prevalence of periprosthetic lucencies in up to 85% of cases has been reported, although their significance to component migration is debated.[4,9,10,23] Regardless, close follow-up is

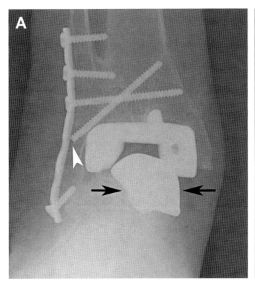

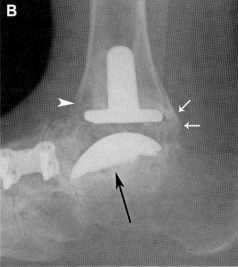

Fig. 10. Component subsidence and migration. (A) AP radiograph of an Agility Ankle depicts marked subsidence and medial tilting of the talar component (*arrows*). The tibiofibular syndesmotic fusion remains solid despite the presence of a fractured syndesmotic screw (*arrowhead*). (B) Lateral radiograph of a Buechel-Pappas total ankle shows advanced subsidence of the talar component (*black arrow*). An ill-defined lucency within the anterior tibia adjacent to the tibial component represents coexistent polyethylene osteolysis (*arrowhead*). Also note the prominent bony overgrowth bridging the posterior aspect of the ankle joint (*white arrows*), which often results in significant impingement.

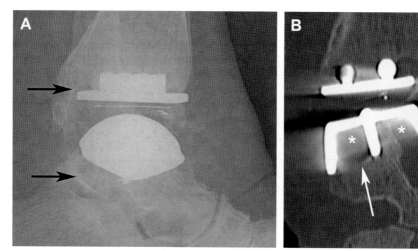

**Fig. 11.** Polyethylene osteolysis. (A) Lateral radiograph of a STAR total ankle shows poorly defined periprosthetic lucencies surrounding the posterior aspect of the tibial component and within the talus posteriorly (*arrows*). (B) Coronal CT examination of the same patient more clearly depicts the extent of polyethylene osteolysis about the tibial and talar components (*thin white arrows*). Note extension of osteolysis immediately inferior to the concave undersurface of the talar component (*asterisks*). Evaluation of this region is clearly inadequate with radiography, highlighting the usefulness of CT in these cases.

recommended for all periprosthetic lucencies to monitor for evidence of progression, which could indicate risk for subsequent component migration.

Long-term stability of the ankle after total ankle arthroplasty requires appropriate ligament balancing to prevent potential varus or valgus instability. This instability can lead to significant component malalignment with migration of the polyethylene spacer in three-component designs (**Fig. 12**). Ligament balancing can often be achieved at surgery, through either ligament repair or reconstruction, or proper selection of the polyethylene spacer (**Fig. 13**).[2] Although considered a rare complication, polyethylene spacer fractures secondary to component malalignment and excessive contact stress have been reported (**Fig. 14**).[24]

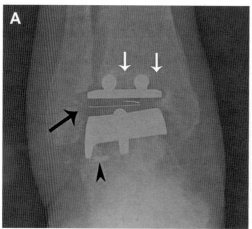
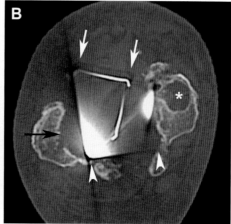

**Fig. 12.** Migration of polyethylene spacer with component malalignment. (A) AP radiograph of a STAR total ankle shows component malalignment with lateral migration of the polyethylene spacer and remodeling of the adjacent fibula (*black arrow*). These changes often occur from ligamentous instability. Note suture anchor from failed lateral ligamentous reconstruction performed at STAR device placement (*arrowhead*). Ill-defined lucencies surrounding the tibial component (*white arrows*) represent evidence of polyethylene osteolysis. (B) Axial CT of the same patient confirms displacement of the polyethylene spacer (*white arrows*) with respect to the tibial component (*arrowheads*). Note associated erosion of the adjacent fibula (*black arrow*) and polyethylene osteolysis in the medial malleolus (*asterisk*).

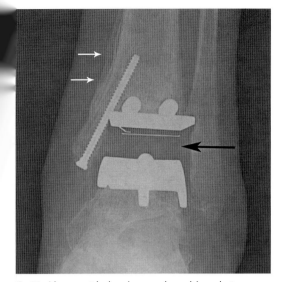

Fig. 13. Ligament balancing can be achieved at surgery through proper selection of the polyethylene spacer. In this patient who has a STAR device, a thick polyethylene spacer (*black arrow*) was used to improve ankle stability. Note periosteal reaction along the medial tibia (*white arrows*) related to healing of prior medial malleolar fracture with fully threaded malleolar screw in place.

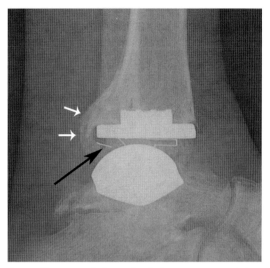

Fig. 14. Fracture of the polyethylene component. Lateral radiograph of a STAR device clearly shows posterior displacement of a wire fragment embedded within the polyethylene (*black arrow*), indicating failure of the polyethylene spacer. Also note the exuberant bony overgrowth bridging the posterior aspect of the ankle joint (*white arrows*). Abnormalities of the polyethylene component are often radiographically occult (especially when dealing with devices lacking an imbedded metallic marker). In these cases, CT can effectively evaluate the integrity and position of the polyethylene component.

One of the most frequently encountered delayed complications leading to revision surgery involves the development of bony overgrowth and subsequent impingement, with a reported revalence of up to 63% (**Figs. 10**B and **14**).[6,13]

Currently available second-generation total ankle devices were developed with similar design philosophies and therefore exhibit many of the same complications. Three-component (mobile-bearing) designs show a slightly increased risk for polyethylene spacer dislocation and may generate more wear particles from the two separate articulations. Two-component (fixed-bearing) designs have only partial conformity involving a single articulation, which increases not only stability but also theoretically polyethylene contact stress and wear. The risk for polyethylene spacer dislocation is much lower with two-component designs because the spacer is fixed to the tibial component.[1]

Individualized component design features account for several unique postoperative complications, which may be anticipated on follow-up imaging. The three-component STAR device permits limited inversion and eversion, which may result in excessive contact stress (edge-loading) on the polyethylene spacer and transfer of increased load to the prosthesis–bone interface.[1] Excessive contact stress accelerates wear on the polyethylene component, ultimately predisposing patients to osteolysis. Revision rates of 24% to 34% have been reported with the uncemented STAR device.[5,6]

The Buechel-Pappas total ankle uses a fully conforming deep-sulcus polyethylene spacer, which allows limited inversion and eversion motion and theoretically reduces contact stress.[1,16] The small AP dimensions of the Buechel-Pappas tibial plate compared with those of the resected distal tibia predisposes this device to bony overgrowth, which may ultimately lead to impingement (**Fig. 10**B).[16] Bony overgrowth limits motion in mobile-bearing ankles and essentially converts them to two-component designs. Reported clinical results of the Buechel-Pappas total ankle show a cumulative survivorship of 93.5% at 10 years.[16] In the same study, the most frequently encountered complication was delayed wound healing (14%) followed by malleolar fractures (6%), infection (4%), talar component subsidence (2%), and severe spacer wear (2%).

Prevalence of delayed syndesmotic union and nonunion (unique to the Agility Ankle) has been reported to be approximately 33% and 10%, respectively.[9] Nonunion or delayed union of the syndesmotic fusion has been associated with the development of circumferential lucencies about the tibial component (**Fig. 8**A). Although the significance of these periprosthetic lucencies (defined as <2 mm in width) has been debated, the rate of component migration and subsidence may be increased in these cases.[4,9,10]

Nonunion of the syndesmosis is also associated with the development of lysis (defined as lucencies >2 mm in width).[9] When lysis occurs in a characteristic location along the lateral margin of the tibial component, it is called *ballooning lysis*. This phenomenon is believed to occur secondary to osseous resorption in a region of persistent micromotion or shear stress between the implant and residual lateral malleolus, and typically stabilizes within 1 year after implantation.[4,9] In contrast, progressive lysis in other locations is considered concerning for osteolysis related to polyethylene particulate disease.

Agility Ankle component subsidence or migration most frequently involves the talar component (**Fig. 10**A).[10,13] This complication may be attributable to the narrow design of the talar component, which only partially covers the cut talar surface.[10] Newer designs incorporate a wider-based talar component to combat subsidence.[2] The 5-year survival rates of the Agility Ankle has been reported at 54% using reoperation and 80% using failure as respective end points.[13] Knecht and colleagues[4] reported a major revision rate of 11% for the Agility Ankle over a mean follow-up period of 9 years.

Limited data are currently available on results of newer total ankle designs, including the INBONE, Salto-Talaris, and Eclipse ankles (and a recent conditional FDA approval of the STAR mobile-bearing design). Nonetheless, continual advances in implant design and surgical technique hold much promise for improved outcomes.

## SUMMARY

Intermediate-term results reported with second-generation total ankle arthroplasty devices are encouraging. Despite recent advancements in implant design and corresponding surgical techniques, the durability of second-generation devices remains under continued scrutiny. An increase in popularity of these devices necessitates a familiarity with basic component design philosophy and an appreciation for both normal and abnormal postoperative imaging features. Serial radiography is integral to the postoperative evaluation of total ankle arthroplasties. CT complements postoperative imaging evaluation of implant components and surrounding bone, specifically regarding occult or equivocal radiographic findings.

## REFERENCES

1. Easley ME, Vertullo CJ, Urban WC, et al. Total ankle arthroplasty. J Am Acad Orthop Surg 2002;10:157–67.
2. DeOrio JK, Easley ME. Total ankle arthroplasty. Instr Course Lect 2008;57:383–413.
3. Berquist TH, DeOrio JK. Reconstructive procedures. In: Berquist TH, editor. Radiology of the foot and ankle. 2nd edition. Philadelphia: Lippincott Williams & Wilkins; 2000. p. 479–85.
4. Knecht SI, Estin M, Callaghan JJ, et al. The Agility total ankle arthroplasty. Seven to sixteen-year follow-up. J Bone Joint Surg Am 2004;86:1161–71.
5. Anderson T, Montgomery F, Carlsson A. Uncemented STAR total ankle prostheses: three to eight-year follow-up of fifty-one consecutive ankles. J Bone Joint Surg Am 2003;85:1321–9.
6. Valderrabano V, Hintermann B, Dick W. Scandinavian total ankle replacement. Clin Orthop 2004;424: 47–56.
7. Bestic JM, Peterson JJ, DeOrio JK, et al. Postoperative evaluation of the total ankle arthroplasty. AJR Am J Roentgenol 2008;190:1112–23.
8. Gruen TA, McNeice GM, Amstutz HC. "Modes of failure" of cemented stem-type femoral components: a radiographic analysis of loosening. Clin Orthop Relat Res 1979;141:17–27.
9. Pyevich MT, Saltzman CL, Callaghan JJ, et al. Total ankle arthroplasty: a unique design. Two to twelve-year follow-up. J Bone Joint Surg Am 1998;80: 1410–20.
10. Kopp FJ, Patel MM, Deland JT, et al. Total ankle arthroplasty with the agility prosthesis: clinical and radiographic evaluation. Foot Ankle Int 2006;27(2): 97–103.
11. Hanna RS, Haddad SL, Lazarus ML. Evaluation of periprosthetic lucency after total ankle arthroplasty: helical CT versus conventional radiography. Foot Ankle Int 2007;28(8):921–6.
12. Lee MJ, Kim S, Lee SA, et al. Overcoming artifacts from metallic orthopedic implants at high-field-strength MR imaging and multidetector CT. Radiographics 2007;27:791–803.
13. Spirt AA, Assal M, Hansen ST. Complications and failure after total ankle arthroplasty. J Bone Joint Surg Am 2004;86:1172–8.
14. Kofoed H. Scandinavian total ankle replacement (STAR). Clin Orthop Relat Res 2004;424:73–9.
15. Anderson T, Montgomery F, Carlsson A. Uncemented STAR total ankle prostheses. J Bone Joint Surg Am 2004;86:103–11.
16. Buechel FF, Buechel FF, Pappas MJ. Ten-year evaluation of cementless Buechel-Pappas meniscal bearing total ankle replacement. Foot Ankle Int 2003;24(6):462–72.
17. Conti SF, Wong YS. Complications of total ankle replacement. Clin Orthop 2001;391:105–14.

18. Haddad SL, Coetzee JC, Estok R, et al. Intermediate and long-term outcomes of total ankle arthroplasty and ankle arthrodesis. A systematic review of the literature. J Bone Joint Surg Am 2007;89:1899–905.

19. Stengel D, Bauwens K, Ekkernkamp A, et al. Efficacy of total ankle replacement with meniscal-bearing devices: a systematic review and meta-analysis. Arch Orthop Trauma Surg 2005;125:109–19.

20. Jackson MP, Singh D. Total ankle replacement. Curr Orthop 2003;17:292–8.

21. Doets HC, Brand R, Nelissen RG. Total ankle arthroplasty in inflammatory joint disease with use of two mobile-bearing designs. J Bone Joint Surg Am 2006;88:1272–84.

22. McGarvey WC, Clanton TO, Lunz D. Malleolar fracture after total ankle arthroplasty: a comparison of two designs. Clin Orthop Relat Res 2004;424: 104–10.

23. San Giovanni TP, Keblish DJ, Thomas WH, et al. Eight-year results of a minimally constrained total ankle arthroplasty. Foot Ankle Int 2006;27:418–27.

24. Assal M, Al-Shaikh R, Reiber B, et al. Fracture of the polyethylene component in an ankle arthroplasty: a case report. Foot Ankle Int 2003;24:901–3.

# Imaging of Tarsal Coalition

Julia Crim, MD

**KEYWORDS**

- C-sign • Talar beak • Subtalar coalition
- Calcaneonavicular coalition

A coalition is a congenital bony, cartilaginous, or fibrous connection (called a bar) between two or more bones. Coalitions are clinically significant because they prevent normal joint motion. They are most frequently seen in the hindfoot (tarsal coalition), but also occur in the wrist and occasionally the elbow.

The existence of tarsal coalition has been recognized since the eighteenth century,[1] but it was not until 1948 that Harris and Beath[2] made the first widely known report identifying tarsal coalition as a cause of a painful, rigid flatfoot, and the condition began to be viewed as a clinically significant entity.

Tarsal coalitions are attributable to congenital failure of segmentation of the tarsal bones.[3] They most commonly occur between the talus and calcaneus (subtalar coalition) and between the anterior process of the calcaneus and the navicular (calcaneonavicular coalition). They may also be seen between talus and navicular, between calcaneus and cuboid, or between multiple tarsal bones. Coalitions are usually an isolated anomaly, and are at least partly familial; review of first-degree relatives of patients who have symptomatic flatfoot found that 39% had asymptomatic coalitions.[4] A small fraction of coalitions are associated with carpal coalition, symphalangism, and fibular hemimelia.[1,3]

The prevalence of tarsal coalition has long been debated in the literature.[5–8] Most studies report a prevalence of 1% to 3% in the adult population. A recent retrospective record review found tarsal coalition had been diagnosed in 0.6% of more than 27,000 ankle MR imaging studies.[9] When the authors performed a second review of 607 MR imaging studies randomly selected from the initial database they diagnosed coalitions, primarily calcaneonavicular, in 12% of patients. Given that this prevalence is at enormous variance with previous reports, and weak diagnostic criteria were used for diagnosis, these results should be viewed with caution.

There are variable clinical presentations of tarsal coalition. Although it is a congenital condition, it is asymptomatic in early life. The classic presentation is in the second decade when the patient complains of chronic pain and is seen to have a rigid, flat foot on clinical examination. Patients who are not highly active often present later in life,[10] and some affected individuals may never become symptomatic. In college-age patients, the most common presentation is repeated ankle sprain. Because of Harris's[2] landmark study, coalitions are sometimes believed to be universally associated with flatfoot deformity. Only about half of coalitions are associated with flatfoot, however,[6] and they may even be associated with a cavus foot deformity.[10–13]

Tarsal coalition may be difficult to identify on clinical and imaging evaluation. Given the high prevalence of coalition, radiologists must be alert to the often subtle imaging findings.

## PERTINENT NORMAL IMAGING FINDINGS IN HINDFOOT

The middle subtalar joint can be evaluated on the anterior-posterior (AP) and axial (Harris) views. The sustentaculum tali is shaped like a flat brick. The middle subtalar facet, above it, has a straight contour. If the lateral radiograph (**Fig. 1**A) is well centered (ie, if the posterior subtalar joint is in profile), then the middle subtalar joint should always be in profile. On the Harris view (see **Fig. 1**B), the sustentaculum tali juts out from the medial margin of the calcaneus, and the

Department of Radiology, University of Utah School of Medicine, 30 North 1900 East #1A71, Salt Lake City, UT 84132-2140, USA

*E-mail address:* julia.crim@hsc.utah.edu

Radiol Clin N Am 46 (2008) 1017–1026
doi:10.1016/j.rcl.2008.09.005
0033-8389/08/$ – see front matter © 2008 Elsevier Inc. All rights reserved.

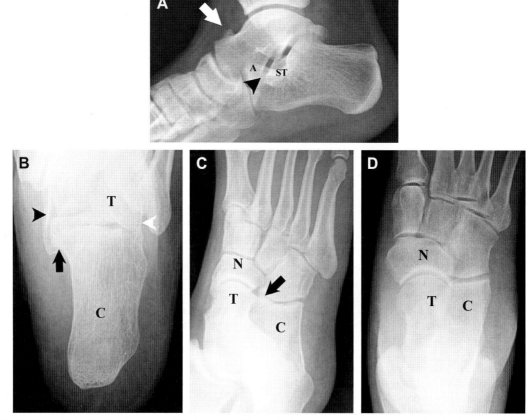

Fig. 1. Normal hindfoot radiographs. (A). Lateral radiograph shows normal appearance of sustentaculum tali (ST), which forms a rectangle below the middle subtalar facet (*arrowhead*). Anterior process of calcaneus (A) forms a triangle. This patient has a large talar ridge (*arrow*), which is a normal variant at the anterior attachment of the ankle joint capsule and not to be mistaken for a talar beak. (B) Harris view shows normal contour of under-surface of sustentaculum tali (*arrow*) and middle subtalar facet (*black arrowhead*) and posterior subtalar facet (*white arrowhead*). C, calcaneus; T, talus. (C) Oblique radiograph shows pointed tip of anterior process of calca-neus (*arrow*) separated from navicular (N). Calcaneus and navicular may approach more closely without a coali-tion being present. (D) Anteroposterior radiograph shows lateral margin of talus (T) and navicular (N) are aligned. Anterior process of calcaneus (C) is not visible on this view.

middle subtalar joint is visible above it and medial to the lateral subtalar joint.

The relationships of the calcaneus and navicular are evaluated on the lateral, oblique, and AP views. On the lateral view (see **Fig. 1**A), the anterior process of the calcaneus is pointed and short. On the oblique view (see **Fig. 1**C), the anterior process is triangular, and a space is present between the anterior process and the navicular. A caveat must be mentioned: in the context of a flatfoot de-formity, the anterior process may come close to the navicular, but it maintains its normal triangular contour as opposed to the squared contour seen in calcaneonavicular coalition. On the AP view (see **Fig. 1**D), the lateral margins of the talar head and the navicular are aligned.

On CT and MR, the anatomic relationships of the subtalar joint are more easily seen. Coronal and sagittal cross-sectional imaging show the normal brick-shaped sustentaculum tali (**Fig. 2**A–C) and the flat contour of the middle subtalar joint. Note that the most posterior portion of the sustentacu-lum tali is nonarticular.

The anterior process of the calcaneus is best seen on sagittal CT and MR images (**Fig. 3**A). It is surprising how closely the anterior process of the calcaneus and the lateral margin of the navic-ular approach each other on axial images in some individuals (see **Fig. 3**B,C). As long as normal contours are maintained and there are no reactive changes in the adjacent bones, one may be confident that there is no coalition.

## RADIOGRAPHIC FINDINGS OF SUBTALAR COALITION

Subtalar coalitions almost always involve the middle subtalar facet, although an isolated coalition of the posterior facet may rarely occur. Osseous and nonosseous subtalar coalitions cause abnormal bone overgrowth of both the sustentaculum tali and the adjacent talus. These changes are readily seen on the Harris view (**Fig. 4**A), and it is on this view that radiographic diagnosis of coalition is traditionally made.[2,14,15] Osseous coalitions are characterized by a continuous bony bar. Nonosseous subtalar coalitions demonstrate bony overgrowth, with the talus and sustentaculum tali separated by a narrow, irregular cleft. Sclerosis and subchondral cysts are often visible.

The Harris view is not part of routine ankle or foot radiographic series, and therefore various radiographic signs of subtalar coalition visible on the routine lateral view have been described. None of these are infallible in isolation, but all raise the suspicion of coalition.

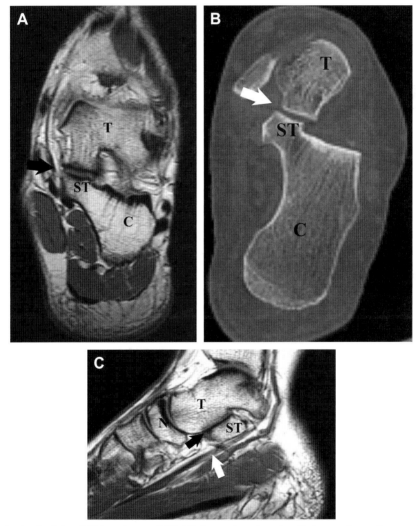

Fig. 2. Normal subtalar joint, MR imaging and CT. (A) Coronal proton density image through normal middle subtalar facet (arrow) shows sustentaculum tali (ST) is medial to body of calcaneus (C). Talus (T) body forms a short pillar, which articulates with sustentaculum tali. (B) Oblique axial CT through middle subtalar joint resembles a Harris view. Middle subtalar joint is marked by arrow. (C) Sagittal T1-weighted MR image shows sustentaculum tali and straight orientation of joint (black arrow). Flexor hallucis longus tendon (white arrow) passing beneath sustentaculum is a useful landmark.

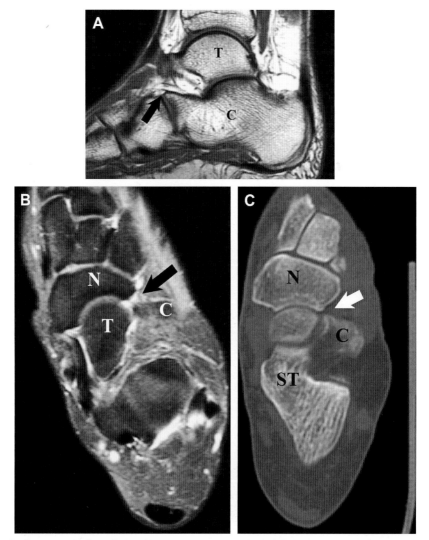

**Fig. 3.** Normal calcaneonavicular relationships, MR imaging and CT. (*A*) Sagittal T1 MR shows normal, triangular tip of anterior process of calcaneus (*arrow*). This plane is usually best for evaluation of suspected calcaneonavicular coalition. (*B*) Axial proton density with fat saturation MR shows small space (*arrow*) between anterior process and navicular. In this case, the gap is easy to see because of fluid from a talonavicular joint effusion; however, if no fluid is present it may be difficult to tell soft tissue fat from bone marrow fat. (*C*) Oblique axial CT shows how narrow the separation may be (*arrow*) between a normal anterior process of the calcaneus and the navicular. There are no alterations in bony contour or subchondral cysts, which would be seen in cases of non-bony coalition.

## C-Sign

Lateur and colleagues[16] first reported the C-sign as an indication of tarsal coalition. The C-sign is formed by continuity of the inferomedial border of the talus with the sustentaculum tali, seen on lateral radiograph (see **Fig. 4**B,C) The C-sign has been reported as having a sensitivity ranging from 40%[17] to 94%[16] and a specificity ranging from 87%[6] to 50%.[17] The C-sign results from close apposition of medial talus and sustentaculum tali, which occurs in most cases of flatfoot deformity. As Brown and coworkers[17] pointed out, C-sign is more indicative of flatfoot deformity than coalition.

## Dysmorphic Sustentaculum Tali

The normal sustentaculum tali appears rectangular on the lateral radiograph, resembling a building brick. When a subtalar coalition is present, the inferior contour becomes enlarged and rounded (see **Fig.** 4B,C). This sign was originally reported to

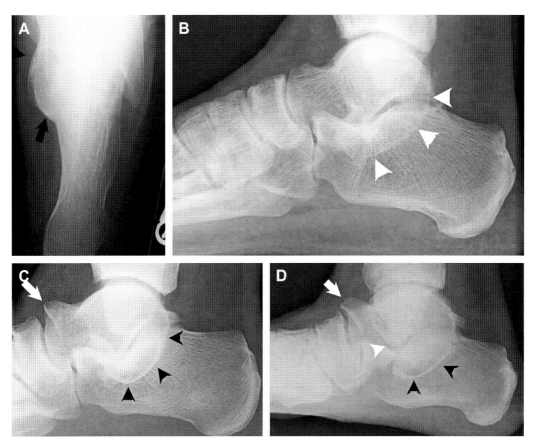

Fig. 4. Radiographs of subtalar coalition. (*A*) Harris view shows bulbous sustentaculum tali, with rounded inferior contour (*arrow*) and overgrowth in expected region of middle subtalar facet (*arrowhead*). (*B*) Lateral radiograph shows dysmorphic sustentaculum tali, with bony overgrowth and rounding of its inferior contour. Continuity of sustentaculum tali contour with that of medial talus is the C-sign (*arrowheads*). (*C*) Lateral radiograph shows talar beak (*arrow*) arising at talonavicular joint and curving away from joint and dysmorphic sustentaculum tali and C-sign (*arrowheads*). (*D*) Lateral radiograph shows rounded lateral process of talus (*white arrowhead*) and dysmorphic sustentaculum tali (*black arrowheads*). Bony prominence (*arrow*) at dorsal margin of talar head has features of both osteophyte and beak, perhaps because this is an older patient who has developed osteoarthritis.

have a sensitivity of 82% and a specificity of 70%,[6] but a more recent report found a sensitivity of 70%.[9]

### Blunted Lateral Process of Talus

Decreased motion of the middle subtalar facet increases stress at the posterior subtalar facet. As a result of the altered stress, the lateral process of the talus, normally triangular with an inferior apex, develops a rounded contour (see **Fig. 4**D).[15] This finding has had limited acceptance in the literature and is not commonly seen but can be a useful corroborating sign.

### Talar Beak

A talar beak may occur with either a subtalar or a calcaneonavicular coalition. Tarsal coalition

decreases normal motion in portions of the hindfoot, with compensatory increase in the range of motion of the talonavicular joint. The articular surface of the talar head flares superiorly to accommodate the increased range of motion. This superior flare is called a talar beak (see **Fig. 4**C). There are three different types of prominences on the dorsal margin of the distal talus: talar beak, talar osteophytes, and talar ridge. Only the talar beak indicates coalition. The distinguishing radiographic features of these three entities were discussed by Resnick.[18] A talar beak, indicating coalition, is a widening of the joint surface, and flares upward away from the navicular. A talar osteophyte attributable to osteoarthritis originates slightly proximal to the joint and arcs forward over the joint. A talar ridge (see **Fig. 1**A), the normal anterior attachment of

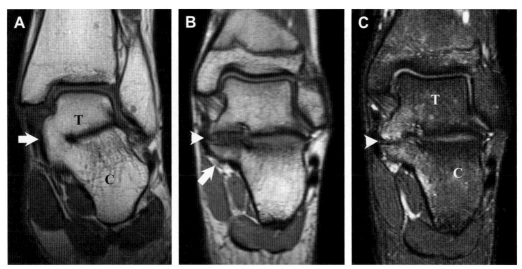

Fig. 5. MR image of subtalar coalition. (*A*) Coronal proton density image shows a bony coalition (*arrow*) with overgrowth of sustentaculum tali and adjacent talus. (*B*) Coronal proton density images shows a non-bony coalition, with a narrow cleft (*arrowhead*) between talus and sustentaculum tali, and a rounded inferior margin of the sustentaculum (*arrow*). (*C*) Coronal T2 with fat saturation image in the same patient as B shows that the cleft (*arrowhead*) is narrow and irregular. Subchondral cysts and bone marrow edema are useful clues for diagnosis.

the tibiotalar joint capsule, is centered more proximally on the talar neck. Occasionally it may be difficult to differentiate a talar beak and talar osteophytes (see **Fig. 4**D).

### Absent Middle Facet Sign

If the lateral radiograph is well centered on the hindfoot, then the middle facet articular surfaces and the joint space between them are visible in

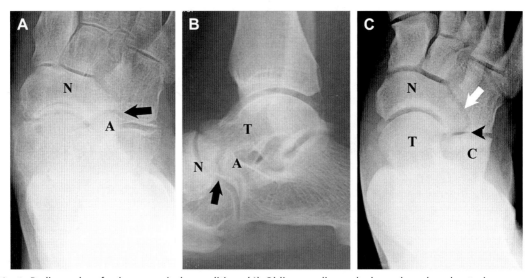

Fig. 6. Radiographs of calcaneonavicular coalition. (*A*) Oblique radiograph shows broadened anterior process (A) forming a connection (*arrow*) with the navicular (N). There is remodeling of both navicular and anterior process to form the closely congruent non-bony bar. (*B*) Lateral radiograph again shows broadened anterior process and non-bony coalition (*arrow*). (*C*) Anteroposterior process shows broadened navicular (reverse anteater sign, *arrow*). Coalition is hard to see (*arrowhead*) because anterior process of calcaneus is not in profile.

he normal foot (see **Fig. 1**A). The joint is not visible in cases of subtalar coalition (see **Fig. 4**A–D) due either to complete bony bar or to the obliquity of the narrow cleft between the bones in nonosseous coalition. This sign has a reported sensitivity and specificity ranging from 75% and 90%, respectively,[19] to 100% and 40%.[6] The absent middle facet sign is useful only in well-positioned radiographs. The posterior subtalar joint can be used as a positioning landmark on lateral radiographs; if the posterior subtalar joint is well seen in profile, then the middle subtalar joint should also be seen unless a coalition is present. If the posterior subtalar joint cannot be seen in profile because of malpositioning, the middle facet is often obscured also.

## CT AND MR IMAGING FINDINGS OF SUBTALAR COALITION

CT and MR imaging are the most reliable methods for diagnosing subtalar coalition.[6,9,20–25] Bony continuity across the middle subtalar facet is easily recognized, but a nonosseous subtalar coalition may be missed on MR if the irregular cleft between the dysmorphic bones is mistaken for a joint (**Fig. 5**A–C). Unlike a true middle subtalar facet, the interosseous space of a fibrous or cartilaginous coalition is narrow, obliquely oriented, and has an undulating contour. Subchondral cysts are often present. Bone marrow edema centered about the coalition is usually seen on fluid-sensitive MR imaging sequences.[26] The sustentaculum

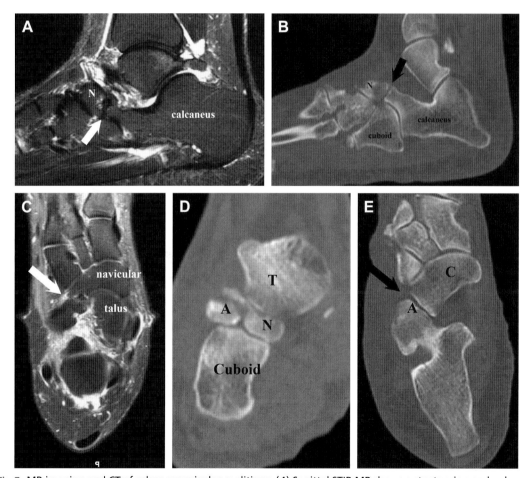

Fig. 7. MR imaging and CT of calcaneonavicular coalitions. (A) Sagittal STIR MR shows anteater sign and enlarged lateral portion of navicular, separated by narrow fibrous bar (arrow). Sclerosis and cysts are seen adjacent to the bar. (B) Sagittal CT shows a similar coalition (arrow). Note irregularity of apposing surfaces and subchondral cysts. (C) Axial proton density with fat saturation image shows that bar (arrow) is difficult to appreciate because marrow and soft tissue fat have same signal intensity. (D) Coronal CT shows fibrous coalition. Elongated anterior process of calcaneus (A) projects superior to cuboid (Cu); it can be seen articulating with enlarged navicular (N). (E) Axial CT in same patient shows non-bony coalition (arrow) bordered by broad anterior process and reverse anteater sign.

tali is typically enlarged and has a rounded contour inferiorly. Associated tenosynovitis may be identified either in peroneal tendons or in flexor tendons, reflecting altered biomechanics.

## RADIOGRAPHIC FINDINGS OF CALCANEONAVICULAR COALITION
### Anteater Sign

This sign was originally described on oblique radiographs of the foot.[15,27] The normally triangular anterior process of calcaneus becomes elongated and its tip is squared like the snout of an anteater (**Fig. 6**A). The elongated anterior process abuts the lateral margin of the navicular. The sign is also visible on lateral radiographs (see **Fig. 6**B) where it has a sensitivity of 72% and a specificity of 90%[6] in one report, but a sensitivity of only 10% in a subsequent report.[9] The sign is more difficult

to see on lateral radiographs because of the superimposition of overlying bones.

### Elongated Navicular Sign (Reverse Anteater)

This sign is visible on AP radiographs of the foot (see **Fig. 6**C). Normally, the lateral margins of the navicular and the head of the talus are aligned. When a calcaneonavicular coalition is present, the navicular extends further laterally, and the anteroposterior dimension of the lateral portion tends to be smaller than at the medial portion of the navicular. The original reported sensitivity of this sign was 50% and specificity was 100%,[6] although a subsequent report found a sensitivity of only 18%.[9]

## CT AND MR IMAGING FINDINGS OF CALCANEONAVICULAR COALITION

A calcaneonavicular coalition is often easier to see using conventional radiography than either MR

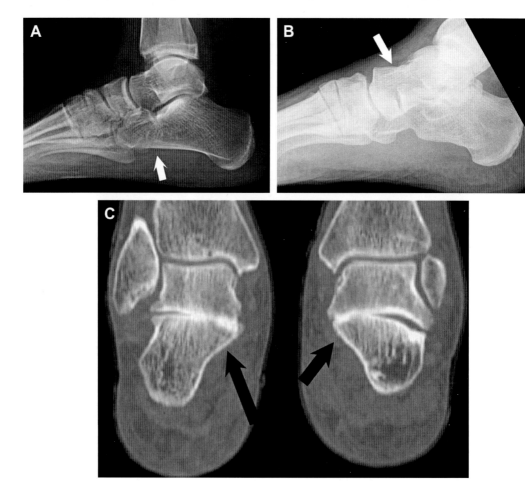

**Fig. 8.** Other coalitions. (*A*) Lateral radiograph shows complete absence of calcaneocuboid joint (*arrow*). (*B*) Lateral radiograph shows complete absence of talonavicular joint (*arrow*). (*C*) Coronal CT shows bilateral bony posterior subtalar facet coalitions (*arrows*). Note that only portions of the joints are fused. This type of coalition is not visible on radiographs.

maging or CT, because of the oblique orientation of the small bar, which can be mistaken for normal bone on cross-sectional imaging. Sagittal images most reliably show the elongated anterior process of the calcaneus and its blunted tip (**Fig. 7**A,B). If images are oblique, or the midfoot is adducted, the bar may be difficult to see. Subchondral cysts or bone marrow edema in the anterior process of the calcaneus are useful hints that a coalition may be present.

For cases in which diagnosis is not definitive on sagittal images, axial and coronal planes are used. To accurately make the diagnosis on these images, it is important to remember that in the normal foot the distance between the anterior process of calcaneus and the navicular is often small. More important than the distance between the calcaneus and navicular are the abnormal shape of the anterior process and adjacent navicular, and the presence of reactive cysts and bone marrow edema. Unfortunately, fatty bone marrow may be difficult to distinguish from fat in soft tissues, making determination of bone outline difficult on MR (see **Fig. 7**C).

It may be difficult to distinguish between calcaneonavicular coalition (see **Fig. 7**D,E) and the normal cuboid-navicular joint (see **Fig. 3**D,E). A calcaneonavicular bar may be mistaken for cuboid-navicular joint because of the sigmoid shape of the calcaneocuboid joint. Axial and coronal images may cut obliquely through portions of each bone. This problem can be avoided by using a localizer to compare between planes and by comparing a single image to adjacent images.

## OTHER TYPES OF COALITION

Other types of coalition are rare. Coalitions are reported in the posterior subtalar facet and between the cuboid and navicular,[28] talus and navicular,[29–31] the navicular and cuneiforms,[32] the calcaneus and cuboid,[33] and between multiple bones.[4,5,34,35] These are generally easily seen on radiographs (**Fig. 8**A,B).

One rare type of coalition, the posterior subtalar coalition, is not visible on radiographs and is difficult to see even on advanced imaging. This coalition was originally described by Harris,[2] who detected it at time of surgical exploration. The posterior subtalar coalition usually involves the anteromedial margin of the posterior subtalar joint, and the posterior, usually nonarticular, portion of the sustentaculum tali (see **Fig. 8**C).

## COALITIONS OF MULTIPLE BONES

Extensive fusions of the hindfoot are often associated with fibular hemimelia or other congenital syndromes. When coalitions of multiple tarsal bones are present, the severe limitation of motion can result in a ball-in-socket configuration of the talus.[36–39] This configuration refers to a talar trochlea, which is convex superiorly from medial to lateral, as opposed to the normal concave configuration. Ball-in-socket talus is not a feature of a simple subtalar or calcaneonavicular coalition.

## REFERENCES

1. Mosier KM, Asher M. Tarsal coalitions and peroneal spastic flat foot [a review]. J Bone Joint Surg Am 1984;66(7):976–84.
2. Harris RI. Rigid valgus foot due to talocalcaneal bridge. J Bone Joint Surg Am 1955;37(1):169–83.
3. Harris BJ. Anomalous structures in the developing human foot [abstract]. Anat Rec 1955;121:1.
4. Leonard MA. The inheritance of tarsal coalition and its relationship to spastic flat foot. J Bone Joint Surg Br 1974;56(3):520–6.
5. Kulik SA Jr, Clanton TO. Tarsal coalition. Foot Ankle Int 1996;17(5):286–96.
6. Crim JR, Kjeldsberg KM. Radiographic diagnosis of tarsal coalition. AJR Am J Roentgenol 2004;182(2):323–8.
7. Percy EC, Mann DL. Tarsal coalition: a review of the literature and presentation of 13 cases. Foot Ankle 1988;9(1):40–4.
8. Stormont DM, Peterson HA. The relative incidence of tarsal coalition. Clin Orthop Relat Res 1983;(181):28–36.
9. Nalaboff KM, Schweitzer ME. MRI of tarsal coalition: frequency, distribution, and innovative signs. Bull NYU Hosp Jt Dis 2008;66(1):14–21.
10. Varner KE, Michelson JD. Tarsal coalition in adults. Foot Ankle Int 2000;21(8):669–72.
11. Barrett SE, Johnson JE. Progressive bilateral cavovarus deformity: an unusual presentation of calcaneonavicular tarsal coalition. Am J Orthop 2004;33(5):239–42.
12. Knapp HP, et al. Tarsal coalition in an adult with cavovarus feet. J Am Podiatr Med Assoc 1998;88(6):295–300.
13. Stuecker RD, Bennett JT. Tarsal coalition presenting as a pes cavo-varus deformity: report of three cases and review of the literature. Foot Ankle 1993;14(9):540–4.
14. Vaughan WH, Segal G. Tarsal coalition, with special reference to roentgenographic interpretation. Radiology 1953;60(6):855–63.
15. Conway JJ, Cowell HR. Tarsal coalition: clinical significance and roentgenographic demonstration. Radiology 1969;92(4):799–811.
16. Lateur LM, et al. Subtalar coalition: diagnosis with the C sign on lateral radiographs of the ankle. Radiology 1994;193(3):847–51.

17. Brown RR, Rosenberg ZS, Thornhill BA. The C sign: more specific for flatfoot deformity than subtalar coalition. Skeletal Radiol 2001;30(2):84–7.

18. Resnick D. Talar ridges, osteophytes, and beaks: a radiologic commentary. Radiology 1984;151(2):329–32.

19. Liu PT, et al. Absent middle facet: a sign on unenhanced radiography of subtalar joint coalition. AJR Am J Roentgenol 2003;181(6):1565–72.

20. Deutsch AL, Resnick D, Campbell G. Computed tomography and bone scintigraphy in the evaluation of tarsal coalition. Radiology 1982;144(1):137–40.

21. Herzenberg JE, et al. Computerized tomography of talocalcaneal tarsal coalition: a clinical and anatomic study. Foot Ankle 1986;6(6):273–88.

22. Pineda C, Resnick D, Greenway G. Diagnosis of tarsal coalition with computed tomography. Clin Orthop Relat Res 1986;(208):282–8.

23. Stoskopf CA, et al. Evaluation of tarsal coalition by computed tomography. J Pediatr Orthop 1984;4(3):365–9.

24. Newman JS, Newberg AH. Congenital tarsal coalition: multimodality evaluation with emphasis on CT and MR imaging. Radiographics 2000;20(2):321–32 [quiz 526–7, 532].

25. Lemley F, et al. Current concepts review: tarsal coalition. Foot Ankle Int 2006;27(12):1163–9.

26. Sijbrandij ES, et al. Bone marrow ill-defined hyperintensities with tarsal coalition: MR imaging findings. Eur J Radiol 2002;43(1):61–5.

27. Chambers CH. Congenital anomalies of the tarsal navicular with particular reference to calcaneo-navicular coalition. Br J Radiol 1950;23(274):580–6.

28. Johnson TR, Mizel MS, Temple T. Cuboid-navicular tarsal coalition—presentation and treatment: a case report and review of the literature. Foot Ankle Int 2005;26(3):264–6.

29. David DR, Clark NE, Bier JA. Congenital talonavicular coalition. Review of the literature, case report and orthotic management. J Am Podiatr Med Assoc 1998;88(5):223–7.

30. Doyle SM, Kumar SJ. Symptomatic talonavicular coalition. J Pediatr Orthop 1999;19(4):508–10.

31. Frost RA, Fagan JP. Bilateral talonavicular and calcaneocuboid joint coalition. J Am Podiatr Med Assoc 1995;85(6):339–41.

32. Gregersen HN. Naviculocuneiform coalition. J Bone Joint Surg Am 1977;59(1):128–30.

33. Pensieri SL, et al. Bilateral congenital calcaneocuboid synostosis and subtalar joint coalition. J Am Podiatr Med Assoc 1985;75(8):406–10.

34. Craig CL, Goldberg MJ. Calcaneocuboid coalition in Crouzon's syndrome (craniofacial dysostosis): report of a case and review of the literature. J Bone Joint Surg Am 1977;59(6):826–7.

35. Pachuda NM, Lasday SD, Jay RM. Tarsal coalition: etiology, diagnosis, and treatment. J Foot Surg 1990;29(5):474–88.

36. Jensen JK. Ball and socket ankle joints. Clin Orthop Relat Res 1972;85:28–31.

37. Pistoia F, Ozonoff MB, Wintz P. Ball-and-socket ankle joint. Skeletal Radiol 1987;16(6):447–51.

38. Ruiz Santiago F, et al. Ball-and-socket ankle joint with hypoplastic sustentaculum tali. Eur Radiol 2002;12(Suppl 3):S48–50.

39. Vichard P, Pinon P, Peltre G. [Ball and socket ankle associated with congenital synostosis of the tarsus. Report of a case (author's transl)]. Rev Chir Orthop Reparatrice Appar Mot 1980;66(6):387–90 [in French].

# Ultrasound of the Hindfoot and Midfoot

David P. Fessell, MD[a],*, Jon A. Jacobson, MD[b]

**KEYWORDS**

- Ultrasound • Hindfoot • Midfoot • Ankle • Tendons
- Ligaments • Masses

Ultrasound (US) is increasingly being used to evaluate musculoskeletal disorders, including foot and ankle pathology.[1–5] Higher frequency transducers and technical advances in recent years have resulted in a higher spatial resolution for sonography compared with MR imaging.[6] Cost saving with US can also be considerable. In many cases the professional and technical cost of an US is approximately 80% less than an MR image of the same anatomy.[7] US has the unique capacity to allow evaluation during dynamic maneuvers which can reveal abnormalities that are not apparent during static imaging. The advantages of an imaging modality that allows visualization during dynamic maneuvers will be highlighted throughout this article. Additional advantages of US include imaging of patients who cannot undergo MR imaging due to pacemakers, hardware, or claustrophobia; direct and real-time evaluation of the site of pain or symptoms with additional history immediately available; flexibility in the field-of-view; ease of contralateral comparison; use of Doppler; and ease of guiding procedures.[8] Disadvantages of US include the learning curve and operator dependence. These disadvantages can be addressed by the simple application of time and effort.

Specialties such as Physical Medicine and Rehabilitation, Rheumatology, and Emergency Medicine are increasingly using US to evaluate musculoskeletal disorders.[9–13] Radiologists, who have years of training in anatomy, pathology, US physics, artifacts, and technical aspects of US imaging, are uniquely suited to apply this versatile modality to foot and ankle pathology. If radiologists are not able to perform musculoskeletal US with great expertise, this business will be taken over by other specialties. If musculoskeletal US is lost, additional modalities such as MR imaging may be lost as well. It is imperative that radiologists continue to be experts in all aspects of musculoskeletal imaging, including US.

The technique for examining the hindfoot and midfoot with US has been described and depicted many recent articles[2,5] and will not be discussed. In this article, normal US anatomy will be shown in all cases before demonstrating the full range of hindfoot and midfoot pathology. Color and power Doppler can aid diagnosis by demonstrating neovascularity in cases of inflammation or fibrosis and will also be discussed.

## HINDFOOT AND MIDFOOT TENDONS: GENERAL COMMENTS

Tendon pathology of the hindfoot and midfoot can be difficult to diagnose. In the acute setting, pain and swelling can limit the physical examination. In the setting of chronic injury it may not be possible to differentiate tendon, ligament, or osseous pathology solely on the basis of the physical examination. US is well tolerated in both the acute and chronic settings. Real-time correlation with the site of pain and symptoms aids diagnosis and is a strength of US. Numerous studies have documented the accuracy of US for detecting tendon pathology[14–19] and these studies will be discussed in each tendon section below. US is not limited to three orthogonal planes, as is MR imaging, and is not subject to magic angle artifact,

[a] Department of Radiology, University of Michigan Hospitals and Health Centers, 1500 E. Medical Center Drive, Taubman Center, Room 2910Q, Ann Arbor, MI 48109-5326, USA
[b] University of Michigan, 1500 E. Medical Center Drive, TC 2910L, Ann Arbor, MI 48109-5326, USA
* Corresponding author.
*E-mail address:* dfessell@umich.edu (D.P. Fessell).

Radiol Clin N Am 46 (2008) 1027–1043
doi:10.1016/j.rcl.2008.08.006
0033-8389/08/$ – see front matter © 2008 published by Elsevier Inc.

which can limit MR evaluation as the tendons curve along their course. Anisotropy is one artifact which can be seen with US when the transducer is not oriented parallel to the structure being evaluated (**Fig. 1**). However, this artifact is easily avoided by rocking the transducer back and forth to alternately show a normal and anisotropic tendon. Normal ankle tendons are round or ovoid in the transverse plane with a speckled, hyperechoic appearance. In the longitudinal plane they demonstrate a fibrillar pattern or echogenic lines. This classic tendon echo signature is seen in all tendons of the body.

Hindfoot and midfoot tendon pathology is most often due to one or more of the following entities: tenosynovitis, tendinosis, and tendon tear. Subluxation and tendon dislocation are also possible, most commonly with the peroneal tendons. Tendinosis is seen as tendon thickening and may show diffuse or more focal regions of hypoechogenicity and loss of the normal fibrillar echotexture.[1] As with MR imaging, with sonography it may be difficult to distinguish tendinosis from low-grade partial thickness tear in some cases. The more severe the tendon thickening and echogenicity alteration, the more likely partial tear is present.[20] Tenosynovitis is noted as increased fluid distending a tendon sheath, with or without hypervascular synovium surrounding the tendon. In the setting of an acute or subacute tendon tear, tenosynovitis is usually present and increases the conspicuity of a tear. Tenosynovitis may not be present in cases of chronic tendon tears. Normal fluid, in the range of 1 to 3 mm, can often be seen partially surrounding the tibialis posterior tendon, flexor digitorum longus, and flexor hallucis longus tendons. Such normal fluid is usually located in the dependent portion of the tendon sheath and at the level of the medial and lateral malleoli.[21]

Partial-thickness tears can be in the longitudinal plane ("longitudinal-type split") or in the transverse plane. Longitudinal splits are the more common type affecting the peroneal tendons and are not uncommonly seen affecting the tibialis posterior tendon as well.[17,22,23] Partial-thickness tears appear as a linear and in some cases globular region of hypoechogenicity, without evidence of retraction of the tendon.[16,17] The transverse plane usually provides the most optimal depiction of partial-thickness tears. Complete tendon rupture is seen as complete fiber disruption in the longitudinal plane, often with retraction of the torn tendon margins and absence of the tendon at the level of the defect in the transverse plane. Fluid, debris, and hematoma are often noted in the tendon gap in the setting of an acute tear, with hypoechoic

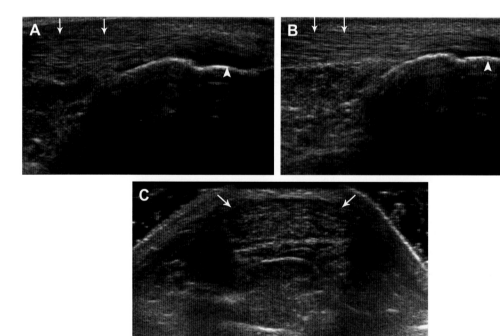

**Fig. 1.** (A) Longitudinal US of a normal Achilles tendon (*arrows*) shows the fibrillar appearance of the tendon. Hypoechogenicity consistent with anisotropy is noted at the insertion on the calcaneus (*arrowhead*). (B) Slight angulation of the transducer "fills-in" the hypoechoic region (*arrowhead*), confirming anisotropy. Arrows denote the normal Achilles tendon. (C) Transverse US of a normal Achilles tendon (*arrows*) shows the echogenic, fibrillar appearance of the normal tendon.

granulation or scar tissue seen at this site in the setting of more chronic tears.

## ACHILLES TENDON

Though the Achilles tendon is the strongest tendon in the body, it is also one of the most frequently injured. Often such injuries are sports related, a fitting irony given that the tendon's name is derived from the great Greek warrior, Achilles.[4,24] The Achilles is also unique because it is surrounded by a paratenon, a thin vascular membrane, rather than a synovial sheath as is seen surrounding the other ankle tendons. Therefore normal fluid is never seen adjacent to the Achilles tendon.[21] A spectrum of pathology can affect the Achilles tendon, ranging from acute or chronic peritendinitis, tendinosis, partial tears, and complete rupture. Tears usually occur in a relatively avascular zone located 2 to 6 cm above the calcaneal insertion, and less commonly at the insertion on the calcaneus.[4]

Numerous reports have used US to assess the Achilles tendon for peritendinitis, tendinosis, and tears.[15,20,25] Peritendinitis is demonstrated as ill-defined tendon margins with or without associated fluid and tendinosis (Fig. 2).[26] Tendinosis can be diffuse or focal and appears as hypoechogenicity with tendon thickening, usually with a fusiform-appearing tendon in the longitudinal plane (see Fig. 2).[20,27] In the transverse plane, tendinosis may manifest as loss of the normal anterior concavity. Tendon calcifications may also be seen with tendinosis, both by US and

radiography.[4] Partial-thickness tears of the Achilles tendon can be diagnosed by a well-defined anechoic or hypoechoic cleft affecting less than the complete cross section of the tendon. As with MR imaging, US may have difficulty distinguishing tendinosis from low- or moderate-grade partial tears; however, all of these entities are usually treated nonoperatively.[15] High-grade partial tears involving more than 50% of the tendon thickness and complete ruptures may be treated operatively or nonoperatively depending on the surgeon and clinical circumstances. Nonoperative treatment of complete ruptures is advocated by some surgeons, especially when the torn tendon ends are approximated or are less than 1 cm separated in plantar flexion (Fig. 3). Dynamic evaluation in dorsiflexion and plantar flexion can be easily performed with US and can directly impact patient management and outcome. Power Doppler evaluation showing hyperemia and neovascularization has been shown to correlate with pain severity but not with clinical outcome.[27]

Acute Achilles tendon rupture may be obvious by clinical examination, however it has been reported as missed in more than 20% of cases, likely due to pain and swelling limiting the clinical examination.[15] The gap between the torn tendon ends is often filled with hematoma and debris in the acute setting; and scar or fibrous tissue in more chronic cases.[4] An additional dynamic maneuver, the sonographic Thompson sign, can also be helpful. The calf is gently squeezed as the Achilles tendon is assessed for synchronous tendon movement from proximal to distal. With

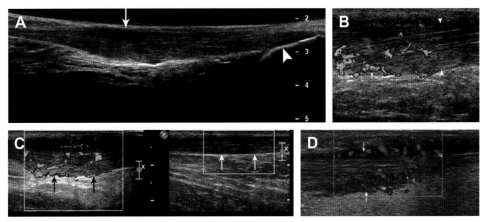

Fig. 2. (A) Longitudinal US of the distal Achilles tendon to the insertion on the calcaneus (arrowhead). The tendon is hypoechoic and enlarged (arrow) consistent with tendinosis. (B) Longitudinal US of the region of tendinosis shows hyperemia (arrows) of the Achilles tendon (between the arrowheads). (C) Split-screen longitudinal US of the hyperemic region of tendinosis with comparison to the contralateral normal Achilles tendon. The region of tendinosis (black arrows) demonstrates thickening and hypernemia compared to the opposite side (white arrows). (D) Longitudinal US of an Achilles tendon with hypoechogenicity (arrows) adjacent to the Achilles. The hypoechoic regions demonstrate hyperemia, consistent with peritendinitis.

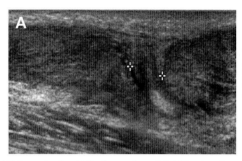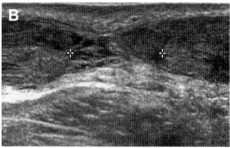

Fig. 3. (*A*) Longitudinal US of a ruptured Achilles tendon during plantar flexion shows less than 1 cm of separation between the torn tendon ends. The patient was successfully treated with casting in plantar flexion. (*B*) Same patient with longitudinal scanning in dorsiflexion shows increased separation and better delineation of the complete tendon rupture.

a complete tear, the proximal torn tendon end will retract proximally but the distal portion of the torn end will not.[4] The foot may also be manually moved from slight dorsiflexion to plantarflexion as an alternate method to show separation of torn tendon ends. Additional helpful signs of a complete tear are herniation of Kager's fat into the site of a tear (**Fig. 4**), refraction artifact (posterior acoustic shadowing) at the site of torn tendon ends (**Fig. 5**), and ease in visualizing the plantaris tendon, which is located medially and may herniate into the site of the tendon tear (**Fig. 6**).[15] An intact plantaris tendon, in the setting of a complete Achilles rupture, should not be mistaken for intact Achilles tendon fibers. Knowledge of the normal anatomy and awareness of this potential pitfall will prevent misdiagnosis.[28] It is also important to assess and report the presence and condition of the plantaris tendon since it may be harvested and used to help reinforce a surgical repair of the Achilles tendon.[29]

The retrocalcaneal bursa is located between the distal Achilles tendon and posterosuperior calcaneal tuberosity. The bursa is reportedly visible in 50% of normal ankles and may contain trace amounts of physiologic fluid, usually less than 3 mm in anteroposterior dimension.[21] This physiologic fluid can be unilateral or asymmetric with the contralateral ankle. Distention of the bursa is consistent with retrocalcaneal bursitis (**Fig. 7**), which may be isolated or seen with rheumatoid arthritis,

Reiter's disease, or other seronegative arthritides. Retrocalcaneal bursitis can also be seen with Achilles tendon pathology and with Haglund's syndrome.[30] Much less commonly seen is retro Achilles or infracalcaneal bursitis which is located posterior to the Achilles tendon and may be seen in association with Haglund's syndrome (**Fig. 8**).

## PERONEAL TENDONS

In experienced hands, US is highly accurate for imaging peroneal tendon tears and can be used as the first imaging test. A sensitivity of 100%, specificity of 85%, and accuracy of 90% is reported in the orthopedic literature, in comparison to surgical findings.[17] Tears of the peroneal tendons are usually of the longitudinal split type, with complete ruptures much less common. The peroneus brevis is more commonly affected, be it by tear, tenosynovitis, or tendinosis.[17,31] This is likely due to its location between the peroneus longus and the fibula, which allows the tendon to be pinched between these two structures. Longitudinal splits may be acute (most frequently in young patients), or chronic (most commonly in the elderly population). Chronic splits may be asymptomatic.[32] Peroneal splits and tears are usually located at the level of the retromalleolar groove and are more frequently, but not exclusively, associated with injury to the superior peroneal retinaculum.[33,34] The axial plane is usually ideal for visualizing

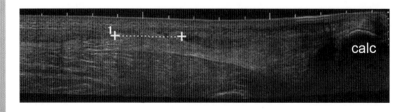

Fig. 4. Longitudinal US of a complete rupture of the Achilles tendon with 2.6 cm of separation between the torn tendon ends and herniation of echogenic Kager's fat into the site of the tear (*dotted line between the crosses*). Calc, calcaneus.

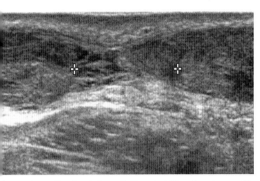

ig. 5. Longitudinal US of the Achilles tendon with complete rupture noted between the proximal tendon end (*single arrowhead*) and distal tendon end (*double arrowhead*). Refraction artifact is noted deep to the torn tendon ends (*arrows*).

ongitudinal splits as an anechoic or hypoechoic cleft (**Fig. 9**). The peroneus longus tendon often insinuates into the split, preventing healing.[4]

As with MR imaging, peroneal tears are more easily visualized when fluid is present distending the tendon sheath, as is usually present in the setting of an acute tear.[4] A potential pitfall that can mimic a peroneal split is the peroneus quartus.

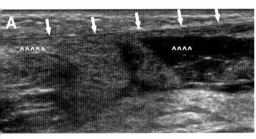

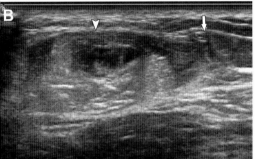

ig. 6. (*A*) Longitudinal US of a complete rupture of the Achilles tendon. The five small arrowheads denote the proximal tendon end and the four small arrowheads denote debris at the site of the tendon tear. The intact plantaris tendon is noted extending through the site of the Achilles tear (*arrows*). (*B*) Transverse US at the site of the complete Achilles rupture demonstrates the plantaris tendon (*arrow*) and debris at the site of the Achilles tear (*arrowhead*).

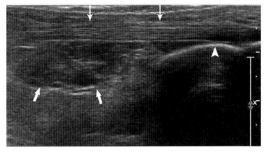

Fig. 7. Longitudinal US shows an intact Achilles tendon (*thin arrows*) to its insertion on the calcaneus (*arrowhead*). The retrocalcaneal bursa is distended and contains debris (*thick arrows*).

This accessory tendon, present in 10% to 20% of individuals, has a variable composition at its insertion, ranging from 100% tendon to predominately or completely muscle. It can be differentiated from a peroneal split by scanning to its distal insertion, usually onto the lateral aspect of the calcaneus (**Fig. 10**).[28,34]

A tear of the peroneus longus can occur in conjunction with a tear of the brevis, or in isolation.[31] Tears of the peroneus longus can occur at the level of the lateral malleolus, at the level of the os peroneum or cuboid groove, or at the level of the midfoot.[4] The os peroneum is located within the peroneus longus tendon. When the ossicle fractures and significantly separates or displaces, the result is usually equivalent to a rupture of the peroneus longus, with retraction of the proximal portion of the fractured os, and often associated peroneal tendon tears.[35]

While tenosynovitis and tendinosis are more common than tendon tears, these entities usually do not require surgical treatment.[4] Tenosynovitis is noted as fluid which completely surrounds the peroneal tendons, while normal fluid is smaller in amount, dependently located, and not circumferential.[21] Peroneal tenosynovitis is more common in the athletic population, in acute inversion injuries, and ankle

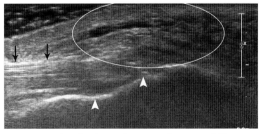

Fig. 8. Longitudinal US shows an intact Achilles tendon (*black arrows*) to its insertion on the calcaneus (*arrowheads*). The retro-Achilles bursa is distended and contains debris (*region within the ellipse*).

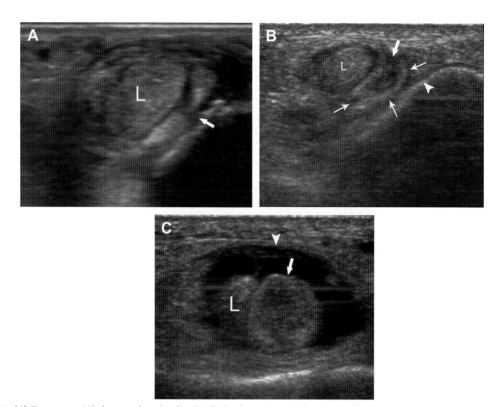

**Fig. 9.** (*A*) Transverse US shows a longitudinal split in the peroneus brevis tendon creating two separate portions of the brevis (*arrow*) at the level of the lateral malleolus. (*B*) Transverse US from a different patient shows a longitudinal split *(thick arrow)* in the peroneus brevis tendon (*thin arrows*) at the level of the lateral malleolus (*arrowhead*). (*C*) Transverse US from a different patient shows marked enlargement and internal hypoechogenicity of the peroneus brevis tendon (*arrow*) with surrounding tenosynovitis (*arrowhead*). L, peroneus longus tendon.

instability.[4,36] If peroneal tenosynovitis is identified, special care should be taken to examine the calcaneofibular ligament, since injury to this ligament can permit pathologic communication of joint fluid into the peroneal tendon sheath.[4]

Several factors have been reported to predispose to peroneal tendon pathology, including anatomic variants such as a peroneus quartus muscle or low-lying peroneal muscle belly. Such variants may cause crowding of the peroneal tendons and promote subluxation. Likewise a flat or convex (rather than concave) retromalleolar groove can also promote subluxation. Hypertrophy of the calcaneal peroneal tubercle or retrotrochlear eminence can abrade the peroneal tendons. Acquired conditions can also predispose to peroneal pathology, the most common being injury to the superior peroneal retinaculum.[34] Additional factors predisposing to peroneal pathology include tarsal coalition, hardware such as orthopedic screws impinging upon the tendons (**Fig. 11**), and fibular or calcaneal osseous spurs.[4,37]

## SUBLUXATION AND DISLOCATION OF THE PERONEAL TENDONS

The peroneal tendons may partially displace (subluxate) or completely displace (dislocate) from their normal position posterior to the fibula. In most cases such abnormal tendon movement occurs intermittently and is not directly visualized by static MR imaging. Only dynamic US can directly visualize the tendons as they subluxate or dislocate laterally and anteriorly over the lateral malleolus. Such subluxation or dislocation is most often posttraumatic, due to dorsiflexion and eversion injury. Typically the superior peroneal retinaculum is injured, allowing recurrent dislocation and leading to tendinosis and tendon tear. Dynamic evaluation of the peroneal tendons adds only a few seconds to the standard ankle US examination. The probe is placed transverse to the tendons, at the level of the retromalleolar groove and the foot is dorsiflexed and everted.[23] The brevis more commonly dislocates, although one or both of the peroneal tendons can dislocate (**Fig. 12**).[3,4,23]

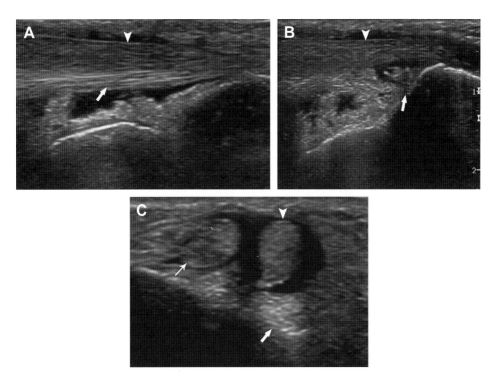

Fig. 10. (A) Longitudinal US shows a peroneus quartus tendon (arrow) deep to the peroneus brevis tendon (arrow-head). Surrounding tenosynovitis is noted. (B) Longitudinal scanning more distally shows the insertion of the peroneus quartus on to the lateral aspect of the calcaneus (arrow) with the peroneus brevis noted more superficially (arrowhead). (C) Transverse US shows the peroneus quartus (thick arrow) deep to the brevis (arrowhead). The peroneus longus is denoted by the thin arrow. Note tenosynovitis.

The peroneal tendons can also remain behind the fibula, in the retromalleolar groove, but transiently "switch" positions during inversion and eversion (**Fig. 13**). This entity has been termed "retromalleolar intrasheath subluxation." It may be symptomatic and surgically treated, or asymptomatic.[23] This entity again requires a dynamic imaging modality which, for all practical purposes, is only possible with US.

## MEDIAL TENDONS

The posterior tibialis tendon (PTT) is also a commonly injured tendon. It serves as a primary inverter of the foot and is an important component of the medial longitudinal arch. When the PTT is ruptured or injured, flatfoot deformity can result. Rupture is, however, less common than tendinosis and partial tears. PTT pathology often begins as tenosynovitis, followed by partial tear and then

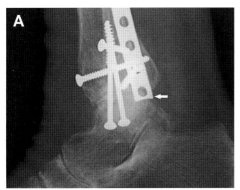
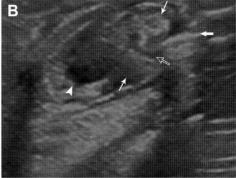

Fig. 11. (A) Lateral radiograph shows multiple screws and a fibular plate extending posterior to the cortex of the fibula (arrow). (B) Transverse US at the level of the lateral fibular plate shows a split (open arrow) creating two portions of the peroneus brevis (thin white arrows) adjacent to the fibular plate (thick white arrow). The arrow-head denotes a small amount of fluid adjacent to the peroneus longus tendon.

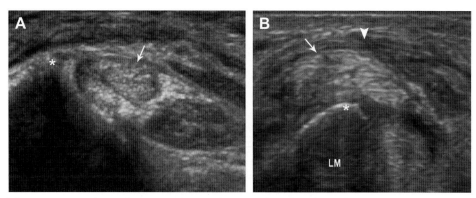

Fig. 12. (A) Transverse US shows the peroneal normal peroneal tendons (*arrow*) posterior to the distal fibula. Asterisk denotes the lateral aspect of the fibula. (B) Transverse US shows the peroneus longus (*arrow*) dislocated lateral to the fibula (*asterisk*) when the ankle is dorsiflexed and everted. Note detached superior peroneal retinaculum (*arrowhead*). LM, lateral malleolus.

complete rupture. Early diagnosis and treatment is the key to preventing severe disability.[38] The accuracy of US for detecting PTT abnormalities is comparable to MR imaging.[16,18,19,39] The os tibiale externum or os naviculare has been reported to be associated with PTT pathology. This is likely due to mechanical strain from altered tendon mechanics.[40]

As with the peroneal tendons, most pathology involving the PTT is at the level of the malleolus (**Fig. 14**). Less commonly, pathology is at the level of the navicular insertion since the tendon has multiple strong slips that fan out and insert broadly over the navicular and plantar aspect of the tarsal bones. Dislocation of the PTT is extremely rare.[41] A unique feature of US is the ability to identify small spurs or cortical irregularity in the medial malleolar groove (**Fig. 15**). Such spurs can abrade the tendon and can be a difficult diagnosis with MR imaging or CT due to their small size and low signal on

MR imaging. With US, direct sonographic and clinical correlation is available for pain or symptoms related to a possible tendon abnormality. Normally the axial diameter of the posterior tibial tendon is approximately twice that of the flexor digitorum longus (FDL) tendon.[4] This "rule of thumb" allows quick assessment of tendon thickening, as seen with tendinosis, or the thinning that can be seen in some partial tears.

A potential pitfall can occur with a complete rupture of the PTT. In this setting the FDL may be displaced anteriorly and potentially be confused with an intact PTT.[28] Making note that each individual tendon is located in its normal position prevents this potential pitfall. The PTT normally has multiple slips at its navicular and plantar insertion and these should not be mistaken for a longitudinal split. The tendon normally curves as it inserts, and in this region it may look artifactually hypoechoic due to anisotropy. Again, direct correlation

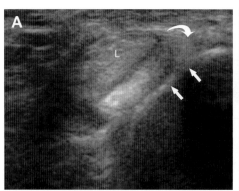
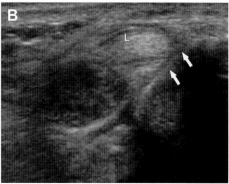

Fig. 13. (A) Transverse US shows the peroneal tendons in their normal location when the ankle is in neutral position. Curved arrow denotes the direction the peroneus longus will move to result in (B). Arrows denote the cortex of the fibular groove. (B) When the ankle is dorsiflexed and everted, the peroneus longus moves anteriorly, adjacent to the fibular cortex (*arrows*). L, peroneus longus.

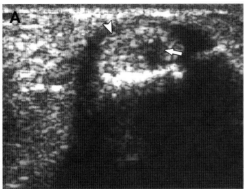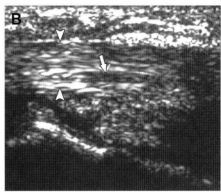

g.14. (A) Transverse US shows the tibialis posterior tendon (arrowhead) with a hypoechoic region extending to he deep surface of the tendon (arrow). (B) Longitudinal US of the posterior tibial tendon (between the arrows) hows a corresponding linear region of hypoechogenicity. Findings are consistent with a longitudinal split of the bialis posterior tendon.

vith symptoms during scanning of this region aids orrect diagnosis.[4]

While pathology of the FDL is extremely rare, pahology affecting the flexor hallucis longus (FHL) an be seen, especially in individuals involved in allet, soccer, or basketball.[4] Friction injuries can ffect the FHL as it courses beneath the

sustentaculum tali and through the fibro osseous tarsal tunnel. Tenosynovitis, stenosing tenosynovitis, and tendinosis can result.[4] An os trigonum and adjacent osseous spurs have been reported to be predisposing factors for FHL pathology. The depth of the FHL can make sonographic evaluation challenging; however, dynamic maneuvers such as

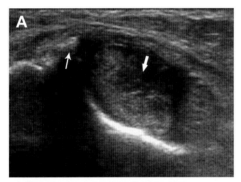

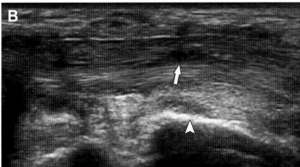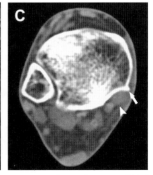

g.15. (A) Transverse US of the tibialis posterior tendon shows a hypoechoic region along the superficial aspect of he tendon (thick arrow) with a spur at the anterior aspect of the medial malleolar groove (thin arrow). (B) Longitudinal US of the tibialis posterior tendon shows a corresponding linear region of hypoechogenicity (arrow) onsistent with a longitudinal split. Arrowhead denotes the medial malleolus. (C) Axial CT in soft tissue windows emonstrates the osseous spur (arrow) at the anterior aspect of the tibialis posterior tendon (arrowhead).

actively or passively flexing the great toe can aid in identification and evaluation.[4]

## ANTERIOR TENDONS

The anterior tendons are the least commonly involved by pathology compared with the medial, lateral, and Achilles tendons. Of the three extensor tendons, the tibialis anterior tendon (ATT) is the most commonly involved by pathology. Though tears of the ATT are uncommon, they classically present with a history of "mass" and evaluation reveals not a mass but rather a torn and retracted tendon (**Fig. 16**). ATT tears typically occur within 3 cm of its insertion.[42] Causes of ATT injury include abrasion by impinging osteophytes from the first tarsal metatarsal joint or talonavicular joint, or from impinging hardware after surgery.[42,43] Impingement may only be noted during dynamic maneuvers such as plantar flexion. US is well suited for such dynamic evaluation. Tendon laceration can occur from penetrating trauma and very rarely from fracture.[44] Discontinuity of the tendon fibers and retraction of the torn tendon ends are noted with US when an ATT rupture is present. A longitudinal "split" of the distal ATT has been noted on MR imaging in asymptomatic volunteers and may be a normal variant as the tendon inserts, similar to the PPT insertion onto the navicular and plantar midfoot.[42]

Tendinosis of the anterior tibial tendon is noted as thickening of the tendon less than or equal to 5 mm at the level of the tarsal bones.[42] Pathology

of the extensor hallucis longus and extensor digitorum longus tendons is less common, compared with the ATT and has been described secondary to ill-fitting shoes or impinging osteophytes. The extensor digitorum longus tendon may be abraded by an osseous ridge at the dorsal aspect of the talus.[37] This can also be the site of a ganglion cyst (see *Masses* below).

## LIGAMENTS

Injury to ankle ligaments is by far the most common type of ankle pathology. A traumatic inversion force is the typical mechanism of injury. The lateral ligaments are most frequently torn; among the components of the lateral collateral ligament complex, the anterior taloficular ligament is most commonly torn. In most cases, ankle ligament ruptures can be diagnosed with high accuracy by physical examination alone.[45] In acute cases with equivocal diagnosis, or in chronic cases with persistent symptoms, US can play a role. In some cases surgical treatment may be needed, with reconstruction of the ligaments to stabilize the ankle and restore pain-free function.[4]

Normal ankle ligaments have a fibrillar echotexture and are sharply marginated, (**Fig. 17**).[46] Anisotropy can be seen with ankle ligaments. As with tendon imaging, this potential artifact is avoided by scanning with the ultrasound beam perpendicular to the ligament. Mild sprain is noted as slight thickening or loss of the normally fibrillar echotexture (**Fig. 18**). With partial tear there is

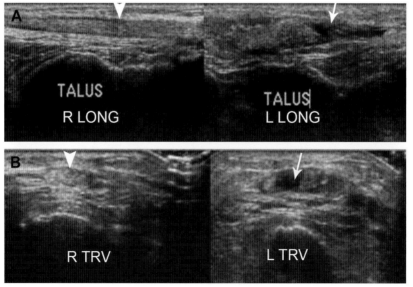

**Fig. 16.** (*A*) Longitudinal split screen US of the normal right (R) tibialis anterior tendon (*arrowhead*) and ruptured left (L) tibialis anterior tendon (*arrow*). (*B*) Transverse split screen US of the normal right tibialis anterior tendon (*arrowhead*) and ruptured left tibialis anterior tendon (*arrow*).

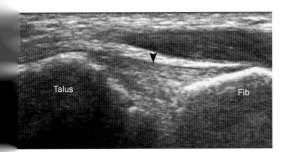

Fig. 17. Longitudinal US of the normal anterior talofibular ligament (*arrowhead*). The normal ligament is echogenic and of uniform thickness. F, fibula.

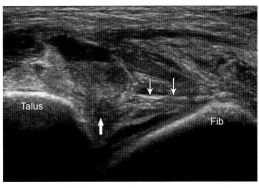

Fig. 19. Longitudinal US of an acutely ruptured anterior talofibular ligament. Thick arrow denotes the site of rupture, at the talar attachment with surrounding hematoma. Thin arrows denote the more normal portion of the ligament at its fibular attachment. Fib, fibula.

discontinuity of the ligament but it remains taut with dynamic maneuvers that place the ligament under tension. With complete tear, a hypoechoic gap is noted and the ligament fibers do not become taut with any maneuver (**Fig. 19**).[47] Osseous avulsion at a ligament attachment site denotes a severe ligament injury.[47] Chronic tears that have undergone scarring may demonstrate thickening of the ligament. Ossification may also be noted within such ligaments.[4] Using a 13-MHz transducer, the reported sonographic accuracy for evaluating the status of the anterior talofibular ligament is 90% to 100%; calcaneofibular ligament, 87% to 92%; and anterior tibiofibular ligament, 85% when compared with MR imaging.[46]

When the anterior talofibular ligament is injured, the calcaneofibular ligament should be carefully assessed since sequential injury of the lateral ligaments, from anterior to posterior, is almost always the norm. The anterior talofibular ligament is examined dynamically during plantar flexion and during inversion stress, or using the anterior drawer test.[4] Lateral talar process fracture can also be assessed when scanning the anterior talofibular ligament by sweeping the probe clockwise to assess the lateral aspect of the talus.[48] The calcaneofibular ligament can be examined

dynamically during dorsiflexion with inversion. The peroneal tendons are located immediately superficial to the calcaneofibular ligament (**Fig. 20**). As noted previously, fluid in the peroneal tendon sheath should prompt careful assessment of the calcaneofibular ligament since ligament injury can allow communication with the peroneal tendon sheath. Visualization of the proximal attachment of the calcaneofibular ligament may be limited by sonography secondary to its position deep to the lateral malleolus.[4]

The anterior tibiofibular ligament is injured in cases of "high ankle sprain." For dynamic imaging, the ankle is placed in dorsiflexion and varus.[4] The deltoid ligament is much less commonly injured but can be examined dynamically with dorsiflexion and eversion stress (**Fig. 21**).[46] If acute deltoid ligament injury is suspected, the lateral malleolus should be assessed for associated fracture and the anterior tibiofibular ligament for associated injury.[47]

## ANKLE JOINT PATHOLOGY

US is well suited for rapid evaluation of joint fluid and can also guide aspiration.[49] It has been reported that static US can detect as little as 2 mL of ankle fluid, versus 1 mL for MR imaging of the ankle.[50] Dynamic maneuvers, such as scanning during dorsiflexion and plantar flexion may aid detection of smaller amounts of fluid. Simple joint fluid appears as anechoic distention of the anterior joint capsule (**Fig. 22**). More complex joint fluid may appear sonographically similar to synovitis. Dynamic maneuvers, including scanning during dorsiflexion and plantar flexion and during compression of the joint capsule by the

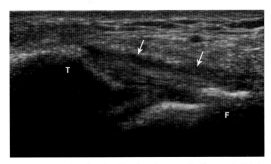

Fig. 18. Longitudinal US of a hypoechoic and thickened anterior talofibular ligament (*arrows*) consistent with sprain. F, fibula; T, talus.

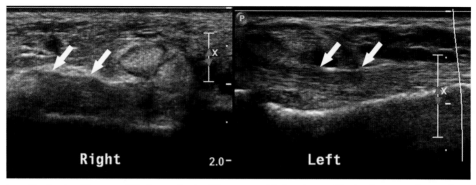

**Fig. 20.** Longitudinal split screen US of a patient with a normal left calcaneofibular ligament (*arrows*) and a ruptured right calcaneofibular ligament (*arrows*). Note the calcaneofibular ligament is located immediately deep to the round, echogenic peroneal tendons.

transducer, can aid evaluation. With dynamic maneuvers, collapse of the joint capsule and visualization of swirling hypoechoic fluid, and joint recess compressibility favors complex joint fluid rather than synovitis. If the complex intra-articular region demonstrates internal flow on Doppler evaluation, the findings are consistent with synovitis or an intra-articular mass such as pigmented villonodular synovitis. Intra-articular bodies can be accurately detected with US and appear as hyperechoic foci, usually with surrounding fluid. The sonographic sensitivity and specificity for detection of intra-articular bodies has been reported to be 100% and 95% respectively.[51]

## PLANTAR FASCIITIS

While plantar fasciitis is often diagnosed clinically, US can be helpful, especially in chronic cases or those recalcitrant to conservative therapies. Plantar fasciitis is the most common cause of heel pain and can be found in young athletes as well as obese and elderly patients.[4,52] The reported sensitivity and specificity of sonography is 80% and 89% compared with MR imaging.[53] The high prevalence of this condition, combined with the

expense of MR imaging, may favor US imaging in many cases.

The normal plantar fascia appears as a fibrillar band measuring 3 to 4 mm in thickness. With plantar fasciitis, fascia is hypoechoic and greater than 5 mm in thickness at the calcaneal attachment **(Fig. 23)**.[54,55]

Rupture of the plantar fascia is much less common but occurs in a similar patient population.[4] Location of these entities is different, with fasciitis at the calcaneal attachment and plantar fascial ruptures at the proximal or middle portion of the fascia. Acute fascial tears are noted as disruption of the fibers with surrounding or intervening fluid. The plantar fascia can be dynamically assessed by extending the toes dorsally, potentially aiding conspicuity of fascial tears.[4] The differential diagnosis of plantar heel pain also includes a foreign body, which is well assessed with US (see foreign bodies below).

## MASSES

US can diagnostically evaluate the most common ankle masses, such as a ganglion cyst, nerve sheath tumor, abscess, and aneurysm; and aid

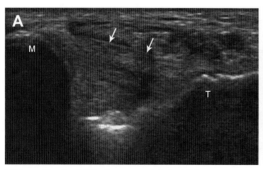
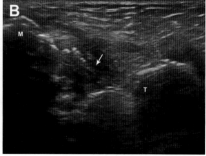

**Fig. 21.** (A) Longitudinal US of a normal deltoid ligament (*arrows*) with components noted coursing from the medial malleolus to the talus. (B) Longitudinal US of a torn deltoid ligament with wavy, echogenic fibers retracted from the talar insertion (*arrow*). M, medial malleolus; T, talus.

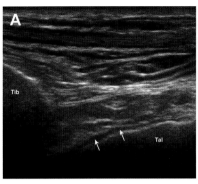
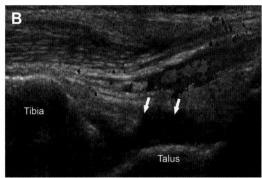

Fig. 22. (A) Longitudinal US of a normal anterior tibiotalar joint without detectable fluid. Arrows denote the hypoechoic cartilage of the talus. Tal, talus; Tib, tibia. (B) Longitudinal US of a joint effusion at the anterior tibiotalar joint (*arrows*). Note Doppler flow in the more superficial dorsalis pedis artery.

diagnosis of other masses. Specific features which aid diagnosis of a mass include location, relationship to adjacent vessels, nerves, joints and tendons, internal blood flow with Doppler evaluation, and compressibility.[43] Dynamic evaluation during joint motion can also be helpful in some cases, such as differentiating joint fluid, which moves with joint motion, from an adjacent ganglion which does not.

Ganglion cysts are often multiloculated and my have internal septations. A neck or communication with an adjacent tendon sheath or joint may be seen and should be searched for diligently to aid surgical resection. Ganglia can be anechoic or, in some cases, hypoechoic and may contain internal debris (**Fig. 24**).[56,57] They are well defined, with no internal Doppler flow.[56,58] An adventitial "medial malleolar bursa" can be seen at the medial malleolus, most commonly seen in ice skaters or hockey players, and thought to be due to poorly fitting footwear.[59]

Infection of the soft tissues of the hindfoot and midfoot ranges from cellulitis to abscess. Subcutaneous edema is noted as a reticular pattern of hypoechogenicity in the subcutaneous tissues.

Clinical correlation is required to separate edema from cellulitis. Soft tissue gas can be seen with an infectious process, sinus tract, or secondary to surgery or intervention. Gas is noted as a focus of hyperechogenicity which may also show comet-tail artifact.[43] An abscess can appear hyperechoic or hypoechoic, often with an echogenic rim and overlying skin thickening. An abscess may demonstrate surrounding hyperemia but does not have internal Doppler flow. Swirling of complex fluid may be seen with transducer pressure. US can also aid aspiration.[49]

Nerve sheath tumors appear as a well-defined fusiform mass, with hypoechoic or mixed echogenicity. They may demonstrate internal hyperemia. Schwannomas and neurofibromas may exhibit a sonographic "target sign" with central hypoechogenicity and peripheral hypoechogenicity.[58] An entering or exiting nerve is a key discriminator and can separate a nerve sheath tumor from other more nonspecific masses.

Lipomas can have characteristic US imaging features including a well-defined ovoid shape parallel to the skin surface, relative

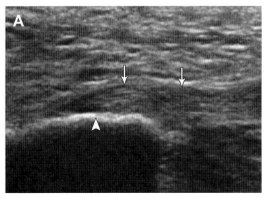
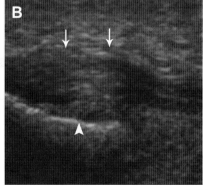

Fig. 23. (A) Longitudinal US of the normal plantar fascia (*arrows*) at the calcaneal origin (*arrowhead*). (B) US of plantar fascitis shows the hypoechoic and thickened plantar fascia (*arrows*) at the calcaneal origin (*arrowhead*).

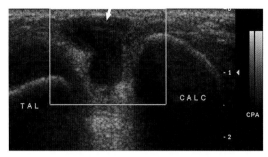

Fig. 24. Transverse US at the lateral ankle shows a hy-poechoic ganglion cyst between the calcaneus (calc) and talus (tal). Note the absence of internal Doppler flow.

hyperechogenicity, and absence of internal blood flow on Doppler evaluation.[58] While the sono-graphic appearance overlaps with that of other masses, in the context of a long-standing, stable, and pliable mass, the diagnosis can be inferred with follow-up to assure stability. MR imaging is diagnostic for a lipoma and can be obtained for corroboration as needed.

An aneurysm, while rare in the hindfoot or mid-foot, has also been described.[43] Ultrasound is well-suited to evaluate an aneurysm and can easily and rapidly identify the mass as originating from a vessel. Doppler evaluation should be used and can demonstrate a focal or fusiform enlargement of the vessel. Several additional uncommon ankle masses have been described by ultrasound including a glomus tumor, epidermal inclusion cyst, and subcutaneous granuloma annulare.[58] Like many masses which are evaluated with MR imaging, these masses have a nonspecific sono-graphic appearance.

## FOREIGN BODIES

Foreign bodies are relatively common in the foot. Ultrasound has shown sensitivity and specificity of 90% to100% for detection of foreign bodies in multiple cadaveric and clinical studies.[60–63] The smallest reported foreign body detected by US is 0.5 mm.[64] False negatives are unusual but can potentially occur if the foreign body is very small, located adjacent to a bone or liga-ment, or is obscured by soft tissue gas. False positives are also rare but can potentially be seen secondary to echogenic gas bubbles, calci-fications, or echogenic scar tissue.[62] Whenever possible, radiographs should be reviewed before US to assess for associated osseous and soft tissue findings. It is optimal to perform US before surgical exploration since soft tissue gas can cause an artifact that limits the sonographic evaluation by obscuring or simulating a foreign body. Tissue harmonics, an optimal scanning mode used in abdominal ultrasound, may de-crease the conspicuity and shadowing of the for-eign body and should be used with caution when assessing for a foreign body.[65] In general, we do not find tissue harmonics to be of great utility in musculoskeletal ultrasound.

All foreign bodies appear echogenic, regardless of their composition.[66] A hypoechoic surrounding halo[62] may be noted, as well as variable posterior shadowing (Fig. 25). These features can aid detec-tion and diagnosis, especially of small foreign bod-ies. Doppler interrogation should always be used when evaluating foreign bodies and can aid detec-tion of the foreign body which may be seen as an echogenic structure surrounded by hyperemia. Low-velocity Doppler settings should be used.[62] Doppler evaluation can help differentiate fluid (no Doppler flow) from phlegmonous tissue (may

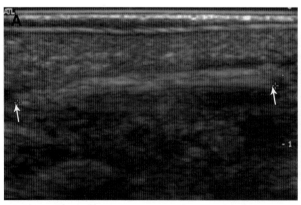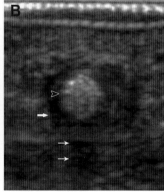

Fig. 25. (A) Longitudinal US of a wooden foreign body (between the arrows) in the foot. (B) Transverse US of the foreign body (arrowhead) with a surrounding hypoechoic halo (thick arrow) and posterior acoustic shadowing (thin arrows).

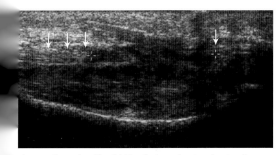

Fig. 26. Longitudinal US of the plantar foot of a patient who stepped on a piece of glass. The flexor hallucis longus tendon has been lacerated and is retracted proximally. The three arrows denote the proximal end of the ruptured tendon and the single arrowhead the distal end of the tendon. The tendon was surgically repaired.

demonstrate Doppler flow). The presence of a foreign body should prompt a diligent search for associated complications such as tendon or neurovascular injury (**Fig. 26**). Associated findings such as tenosynovitis, joint effusion, abscess (**Fig. 27**), and periostitis should prompt immediate notification of the referring clinician so that timely treatment for infection can be instituted.

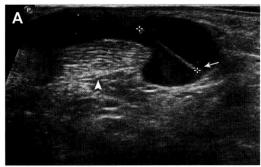

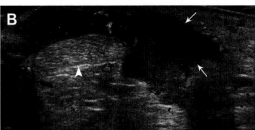

Fig. 27. (*A*) US performed transverse to the Achilles tendon (*arrowhead*) shows an abscess superficial to the Achilles with a linear echogenic foreign body (*arrow, between the cursors*). (*B*) Transverse US performed at an adjacent level with Doppler demonstrates hyperemia surrounding the abscess (*arrows*). Arrowhead denotes the Achilles tendon.

## SUMMARY

US offers several advantages for imaging the hind and midfoot, including its unique capacity to allow evaluation during dynamic maneuvers. This feature can reveal abnormalities that are not apparent during static imaging. US permits imaging of patients who cannot undergo MR imaging and provides real-time evaluation of the symptomatic site. Additional history can be obtained from the patient during US evaluation and the contralateral anatomy can be quickly assessed as needed. US has demonstrated great utility and accuracy for imaging the hindfoot and midfoot, including tendon, ligament, joint, and soft tissue pathology. It is imperative that radiologists provide expertise in all aspects of musculoskeletal imaging, including US.

## REFERENCES

1. Jacobson JA. Ultrasound clinics. Philadelphia: W.B. Saunders Company; 2007;765.
2. Jacobson JA. Fundamentals of musculoskeletal ultrasound. Philadelphia: Saunders Elsevier; 2007;345.
3. Khoury V, Cardinal E, Bureau NJ. Musculoskeletal sonography: a dynamic tool for usual and unusual disorders. AJR Am J Roentgenol 2007;188:W63–73.
4. Khoury V, Guillin R, Dhanju J, et al. Ultrasound of ankle and foot: overuse and sports injuries. Semin Musculoskelet Radiol 2007;11:149–61.
5. Bianchi S, Martinoli C, Gaignot C, et al. Ultrasound of the ankle: anatomy of the tendons, bursae, and ligaments. Semin Musculoskelet Radiol 2005;9:243–59.
6. Erickson SJ. High-resolution imaging of the musculoskeletal system. Radiology 1997;205:593–618.
7. Parker L, Nazarian LN, Carrino JA, et al. Musculoskeletal imaging: medicare use, costs, and potential for cost substitution. J Am Coll Radiol 2008;5:182–8.
8. Nazarian LN. The top 10 reasons musculoskeletal sonography is an important complementary or alternative technique to MRI. AJR Am J Roentgenol 2008;190:1621–6.
9. Lew HL, Chen CP, Wang TG, et al. Introduction to musculoskeletal diagnostic ultrasound: examination of the upper limb. Am J Phys Med Rehabil 2007; 86:310–21.
10. Chew K, Stevens KJ, Wang TG, et al. Introduction to diagnostic musculoskeletal ultrasound: part 2: examination of the lower limb. Am J Phys Med Rehabil 2008;87:238–48.
11. Brown AK, O'Connor PJ, Roberts TE, et al. Recommendations for musculoskeletal ultrasonography by rheumatologists: setting global standards for best practice by expert consensus. Arthritis Rheum 2005;53:83–92.

12. Grassi W, Filippucci E. Ultrasonography and the rheumatologist. Curr Opin Rheumatol 2007;19:55–60.

13. Legome E, Pancu D. Future applications for emergency ultrasound. Emerg Med Clin North Am 2004;22:817–27.

14. Rawool NM, Nazarian LN. Ultrasound of the ankle and foot. Semin Ultrasound CT MR 2000;21:275–84.

15. Hartgerink P, Fessell DP, Jacobson JA, et al. Full-versus partial-thickness Achilles tendon tears: sonographic accuracy and characterization in 26 cases with surgical correlation. Radiology 2001;220:406–12.

16. Waitches GM, Rockett M, Brage M, et al. Ultrasonographic-surgical correlation of ankle tendon tears. J Ultrasound Med 1998;17:249–56.

17. Grant TH, Kelikian AS, Jereb SE, et al. Ultrasound diagnosis of peroneal tendon tears. A surgical correlation. J Bone Joint Surg Am 2005;87:1788–94.

18. Chen YJ, Liang SC. Diagnostic efficacy of ultrasonography in stage I posterior tibial tendon dysfunction: sonographic–surgical correlation. J Ultrasound Med 1997;16:417–23.

19. Gerling MC, Pfirrmann CW, Farooki S, et al. Posterior tibialis tendon tears: comparison of the diagnostic efficacy of magnetic resonance imaging and ultrasonography for the detection of surgically created longitudinal tears in cadavers. Invest Radiol 2003;38:51–6.

20. Astrom M, Gentz CF, Nilsson P, et al. Imaging in chronic Achilles tendinopathy: a comparison of ultrasonography, magnetic resonance imaging and surgical findings in 27 histologically verified cases. Skeletal Radiol 1996;25:615–20.

21. Nazarian LN, Rawool NM, Martin CE, et al. Synovial fluid in the hindfoot and ankle: detection of amount and distribution with US. Radiology 1995;197:275–8.

22. Diaz GC, van Holsbeeck M, Jacobson JA. Longitudinal split of the peroneus longus and peroneus brevis tendons with disruption of the superior peroneal retinaculum. J Ultrasound Med 1998;17:525–9.

23. Neustadter J, Raikin SM, Nazarian LN. Dynamic sonographic evaluation of peroneal tendon subluxation. AJR Am J Roentgenol 2004;183:985–8.

24. Kannus P, Natri A. Etiology and pathophysiology of tendon ruptures in sports. Scand J Med Sci Sports 1997;7:107–12.

25. Paavola M, Paakkala T, Kannus P, et al. Ultrasonography in the differential diagnosis of Achilles tendon injuries and related disorders. A comparison between pre-operative ultrasonography and surgical findings. Acta Radiol 1998;39:612–9.

26. Kainberger FM, Engel A, Barton P, et al. Injury of the Achilles tendon: diagnosis with sonography. Am J Roentgenol 1990;155:1031–6.

27. Zanetti M, Metzdorf A, Kundert HP, et al. Achilles tendons: clinical relevance of neovascularization diagnosed with power Doppler US. Radiology 2003;227:556–60.

28. Patel S, Fessell DP, Jacobson JA, et al. Artifacts anatomic variants, and pitfalls in sonography of the foot and ankle. AJR Am J Roentgenol 2002;178:1247–54.

29. Lui TH. Endoscopic-assisted Achilles tendon repair with plantaris tendon augmentation. Arthroscopy 2007;23:556.e551–5.

30. Lee JC, Calder JD, Healy JC. Posterior impingement syndromes of the ankle. Semin Musculoskelet Radiol 2008;12:154–69.

31. Saxena A, Cassidy A. Peroneal tendon injuries: an evaluation of 49 tears in 41 patients. J Foot Ankle Surg 2003;42:215–20.

32. Sammarco GJ. Peroneal tendon injuries. Orthop Clin North Am 1994;25:135–45.

33. Sobel M, Geppert MJ, Olson EJ, et al. The dynamics of peroneus brevis tendon splits: a proposed mechanism, technique of diagnosis, and classification of injury. Foot Ankle 1992;13:413–22.

34. Wang XT, Rosenberg ZS, Mechlin MB, et al. Normal variants and diseases of the peroneal tendons and superior peroneal retinaculum: MR imaging features. Radiographics 2005;25:587–602.

35. Brigido MK, Fessell DP, Jacobson JA, et al. Radiography and US of os peroneum fractures and associated peroneal tendon injuries: initial experience. Radiology 2005;237:235–41.

36. Gray JM, Alpar EK. Peroneal tenosynovitis following ankle sprains. Injury 2001;32:487–9.

37. Shetty M, Fessell DP, Femino JE, et al. Sonography of ankle tendon impingement with surgical correlation. AJR Am J Roentgenol 2002;179:949–53.

38. Johnson KA, Strom DE. Tibialis posterior tendon dysfunction. Clin Orthop Relat Res 1989;239:196–206.

39. Nallamshetty L, Nazarian LN, Schweitzer ME, et al. Evaluation of posterior tibial pathology: comparison of sonography and MR imaging. Skeletal Radiol 2005;34:375–80.

40. Schweitzer ME, Caccese R, Karasick D, et al. Posterior tibial tendon tears: utility of secondary signs for MR imaging diagnosis. Radiology 1993;188:655–9.

41. Ouzounian TJ, Myerson MS. Dislocation of the posterior tibial tendon. Foot Ankle 1992;13:215–9.

42. Mengiardi B, Pfirrmann CWA, Vienne P, et al. Anterior tibial tendon abnormalities: MR imaging findings. Radiology 2005;235:977–84.

43. Fessell DP, Jamadar DA, Jacobson JA, et al. Sonography of dorsal ankle and foot abnormalities. AJR Am J Roentgenol 2003;181:1573–81.

44. Din R, Therkilsden L. Rupture of tibialis anterior associated with a closed midshaft tibial fracture. J Accid Emerg Med 1999;16:459.

45. van Dijk CN, Mol BW, Lim LS, et al. Diagnosis of ligament rupture of the ankle joint. Physical

examination, arthrography, stress radiography and sonography compared in 160 patients after inversion trauma. Acta Orthop Scand 1996;67:566–70.

6. Peetrons P, Creteur V, Bacq C. Sonography of ankle ligaments. J Clin Ultrasound 2004;32:491–9.

7. Morvan G, Busson J, Wybier M, et al. Ultrasound of the ankle. Eur J Ultrasound 2001;14:73–82.

8. Copercini M, Bonvin F, Martinoli C, et al. Sonographic diagnosis of talar lateral process fracture. J Ultrasound Med 2003;22:635–40.

9. Fessell DP, van Holsbeeck M. Ultrasound guided musculoskeletal procedures. In: Jacobson JA, editor. Ultrasound clinics. Philadelphia: W.B. Saunders Company; 2007. p. 737–57.

0. Jacobson JA, Andresen R, Jaovisidha S, et al. Detection of ankle effusions: comparison study in cadavers using radiography, sonography, and MR imaging. AJR Am J Roentgenol 1998;170:1231–8.

1. Frankel DA, Bargiela A, Bouffard JA, et al. Synovial joints: evaluation of intraarticular bodies with US. Radiology 1998;206:41–4.

2. Schepsis AA, Leach RE, Gorzyca J. Plantar fasciitis. Etiology, treatment, surgical results, and review of the literature. Clin Orthop Relat Res 1991;266: 185–96.

3. Sabir N, Demirlenk S, Yagci B, et al. Clinical utility of sonography in diagnosing plantar fasciitis. J Ultrasound Med 2005;24:1041–8.

4. Kane D, Greaney T, Shanahan M, et al. The role of ultrasonography in the diagnosis and management of idiopathic plantar fasciitis. Rheumatology 2001; 40:1002–8.

5. Cardinal E, Chhem RK, Beauregard CG, et al. Plantar fasciitis: sonographic evaluation. Radiology 1996;201:257–9.

6. Ortega R, Fessell DP, Jacobson JA, et al. Sonography of ankle Ganglia with pathologic correlation in 10 pediatric and adult patients. AJR Am J Roentgenol 2002;178:1445–9.

57. Wang G, Jacobson JA, Feng FY, et al. Sonography of wrist ganglion cysts: variable and noncystic appearances. J Ultrasound Med 2007;26:1323–8 [quiz: 1330–21].

58. Pham H, Fessell DP, Femino JE, et al. Sonography and MR imaging of selected benign masses in the ankle and foot. AJR Am J Roentgenol 2003;180: 99–107.

59. Brown RR, Sadka Rosenberg Z, Schweitzer ME, et al. MRI of medial malleolar bursa. AJR Am J Roentgenol 2005;184:979–83.

60. Jacobson JA, Powell A, Craig JG, et al. Wooden foreign bodies in soft tissue: detection at US. Radiology 1998;206:45–8.

61. Schlager D, Sanders AB, Wiggins D, et al. Ultrasound for the detection of foreign bodies. Ann Emerg Med 1991;20:189–91.

62. Davae KC, Sofka CM, DiCarlo E, et al. Value of power Doppler imaging and the hypoechoic halo in the sonographic detection of foreign bodies: correlation with histopathologic findings. J Ultrasound Med 2003;22:1309–13 [quiz: 1314–6].

63. Crawford R, Matheson AB. Clinical value of ultrasonography in the detection and removal of radiolucent foreign bodies. Injury 1989;20:341–3.

64. Failla JM, Holsbeeck Mv, Vanderschueren G. Detection of a 0.5-mm-thick thorn using ultrasound: a case report. J Hand Surg 1995;20:456–7.

65. Gibbs TS. The use of sonography in the identification, localization, and removal of soft tissue foreign bodies. Journal of Diagnostic Medical Sonography 2006;22:5–21.

66. Horton LK, Jacobson JA, Powell A, et al. Sonography and radiography of soft-tissue foreign bodies. AJR Am J Roentgenol 2001;176:1155–9.

# Imaging of Lisfranc Injury and Midfoot Sprain

Stephen F. Hatem, MD

**KEYWORDS**

• Lisfranc injury • Midfoot sprain • MRI

"Lisfranc" is one of the best known orthopedic eponyms. Unfortunately, the term is imprecise. Lisfranc is applied to a multitude of normal structures and various injuries: the Lisfranc joint, Lisfranc ligament, Lisfranc injury, and Lisfranc fracture-subluxation or dislocation. Jacques Lisfranc, a field surgeon in Napolean's army, described none of these; rather, he described a forefoot amputation technique that could be performed in less than 1 minute.[1] The site of that amputation, the tarsometatarsal joint, is now known as the Lisfranc joint, and is the common denominator among the various eponyms. The strong interosseous ligament between the first cuneiform (C1) and second metatarsal (M2), is known as the Lisfranc ligament, and is vital to the support of the tarsometatarsal joint. Injuries to the tarsometatarsal joint can be caused by low or high impact. The low-impact midfoot sprain is called a Lisfranc injury; the high-impact injuries are called Lisfranc fracture-subluxation or Lisfranc fracture-dislocation. Only recently has the orthopedic and radiology literature emphasized this distinction and investigated the imaging and clinical differences, highlighting the often-subtle midfoot sprain.

These distinctions are important for more than accurate and precise communication. Lisfranc fracture dislocations are uncommon, with an estimated incidence of 1 per 55,000, and account for only 0.2% of all fractures.[1] Yet midfoot sprains are common in athletes and occur in up to 4% of American football linemen per season.[2]

Up to 35% of Lisfranc injuries are initially misdiagnosed or overlooked.[3] Delays in diagnosis may be related to multiple factors, including a low index of suspicion,[4,5] distracting injuries in patients who have polytrauma,[4] or the subtlety or masking of radiographic findings.[5] Numerous authors have emphasized the importance of prompt diagnosis in minimizing the risk for long-term complications, such as residual ligamentous instability or posttraumatic degenerative arthritis.[1,6–8] Perhaps not surprisingly, Calder and colleagues[4] have shown that poor patient outcomes are associated with a delay in diagnosis of more than 6 months and presence of a compensation claim. Lisfranc injuries are reportedly the second most common injury in malpractice litigation against radiologists and emergency physicians.[9]

Injuries to the tarsometatarsal joint and of the Lisfranc ligament present a challenge.[1] They are difficult to diagnose and[2] outcomes worsen as diagnosis is delayed.[10] As a result, radiologists and clinicians must have a clear understanding of the relevant nomenclature, anatomy, injury mechanisms, and imaging findings.

## ANATOMY

The Lisfranc joint, or tarsometatarsal joint, defines the junction of the midfoot and forefoot, consisting of the following articulations between nine bones (**Fig. 1**):

- The medial, or first cuneiform (C1), with the hallux, or first metatarsal (M1)
- The middle, or second cuneiform (C2), with the second metatarsal (M2)
- The lateral, or third cuneiform (C3), with the third metatarsal (M3)
- The cuboid (Cu), with the fourth (M4) and fifth metatarsals (M5)

Department of Musculoskeletal and Emergency Radiology, Cleveland Clinic, Cleveland Clinic Main Campus, Mail Code A21, 9500 Euclid Avenue, Cleveland, OH 44195, USA
*E-mail address:* hatems@ccf.org

Radiol Clin N Am 46 (2008) 1045–1060
doi:10.1016/j.rcl.2008.09.003

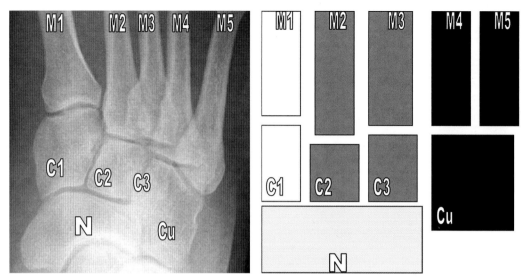

Fig. 1. Normal AP radiograph and schematic of the osseous relationships of the Lisfranc joint. Note how M2 is recessed in a mortise formed by C1 and C3. White shading indicates the medial column, gray the middle column, and black the lateral column. C1, first (medial) cuneiform; C2, second (middle) cuneiform; C3, third (lateral) cuneiform; Cu, cuboid; M1, first metatarsal; M2, second metatarsal; M3, third metatarsal; M4, fourth metatarsal; M5, fifth metatarsal; N, navicular.

These articulations occur within three separate synovial compartments. The first tarsometatarsal joint forms the medial compartment. The second and third tarsometatarsal joints share a capsule that communicates with the first and second intercuneiform and naviculocuneiform joints to form the central compartment. The articulations of the cuboid with the fourth and fifth metatarsals share a capsule, creating the lateral compartment.[11] These joints contribute to the columnar description of the foot: the medial column is defined as the first ray, including the medial cuneiform; the middle column includes the second and third rays and cuneiforms; and the lateral column includes the fourth and fifth rays with the cuboid.[12]

Additional osseous relationships are also important in the assessment of imaging and injury of the Lisfranc joint. These include the intercuneiform joints, especially C1-C2, the naviculocuneiform joint (N-C1C2), and those between the bases of the metatarsals.

These osseous relationships contribute to the intrinsic stability of the tarsometatarsal joint, with M2 the key structure.[13] It has been reported that up to 90% of patients who have Lisfranc injuries have a fracture, typically of the plantar aspects of the medial base of M2 or distal lateral aspect of C2.[3,14] In the coronal (short axis) plane, the osseous structures form a so-called "Roman arch." M2 represents the "keystone" because of its dorsal-most position and trapezoidal articular surface, broad base dorsally, and apex at its plantar surface. This transverse arch is an inherently stable configuration mechanically[13] but predisposes to dorsal displacement (Fig. 2).[15]

When viewed in the axial (long axis) plane, as on an anteroposterior (AP) radiograph, the tarsometatarsal joint is S-shaped.[16] The second metatarsal is recessed proximally with respect to the bases of the hallux and third metatarsals with a resultant mortise configuration. Peicha and colleagues[16] evaluated this configuration in 33 patients who suffered Lisfranc injuries, mostly low-impact sports-related injuries. The depth of the mortise was measured on routine foot radiographs in injured patients. The medial depth was measured on the AP view and the lateral depth on the oblique projection. Comparison was to a control group of measurements from cadavers without Lisfranc injuries. The mortise depth was significantly shallower medially in injured patients (8.95 mm versus 11.61 mm) than in controls ($P<.00001$). They theorized that a longer medial mortise depth allows for a broader and presumably stronger Lisfranc ligament at C1-M2, which protects against injury.

The ligamentous anatomy is complex and variable in course, number, and insertions (Fig. 3).[11] This complexity is reflected in the literature, both orthopedic and radiologic, which is inconsistent with respect to nomenclature and description.[17] A simplified description of the ligamentous constraints (see Fig. 3A) is commonly described,

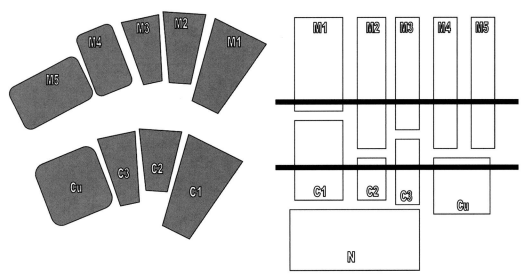

**Fig. 2.** Asymmetric Roman arch of the tarsometatarsal region in the short axis. Note the keystone position of the second metatarsal (M2) and cuneiform (C2). Also note how an image slice between these variably includes both cuneiforms and metatarsal bases. On cross-sectional imaging, cross referencing using a longitudinal plane allows confident localization.

which emphasizes the presence of tarsometatarsal ligaments at each articulation (C1-M1, C2-M2, C3-M3, Cu4-M4, Cu-M5) and three intermetatarsal ligaments (M2-M3, M3-M4, M4-M5). In general, these are described as having weaker dorsal and stronger plantar components. Most importantly, a point of weakness occurs between M1 and M2 where there is no intermetatarsal ligament. Rather, an additional tarsometatarsal ligament that courses obliquely from C1-M2 (the Lisfranc ligament)[18] plays the crucial role of supporting the base of C2 in its mortise between C1 and C3 and in its dorsal, keystone position in the transverse arch.

The detailed anatomic study by De Palma and colleagues in 1997[11] further elucidated the ligamentous relationships of the Lisfranc joint and has served as the anatomic model for subsequent biomechanical studies.[19,20] De Palma and colleagues emphasized a ligamentous system based on location (dorsal, interosseous, or plantar) and course (transverse, longitudinal, or oblique,). Transverse ligaments connect adjacent tarsal (intertarsal) or metatarsal (intermetatarsal) bones. Longitudinal ligaments extend from the tarsal to its corresponding metatarsal bone. Oblique ligaments extend from one tarsometatarsal ray to an adjacent one.

The dorsal ligaments (see **Fig. 3**B) include a variable number of short, flat, ribbonlike horizontal, oblique, or longitudinal bands across the tarsometatarsal joint, including one from each cuneiform to the base of M2, three fine intertarsal ligaments

(transverse at C1-C2 and C2-C3, and oblique from C3-Cu) and three fine ribbonlike transverse intermetatarsal ligaments (M2-M3, M3-M4, and M4-M5). No substantial M1-M2 fibers were observed.

Interosseous ligaments (see **Fig.** 3C) include three cuneometatarsal ligaments (the Lisfranc ligament, the central ligament, and the lateral longitudinal ligament), three intermetatarsal ligaments (M2-M3, M3-M4, M4-M5), and three intertarsal ligaments (C1-C2, C2-C3, and C3-Cu).

The Lisfranc ligament (first interosseous ligament, medial interosseous ligament, or interosseous C1-M2 ligament) is the largest of the ligaments supporting the Lisfranc joint. It has an oblique distal, lateral, and plantar course from the lateral wall of C1, adjacent to the C1-C2 intercuneiform ligament, to the medial base of M2 just beyond the articular surface. The plantar surface is intimately associated with the adjacent C1-C2 interosseous ligament, plantar ligaments, and the peroneus longus tendon. The central ligament (second cuneometatarsal ligament) extends from C2-C3 anteriorly to M2-M3 in most, but was variable. The lateral longitudinal ligament (third cuneometatarsal ligament) extends between C3 and M3 laterally.

The intertarsal interosseous ligaments are thick strong ligaments between C1-C2 (medial intercuneiform interosseous ligament), C2-C3 (lateral intercuneiform interosseous ligament), and C3-Cu (cuneocuboid interosseous ligament). Medial (M2-M3), central (M3-M4), and lateral (M4-M5)

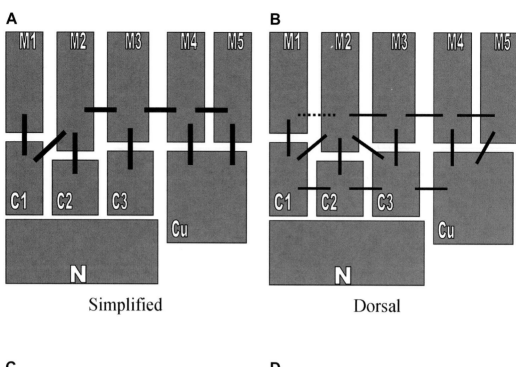

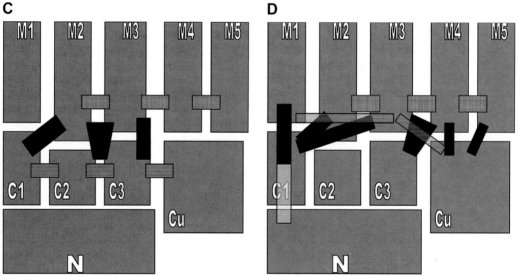

Fig. 3. Ligamentous constraints. (A) Simplified approach to the Lisfranc ligamentous constraints emphasizes absence of M1-M2 intermetatarsal ligament and presence of C1-M2 Lisfranc ligament. (B) Dorsal ligaments are thinner and weaker than the interosseous and plantar ligaments. Insignificant M1-M2 ligaments are occasionally identified (*dashed line*). (C) Interosseous ligaments, including the C1-M2 Lisfranc ligament, are substantial on gross inspection and mechanical evaluation. (D) Plantar ligaments are also substantial. The plantar C1-M2M3 ligament is an important contributor to Lisfranc stability. Refer to text for detailed description. Solid lines in B–D indicate tarsometatarsal ligaments, grid indicates intermetatarsal ligaments, stripes indicate intertarsal ligaments, and dashes indicate an inconstant relationship.

intermetatarsal interosseous ligaments tie the lesser metatarsals to each other.

Plantar ligaments (see **Fig. 3**D) were also found to be variable in size, number, and course. These were strong medially and weaker laterally. The first plantar ligament extended between C1-M1 and variably was in continuity with the more proximal ligament between the navicular and C1. The second ligament was oblique and coursed from C1 to the bases of M2 (thin and deep) and M3 (thick and superficial); this was the strongest of the plantar ligaments. No C2-M2 plantar ligaments were found. The third plantar ligament connected C3 to M3, M4, or both. The fourth and fifth ligaments connected the cuboid to the fourth and fifth, respectively, but were absent in roughly one third. Plantar intermetatarsal and intertarsal ligaments were stronger than the dorsal ligaments. The three intermetatarsal plantar ligaments course transversely and are the medial (M2-M3), central (M3-M4), and lateral (M4-M5); no ligaments extend from M1-M2. The plantar intertarsal ligaments consist of a single band from the base of M1 to M3 (without significant M2 attachment) and a band from M3-Cu.

Solan and colleagues[19] in 2001 reported results of their ex vivo biomechanical investigation of the ligaments of the second tarsometatarsal joint. They used paired cadaver feet and restricted their evaluation to the dorsal C1-M2, interosseous Lisfranc C1-M2, and plantar C1-M2M3 ligaments, and the adjacent bony structures C1, M2, and M3. Initial comparisons showed that the dorsal ligaments were weaker than the Lisfranc/plantar ligamentous complex. Subsequent evaluation revealed that the Lisfranc ligament was significantly stronger and stiffer than the plantar ligaments. These findings were consistent with earlier morphologic anatomic observations.[11,21]

In 2007, Kaar and colleagues[20] reported the results of their cadaveric study in which they sequentially sectioned the ligamentous stabilizers of the Lisfranc joint and evaluated simulated weightbearing (WB) and stress radiographs to assess stability. After initial sectioning of the Lisfranc (interosseous C1-M2) ligament, only 10% of specimens showed C1-M2 instability on simulated WB radiographs, 40% on abduction stress views, and none with adduction stress. They then sectioned either the plantar C1-M2M3 ligament or the C1C2 intercuneiform ligament. After additional sectioning of the plantar C1-M2M3 ligament, 20% showed instability based on C1-M2 widening (0% based on C2-M2) on WB and 100% displaced at both C1-M2 and C2-M2 with abduction stress. The second subgroup, after sectioning of the Lisfranc and then first intercuneiform interosseous

ligament (C1-C2), showed instability at C1-M2 in 20% and C1-C2 in 20%. With adduction stress, 20% showed C1-M2 widening and 80% showed C1-C2 instability. They concluded that transverse instability (C2-M2 tarsometatarsal widening) required section of the Lisfranc and plantar ligaments and was best appreciated under abduction stress. On the other hand, longitudinal instability (C1-C2 intercuneiform widening) required sectioning of the Lisfranc and C1-C2 ligaments and was best appreciated under adduction stress. Presumably working from the assumption that the Lisfranc ligament had to be injured to develop either longitudinal or transverse instability, they did not section either the plantar or intercuneiform ligaments in isolation, nor did they evaluate the combination of plantar and intercuneiform disruption.

Additional support of the tarsometatarsal joints is provided by soft tissues of the plantar foot, including the tendons of the peroneus longus, anterior and posterior tibialis, the long plantar ligament, the plantar fascia, and intrinsic muscles.[20,22] The relative support provided by these and the extent to which their disruption contributes to Lisfranc injuries has not yet been established.

## INJURY MECHANISM

Injuries to the joint can be due to direct forces applied to the tarsometatarsal joint but much more commonly result from indirect forces applied away from the joint, which act on it secondarily. The former account for some high-velocity injuries and the latter for most low-energy injuries.[23] High-velocity injury mechanism may be related to crush injury. As a result, displacement can be either dorsal or plantar depending on the direction of force and the site of application.[14] There are often numerous associated fractures within the foot and at distant sites.[3] Extensive associated soft tissue injuries are common, including vascular compromise and compartment syndrome.[22] These distracting injuries may contribute to missed or delayed diagnosis in this patient group.

Indirect forces account for most athletic injuries and typically occur as a result of forced plantar flexion or forefoot abduction, nearly always resulting in dorsal displacement of the metatarsals.[14] Other mechanisms include rolling the foot when stepping off a step or curb.[10,23]

Plantar flexion injuries can occur in several different ways. In the tiptoe position of full ankle and metatarsophalangeal plantar flexion, full body weight loads the Lisfranc joint along an elongated lever arm, resulting in failure of the joint dorsally and plantar flexion. This mechanism occurs in dancers and is similar to what happens during a misstep off of a curb or step, with the forefoot being "rolled over" by the entire body. Alternatively, if the ankle is plantar flexed while the knee is on the ground, a force directed along the axis of the foot can cause similar plantar flexion and dorsal failure; this is the purported mechanism in the football pileup where a player lands with full body weight on another's heel while the ankle is plantar flexed and the knee is on the ground.[23,24]

Forefoot abduction injuries occur when an athlete, typically wearing cleats, plants his foot and rotates to change direction.[10] Similar mechanism occurs in sailboarders and equestrians whose forefoot is fixed by a strap or stirrup.[25]

## INJURY CLASSIFICATION

There has been an evolution in the classification of Lisfranc injuries over the past century; Quenu and Kuss[26] in 1909 placed Lisfranc injuries into three categories: homolateral, isolated, and divergent. In homolateral injuries all five metatarsals are displaced in one direction. Divergent injuries occur when metatarsals are displaced in different directions in the sagittal and coronal planes. Isolated injuries do not involve all five metatarsals.

First Hardcastle and colleagues in 1982[27] and then Myerson and colleagues in 1986[14] expanded on the Qenu and Kuss classification to more comprehensively describe the spectrum of injuries at the Lisfranc joint (**Fig. 4**).

> Type A: total incongruity of the Lisfranc joint, typically either lateral or dorsoplantar
> Type B: partial incongruity
> > B1: partial medial dislocation, essentially involving the first ray in isolation, with or without displacement of the medial cuneiform
> > B2: partial lateral dislocation, involving any of the other four metatarsals
> Type C: divergent displacement
> > C1: partial
> > C2: total

Although useful for standardizing terminology, and applicable to low- and high-impact injuries, these classifications have not been found to predict outcome.[10,14]

Curtis and colleagues[10] in 1993 reported the first series limited to athletic midfoot injuries and used the American Medical Association's *Standardized Nomenclature of Athletic Injuries* to classify injuries. First- and second-degree injuries were partial tears of the tarsometatarsal ligaments

without instability on examination or fluoroscopic evaluation. Third-degree sprains were defined as complete ligamentous rupture with radiographic diastasis. The Myerson classification was applied to fracture-dislocations. This classification did not predict return to sport: 3 of 19 patients were unable to return to their sport and 2 of these had been classified as low-grade sprains.

Nunley and Vertullo[28] reviewed their experience with athletic midfoot injuries in 2002 and staged them based on a combination of clinical findings, bilateral AP, oblique and lateral WB radiographs, and radionuclide bone scans. Patients who had stage I injuries were unable to continue to play, had pain at the Lisfranc complex, and were nondisplaced radiographically, but demonstrated increased uptake on bone scan. Stage II injured athletes showed M1-M2 diastasis 1 to 5 mm greater than the uninjured foot but no loss of midfoot arch height. Stage III injuries had more than 5 mm of M1-M2 diastasis and arch height loss revealed by decrease in the C1-M5 distance on lateral view compared with the uninjured foot. Displaced injuries were further classified using the Myerson classification. This staging system drove patient management and they achieved excellent outcomes in 93% with nonoperative management of Stage I and operative management of Stage II and III injuries.

## IMAGING

The initial imaging evaluation of the Lisfranc joint should be by radiography. At the Cleveland Clinic the initial radiographic series for injury or trauma is performed unilaterally and consists of non-weightbearing (NWB) AP, internal oblique, and lateral views. Although these radiographs may readily demonstrate fracture or malalignment, often Lisfranc injuries are inapparent or subtle. Nunley and Vertullo[28] found that 50% of their athletes who had midfoot sprains had normal NWB radiographs. In patients who had subtle abnormalities on NWB films, or in patients who had a high clinical concern for midfoot sprain, WB radiographs are advised, with pain control as necessary.[9] A standing AP including both feet should be obtained, along with a WB lateral of the injured foot. Some authors advocate obtaining a comparison contralateral WB lateral view also (**Fig. 5**).[29]

Radiographic assessment of the Lisfranc joint requires a careful search for fracture on all views. In particular, fractures are common at the plantar medial base of M2 and plantar lateral base of C1. Myerson[14] coined the term "fleck sign" to describe these subtle cortical avulsion fractures from either

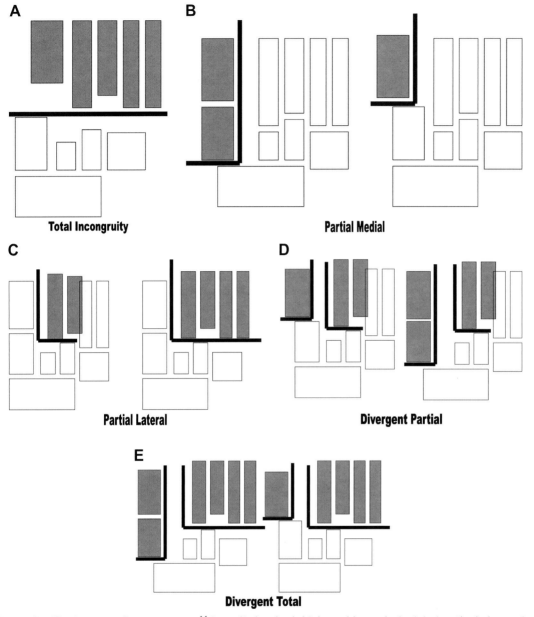

**Fig. 4.** Classification according to Myerson[14] is applied to both high- and low-velocity injuries. Shaded areas indicate displaced segments and black lines indicate lines of force. (*A*) A, total incongruity can result in displacement of all five metatarsal in any one direction (homolateral) but is typically dorsolateral. (*B*) B, partial incongruity. B1, Medial column disruption can occur either through C1-M1 or N-C1 joints. (*C*) B2, middle, or both middle and lateral column subluxation. (*D*) C1, divergent partial incongruity involves medial and middle columns. (*E*) C2, divergent total incongruity involves all metatarsals with medial column displaced medially and middle and lateral columns displaced laterally.

ttachment of the Lisfranc ligament. These are hree times more common in polytrauma patients han athletes,[10,14] and must be differentiated from he normal variant accessory ossicle (os intermetarseum) that occurs slightly more distally in the first ntermetatarsal web site, and which is typically moothly corticated (**Fig. 6**).

Careful attention should also be directed to tarsometatarsal alignment, because even the subtlest of malalignments may portend a significant injury. The asymmetry of the dorsoplantar Roman arch of the cuneiforms, which is elongated laterally, leads to visualization of different portions of the joint on the anteroposterior versus

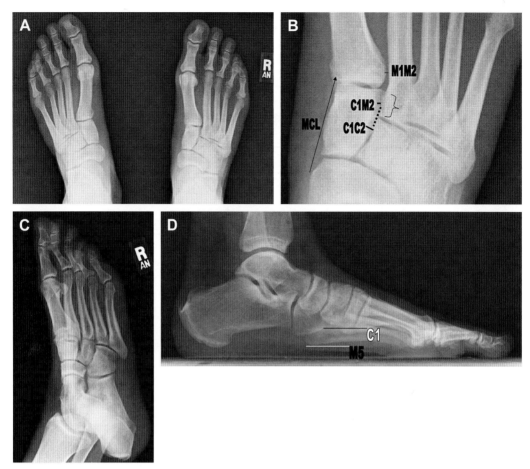

**Fig. 5.** Normal three-view foot series. (*A*) WB AP of both feet. (*B*) Magnification of A annotated with relationships to evaluate for suspected Lisfranc injury. Dashed line indicates second tarsometatarsal alignment. Bracket indicates depth of medial recess of the M2. (*C*) Oblique view. Note near-perfect alignment of medial and lateral margins of C2-M2, lateral margin of C3-M3, and medial margin of Cu-M4. (*D*) WB lateral. Note dorsal position of the plantar aspect of C1 with respect to plantar aspect of M5, perfect dorsal alignment of C1-M1 and C2-M2, and near-neutral talometatarsal angle.

oblique projections. On the AP view, the lateral margin of the first tarsometatarsal and medial margins of the second[30] and third[31] tarsometatarsals should each align nearly perfectly. On the oblique view, the lateral margins of C2-M2 and C3-M3 should align. The alignment of the fourth TMT is more variable but should be within 2 to 3 mm.[30–32]

On the WB lateral radiograph, images should be scrutinized for dorsoplantar subluxation or angulation and loss of the medial plantar arch:

> There should be no step-off at the dorsal margins of the tarsometatarsal joints[9]
> The talometatarsal angle is normally less than 10 degrees[14]
> The plantar surface of the medial cuneiform should project dorsal to the plantar aspect of M5[29]

Various authors have used differing thresholds for measurements related to these alignments and relationships, whereas others emphasize additional measurements:

> M1-M2 asymmetry with widening >1 mm on AP of the injured foot[28]
> Any disruption of the medial C2-M2 line on the AP[28]
> C1-C2 asymmetry with widening >1 mm on AP of the injured foot[28]
> C1-M2 asymmetry with widening >2 mm on WB AP[33]
> Failure of a line drawn on an AP along the medial margins of the navicular and C1 (medial column line) to intersect M1[34]
> C1-M5 asymmetry with narrowing >1.5 mm, or reversal, on the affected side on the WB lateral view[29] (**Fig. 7**)

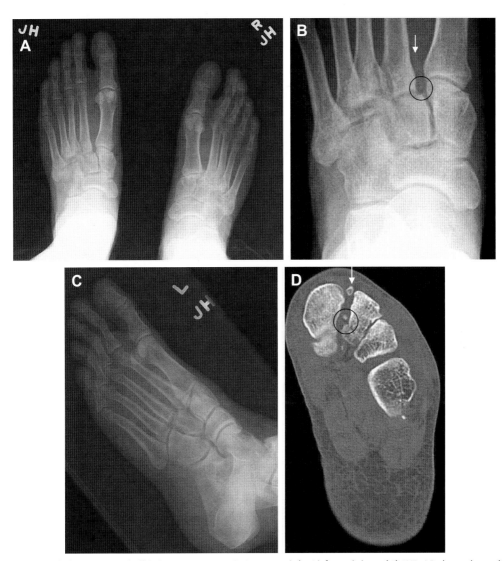

Fig. 6. Acute left foot racquetball injury, Myerson B2. Remote right Lisfranc injury. (*A*) WB AP shows lateral sub-luxation of the left C2M2 joint with diastasis of M1M2, C1M2, and C1C2. Note shallow depth of recession of each M2, perhaps predisposing him to injury. (*B*) Magnified and coned image show smoothly corticated and distal os intermetatarseum (*white arrow*) and proximal fleck fracture (*circled*). (*C*) Oblique view shows C2-M2 and C3-M3 malalignment and additional fracture lateral to the M2 base. (*D*) Oblique axial CT image shows both the os in-termetatarseum (*white arrow*) and fleck fracture (*circled*). (*E*) Oblique axial CT image shows numerous radio-graphically occult fracture fragments from the dorsum of C3. (*F*) Long axis CT reconstruction shows subtle malalignment of the C2-M2 and C3-M3 joints. (*G*) Despite operative reduction and fixation, WB AP 10 months later shows early C2-M2 arthrosis.

Talometatarsal angle >15 degrees on the lateral view[14]

Radiographic assessment is limited by difficulties with accuracy and reproducibility.[33–36] In general, however, lateral step-off at the second tarsometatarsal joint is accepted as the most common and reliably detected abnormality in Lisfranc injuries,[17] with diastasis of 2 mm or more indicating instability.[14,20,28]

In addition, normal WB views have been reported in patients who have midfoot sprains and Lisfranc injuries even on retrospective review.[24,28,33,36] False-negative WB views may be related to soft tissue swelling or pain limiting the degree of WB.[36] Stress radiographic views, radionuclide bone scan, CT, and MR imaging may each have a role in evaluating these injuries. At the present time no consensus imaging algorithm exists.

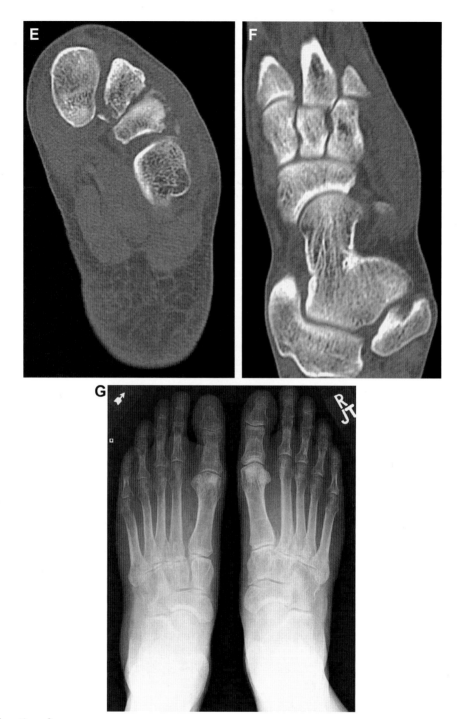

**Fig. 6.** (*continued*).

Stress views are advocated for their ability to directly demonstrate instability when initial radiographs are normal or show minimal diastasis.[6,10,20,34,37] Anesthesia may be necessary to achieve adequate pain control.[10] Pronation-abduction stress is most commonly advocated, although Kaar and colleagues emphasized the importance of adduction stress views in identifying longitudinal instability patterns of the first ray.[20]

Radionuclide bone scans are advocated for their ability to identify a midfoot sprain in the absence of radiographic findings,[28] particularly in patients presenting long after the initial injury.[6,8]

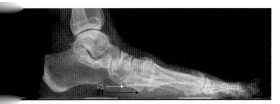

Fig. 7. WB lateral shows reversal of the normal relationship of C1 and M5, with C1 plantar to M5. Note severe tarsometatarsal osteoarthritis in this patient who had chronic Lisfranc injury.

Multidetector CT exquisitely depicts osseous anatomy and articular alignment in essentially any plane (see **Fig. 6**D–F).[36] Direct visualization of ligaments is limited, however, and WB or stress imaging is not practically feasible.[17] Tarsal fractures[36,38] and tarsometatarsal malalignment[38,39] are more readily identified on CT than radiographs. Tarsal fractures, in addition to the cuneiforms, can involve any of the bones of the feet but most frequently the cuboid.[36] The principle role of CT in the assessment of tarsometatarsal injuries is improved detection and delineation of fractures and their degree of comminution, intra-articular extension, displacement,[40] and any interposed soft tissues, typically tendons, that could preclude reduction.[1] As a result, CT is particularly recommended in patients who have high-velocity midfoot injuries or when fractures other than simple fleck signs are identified on initial radiographs.[7,36,38,41]

In contradistinction, MR imaging excels at depiction of soft tissues (see **Fig. 7; Figs. 8** and **9**); in the author's experience and literature review there are no reports of falsely positive or negative MR imaging with respect to Lisfranc ligament injuries. Preidler and colleagues[36,42,43] published a series of three papers investigating MR imaging of the normal and injured Lisfranc joint from 1996 to 1999. In a cadaver study, they initially established that MR imaging reliably depicted the anatomy of the tarsometatarsal joint and promoted oblique axial images (proscribed along the long axis of the foot parallel to the dorsum) to evaluate bony alignment and the interosseous Lisfranc ligament. Tarsometatarsal ligaments were best visualized in the sagittal plane. Intermetatarsal ligaments were seen best in the coronal (short axis of foot) images, and were thicker plantarly. MR arthrography performed after injection of each tarsometatarsal compartment did not improve visualization of the ligamentous anatomy.[42]

Shortly thereafter, Preidler and colleagues[43] reported their experience with MR imaging of Lisfranc injuries in 11 patients. MR imaging identified malalignment in all 11 patients at the second tarsometatarsal joint, confirming the radiographic findings in all 5 patients for whom radiographs were available. The interosseous Lisfranc ligament was disrupted in 8 patients and the remaining 3 had fractures of either the M2 base or lateral wall of C1. Additionally, intermetatarsal ligament injuries, other metatarsal fractures, and tarsal fractures were identified. In the 9 patients who were treated surgically, all MR imaging findings were confirmed.

Subsequently, Preidler and colleagues[36] reported results from a prospective study of 49 patients who had acute midfoot hyperflexion injuries attributable to low- and high-impact mechanisms and proved the impact of additional imaging beyond radiographs on patient management. Each patient underwent routine and WB radiographs the day of injury, CT within 2 days, and MR imaging within 5 days. Eight patients had tarsometatarsal malalignment on routine and WB views; an additional 8 showed malalignment on CT and MR imaging. CT and MR imaging also each demonstrated more fractures than were seen on radiographs: CT revealed more than 50% more metatarsal and twice as many tarsal fractures; MR imaging showed about 25% more metatarsal fractures and just under twice as many tarsal fractures, and numerous additional bone bruises. Some of these bone bruises correlated with nondisplaced cortical fractures seen on CT but misdiagnosed as bone bruises on MR imaging. Imaging findings were confirmed in the 11 patients who went to surgery. The authors concluded that management changed in 8 patients because of findings on CT scan and that MR imaging did not further change treatment in these or change management in any other patient. They did not specifically address whether MR imaging in the absence of a prior CT would have changed management compared with radiographs alone. Their results strongly suggest that it would have had a similar impact as CT, however, because all malalignments were identified on both modalities, MR demonstrated more bony injuries (although some nondisplaced fractures were misdiagnosed as bone bruises), and MR afforded direct visualization of Lisfranc ligament disruption.

Potter and colleagues[33] reported their experience evaluating the Lisfranc ligament in 23 patients who suffered midfoot injury and had radiographs and MR imaging. Most were athletes who had suffered low-impact injuries. The study was not designed to evaluate the impact of particular radiographic or MR imaging findings on patient management or outcome. A cadaver study of anatomic–MR imaging correlation was also performed. They described the Lisfranc ligament as having two bands, dorsal and plantar.

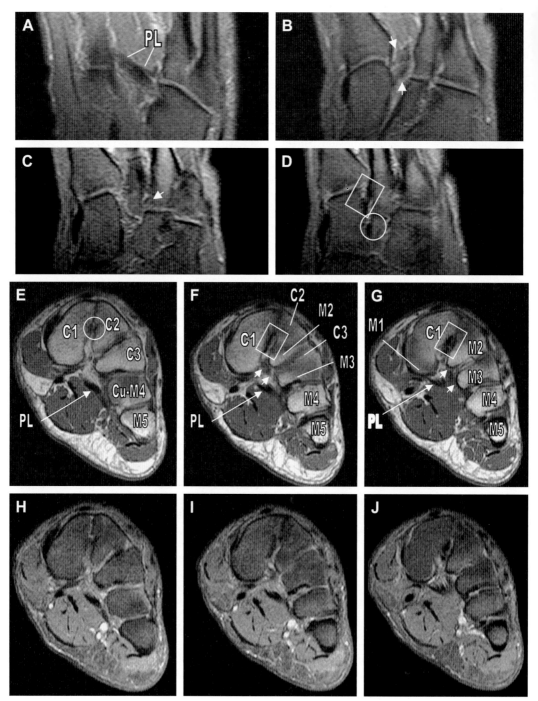

**Fig. 8.** Normal MR imaging of the Lisfranc Joint. (*A–D*) Consecutive plantar to dorsal fluid-sensitive oblique long axis images (fat-suppressed turbo spin echo PD TR4000/TE13). (*A*) The peroneus longus (PL) is immediately deep and orthogonal to the plantar C1-M2M3 ligament (*arrows*) in B and C. The interosseous C1-M2 Lisfranc ligament (*rectangle*) and C1-C2 interosseous ligament (*circle*) are seen in D. (*E–G*) T1 (TR687/TE15), and (*H–J*) fat-suppressed TSE T2 (TR5200/TE14) short axis images from proximal to distal. (*E*) The C1-C2 interosseous ligament (*circle*) is seen at the midportion of the cuneiforms which are closely apposed without fluid or edema. (*B*) Immediately distal is the C1 attachment of the Lisfranc C1M2 interosseous ligament (*rectangles*), which courses obliquely to attach to M2 (*G*). The plantar C1-M2M3 ligament is seen to have a slightly more longitudinal course from the base of C1 to the tip of M1 and the medial base of M3 (*F, G, short arrows*). Note the underlying peroneus longus tendon as it courses from proximal lateral to distal medial to insert on the base of M1. Fluid-sensitive images H–J show no abnormal signal within the ligaments, PL, and adjacent osseous structures.

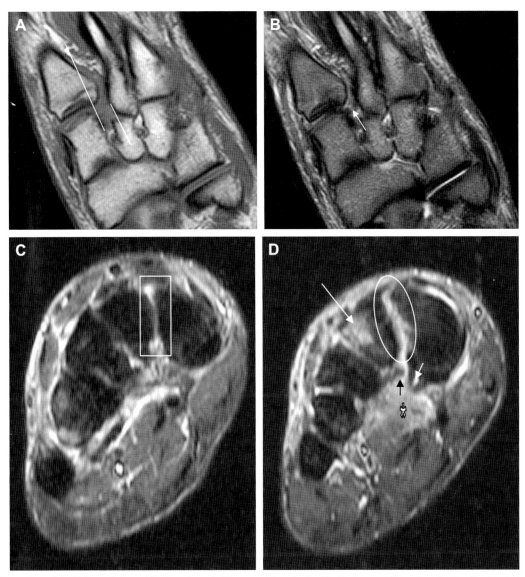

Fig. 9. Unstable Lisfranc injury, MR imaging. A 16-year-old male football player suffered a plantar flexion injury when a player landed on his heel after he had been tackled. (*A*) T1 (TR600/TE14) oblique long axis shows subtle C1-M1 and C2-M2 lateral subluxations (*lines*). (*B*) TSE T2 (TR3458/TE96) in the same plane shows complete tear of the interosseous Lisfranc ligament (*arrow*) with adjacent edema. (*C, D*) Inversion recovery (TR7000/TE22/TI150) short axis images. There is fluid at the first intercuneiform space and nonvisualization of the C1-C2 ligament (*rectangle*) (*C*). At the level of C1-M2 (*D*), there is abnormal increased signal in the interspace, and nonvisualization of the Lisfranc ligament (*oval*), disruption of the plantar C1-M2M3 ligament (*short black arrow*), injury to the plantar musculature (*\**) and peroneus longus at its insertion (*short white arrow*), and M2 base bone bruise (*long white arrow*).

The dorsal corresponded to the interosseous Lisfranc ligament, whereas the plantar corresponded by description and the limited images published with the C1-M2M3 ligament described by DePalma[11] and evaluated by Kaar and colleagues.[20] Disruption of either band was considered a partial tear (18 of 23) and disruption of both, a complete tear (3 of 23) of the Lisfranc ligament. All patients who had radiographic diastasis at C1-M2 or C2-M2 of 2 mm or more when compared with the uninjured side had partial or complete rupture of the Lisfranc ligament. All patients who had rupture of both bands had at least 2 mm diastasis at C1-M2. Radiographic abnormalities were not consistently seen in patients who subsequently had a partial tear

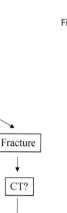

Fig. 10. Proposed imaging decision tree.

identified on MR imaging, however. Because none of this latter subset had surgery and no follow-up information was provided, the significance of identification of these partial tears involving either the interosseous or plantar ligament is uncertain. In the 7 patients who underwent surgery for partial or complete tears, the MR imaging findings were confirmed. Interestingly, additional tears were described of the intercuneiform and intermetatarsal ligaments on MR imaging in the absence of radiographic widening. Although the impact of these findings on patient management was beyond the scope of the study, it is noteworthy that all 4 patients who had C1C2 intercuneiform ligament tears also had full or essentially full-thickness tears of the Lisfranc ligament, radiographic asymmetric C1C2 diastasis of at least 1 mm, and went to surgery. They concluded that MR imaging is not indicated if radiographs are clearly abnormal, but can reveal the extent of ligament injury when radiographs are equivocal.

A recent case report by Hatem and colleagues[24] supported this assertion. Lisfranc ligament disruption was diagnosed with MR imaging despite normal WB radiographs; instability was confirmed by intraoperative stress view before surgical fixation.

Delfaut and colleagues[35] sounded a note of caution with respect to MR imaging interpretation in their study of tarsometatarsal joint alignment in cadavers and asymptomatic volunteers. All had intact Lisfranc ligaments, but step-offs were commonly identified at the first three tarsometatarsal joints, lateral more so than medial. These were typically identified on only a single or limited number of slices, and were believed to be related

to the complexity of the anatomy in this region, joint laxity, and partial volume averaging. They cautioned that care should be taken to not overstate the significance of malalignment identified on MR imaging in the absence of ligamentous or osseous signal abnormality.

MR imaging protocols should be optimized to the scanner being used, institutional demands, and history available at the time of the examination. In general, I find useful sequences include fluid-sensitive (fat-suppressed turbo spin echo proton density/T2 or STIR) short axis (perpendicular to the tarsometatarsal joints), fluid-sensitive oblique long axis oriented parallel to the dorsum of the foot, fluid-sensitive and T1 sagittal. I have at times found a T2* weighted three-dimensional gradient echo sequence helpful because of the ability to reconstruct thin slices in multiple planes and perhaps improved visualization of cortical avulsion fragments by their susceptibility artifacts. Sagittal sequences are useful for cross-referencing exact slice positions for the other planes and assessing the dorsal tarsometatarsal ligaments. Oblique long axis images optimally visualize the interosseous Lisfranc and plantar tarsometatarsal ligaments. Short axis images also show these structures, typically over multiple slices because of the oblique courses of the ligaments, and the C1C2 intercuneiform interosseous ligament and supporting plantar structures, such as the peroneus longus and intrinsic musculature.

## SUMMARY

Although there is no consensus diagnostic imaging approach in suspected Lisfranc injuries, several important points can be garnered and are reflected in the proposed imaging flow chart (Fig. 10).

First, anatomic considerations, both constant and variable, contribute to tarsometatarsal injuries. The effective absence of an intermetatarsal ligament between the first two metatarsal bases, and unique osseous and capsuloligamentous anatomy of the first and second tarsometatarsal joints, accounts for the injuries sustained. Less recession of the second metatarsal base relative to the medial cuneiform predisposes to Lisfranc injury. Weaker dorsal ligaments fail first, but development of instability and its pattern seems to depend on disruption of the interosseous Lisfranc ligament, plantar tarsometatarsal ligaments, supporting plantar forefoot structures, and intercuneiform ligaments.

Second, radiographs should be carefully scrutinized for subtle malalignment or asymmetries. Asymmetric diastasis of more than 2 mm at the involved joints and spaces predicts instability and is usually an indication for prompt surgical reduction and fixation.

Third, initial normal radiographs, routine or WB, do not exclude significant Lisfranc injury and further assessment is advised when there is high clinical concern for injury or symptoms persist.

Fourth, CT's excellence in depicting malalignment and fractures makes it a useful advanced imaging technique in high-energy injuries with fractures.

Finally, the excellence of MR imaging in depicting soft tissue anatomy affords direct visualization of the Lisfranc ligament and additional capsuloligamentous structures, rendering it useful in evaluating suspected low-impact Lisfranc injuries, particularly in the setting of equivocal radiographic studies.

## REFERENCES

1. Philbin T, Rosenberg G, Sferra JJ. Complications of missed or untreated Lisfranc injuries. Foot Ankle Clin N Am 2003;8:61–71.

2. Meyer SA, Callaghan JJ, Albright JP, et al. Midfoot sprains in collegiate football players. Am J Sports Med 1994;22:392–401.

3. Vuori JP, Aro HT. Lisfranc joint injuries: trauma mechanisms and associated injuries. J Trauma 1993; 35:40–5.

4. Calder JDF, Whitehouse SL, Saxby TS. Results of isolated Lisfranc injuries and the effect of compensation claims. J Bone Joint Surg Br 2004;86:527–30.

5. Sherief TI, Mucci B, Greiss M. Lisfranc injury: how frequently does it get missed? And how can we improve? Injury 2007;38:856–60.

6. Aronow MS. Treatment of missed Lisfranc injury. Foot Ankle Clin N Am 2006;11:127–42.

7. Hunt SA, Ropiak C, Tejwani NC. Lisfranc joint injuries: diagnosis and treatment. Am J Orthop 2006;35:376–85.

8. Latterman C, Goldstein J, Wukich DK, et al. Practical management of Lisfranc injuries in athletes. Clin J Sports Med 2007;17:311–5.

9. Gupta RT, Wadhwa RP, Learch TJ, et al. Lisfranc injury: imaging findings for this important but often-missed diagnosis. Curr Probl Diagn Radiol 2008; 37:115–26.

10. Curtis MJ, Myerson M, Szura B. Tarsometatarsal injuries in the athlete. Am J Spts Med 1993;21: 497–502.

11. dePalma L, Santucci A, Sabetta SP, et al. Anatomy of the Lisfranc joint complex. Foot & Ankle Int 1997;18:356–64.

12. Komenda GA, Myerson MS, Biddinger KR. Results of arthrodesis of the tarsometatarsal joints after traumatic injury. J Bone Joint Surg Am 1996;78: 1665–76.

13. Arntz CT, Hansen ST. Dislocations and fracture dislocations of the tarsometatarsal joints. Orthop Clin N Am 1987;18:105–14.

14. Myerson MS, Fisher RT, Burgess AR, et al. Fracture dislocations of the tarsometatarsal joints: end results correlated with pathology and treatment. Foot & Ankle 1986;6:225–42.

15. Bassett FH III. Dislocations of the tarsometatarsal joints. South Med J 1964;57:1294–302.

16. Peicha G, Labovitz, Seibert FJ, et al. The anatomy of the joint as a risk factor for Lisfranc dislocation and fracture-dislocation. J Bone Joint Surg Br 2002;84: 981–5.

17. Crim JS. MR imaging evaluation of subtle Lisfranc injuries: the midfoot sprain. Magn Reson Imaging Clin N Am 2008;16:19–27.

18. Wiley JJ. The mechanism of tarso-metatarsal joint injuries. J Bone Joint Surg Br 1971;53:474–82.

19. Solan MS, Moorman CT, Miyamoto RG, et al. Ligamentous restraints of the second tarsometatarsal joint: biomechanical evaluation. Foot & Ankle Int 2001;22:637–41.

20. Kaar S, Femino J, Morag Y. Lisfranc joint displacement following sequential ligament sectioning. J Bone Joint Surg Am 2007;89:2225–32.

21. Sarrafian SK. Syndesmology. In: Anatomy of the foot and ankle. Philadelphia: JB Lippincott; 1993. p. 159–217.

22. Myerson MS. The diagnosis and treatment of injury to the tarsometatarsal joint complex. J Bone Joint Surg Br 1999;81:756–63.

23. Mantas JP, Burks RT. Lisfranc injuries in the athlete. Clin Spts Med 1994;13:719–30.

24. Hatem SF, Davis A, Sundaram M. Midfoot sprain: Lisfranc ligament disruption. Orthopedics 2005;28: 75–7.

25. Mullen JE, O'Malley MJ. Sprains-residual instability of subtalar, Lisfranc joints, and turf toe. Clin Sports Med 2004;23:97–121.

26. Quenu E, Kuss G. [Etude sur les luxations du metatarse (luxations metatarsotarsiennes) du diastasis entre le 1er et le 2e metatarsien]. Rev Chir 1909; 39:281–336, 720–91, 1093–134 [in French].

27. Hardcastle PH, Reschauer R, Kutscha-Lissberg E, et al. Injuries to the tarsometatarsal joint: incidence, classification and treatment. J Bone Joint Surg Br. 1982;64:349–56.

28. Nunley JA, Vertullo CJ. Classification, investigation and management of midfoot sprains. Am J Spts Med 2002;30:871–8.

29. Faciszewski T, Burks RT, Manaster BJ, et al. Subtle injuries of the Lisfranc joint. J Bone Joint Surg Am 1990;72:1519–22.

30. Foster SC, Foster RR. Lisfranc's tarsometatarsal fracture-dislocation. Radiology 1976;120:79–83.

31. Norfray JF, Geline RA, Steinberg RI, et al. Subtleties of Lisfranc fracture-dislocations. AJR 1981;137: 1151–6.

32. Goiney RC, Connell DG, Nichols DM. CT evaluation of tarsometatarsal fracture-dislocation injuries. AJR 1985;144:985–90.

33. Potter HG, DeLand JT, Gusmer PB, et al. Magnetic resonance imaging of the Lisfranc ligament of the foot. Foot Ankle Int 1998;19:438–46.

34. Coss HS, Manos RE, Buoncristiani A, et al. Abduction stress and AP weightbearing radiography of purely ligamentous injury in the tarsometatarsal joint. Foot Ankle Int 1998;19:537–41.

35. Delfaut EM, Rosenberg ZS, Demondion X. Malalignment at the Lisfranc joint: MR features in asymptomatic patients and cadaveric specimens. Skeletal Radiol 2002;31:499–504.

36. Preidler KW, Peicha G, Lajtai G, et al. Conventional radiography, CT, and MR imaging in patients with hyperflexion injuries of the foot: diagnostic accuracy in the detection of bony and ligamentous changes. AJR Am J Roentgenol 1999;173:1673–7.

37. Arntz CT, Veith RG, Hansen ST. Fractures and fracture-dislocations of the tarsometatarsal joint. J Bone Joint Surg Am 1988;70:173–81.

38. Haapamaki V, Kiuru M, Koskinen S. Lisfranc fracture-dislocation in patients with multiple trauma: diagnosis with multidetector computed tomography. Foot Ankle Int 2004;25:614–9.

39. Lu J, Ebraheim NA, Skie M, et al. Radiographic and computed tomographic evaluation of Lisfranc dislocations: a cadaver study. Foot Ankle Int 1997;18:351–5.

40. Thordarsen DB. Fractures of the midfoot and forefoot. In: Myerson MS, editor. Foot and ankle disorders, vol. 2. Toronto: WB Saunders; 1999. p. 1265–96.

41. Engalnoff G, Anglin D, Hutson HR. Lisfranc fracture-dislocation: a frequently missed diagnosis in the emergency department. Ann Emerg Med 1995;26: 229–33.

42. Preidler KW, Wang Y, Brossman J, et al. Tarsometatarsal joint: anatomic details on MR images. Radiology 1996;199:733–6.

43. Preidler KW, Brossman J, Daenen B, et al. MR imaging of the tarsometatarsal joint: analysis of injuries in 11 patients. AJR 1996;267:1217–22.

# MR Imaging and Ultrasound of Metatarsalgia—The Lesser Metatarsals

Julie M. Gregg, GDU, PhD[a],*, Timothy Schneider, MD[b],
Paul Marks, MD[c]

## KEYWORDS

- Musculoskeletal • Metatarsalgia
- Instability • Bursitis • Neuroma

Metatarsalgia is a general term used to describe pain in the metatarsal region, which is a common clinical problem. Metatarsalgia accompanies many different entities, such as interdigital neuroma, metatarsophalangeal (MTP) joint synovitis or instability, Freiberg infarction, stress fractures and systemic disorders.

## IMAGING PROTOCOLS
### MR Imaging

To achieve high-resolution diagnostic MR images of the forefoot, small field-of-view dedicated surface coils are required. We use a quadrature send-receive wrist coil, which can accommodate all but the largest feet. Images should be taken in three planes using a small field of view. We favor three planes proton density (PD) and two planes of T2 fat-suppressed sequences.[1] A contiguous slice thickness of 2 mm is optimal. The T1 sequence is helpful for delineating fractures and assessing masses with a view to occasionally injecting contrast. Intravenous contrast is typically reserved for assessment of osteomyelitis and unusual masses but is not necessary for imaging Morton neuroma.

### Ultrasound

A high-frequency linear array probe with settings to detect small variations in soft tissue densities is important (ie, a 13–5 MHz probe with a dynamic range of 45–50 dB and a single focal zone).[1] The MTP joints are evaluated with the highest frequency possible and shallowest depth. Dorsally, this is between 1.5 and 2 cm depth; plantarly this is 1.5 to 2.5 cm depth. Transducer pressure must be light when assessing vascularity, but dynamic compression is useful to assess and characterize effusions and synovitis, or to assess subcutaneous masses. To achieve greater depth penetration in the web spaces, the frequency typically needs to be lowered and depth adjusted to between 2 and 4 cm. Web spaces are interrogated from both dorsal and plantar approaches, with pressure manually applied from the opposing surface to splay the metatarsals and dynamically evaluate the compressibility of tissues. Medial to lateral parasagittal evaluation of the plantar plate with and without toe dorsiflexion is critical for assessing the integrity of the plate and MTP joint stability.

## METATARSOPHALANGEAL JOINT INSTABILITY—PLANTAR PLATE DISRUPTION
### Anatomy

The major longitudinal bands of the plantar aponeurosis blend with the plantar capsule, firmly inserting into the plantar plate. The lesser MTP joint plantar plate is situated deep to the metatarsal head, providing strength and support during

[a] Symbion Imaging, Vaucluse Hospital, 82 Moreland Road, Brunswick, 3056, Victoria, Australia
[b] Melbourne Orthopaedic Group, 33 The Avenue, Windsor, 3181, Victoria, Australia
[c] Symbion Imaging, The Avenue Hospital, 40 The Avenue, Windsor, 3181, Victoria, Australia
* Corresponding author.
*E-mail address:* drjules@optusnet.com.au (J.M. Gregg).

Radiol Clin N Am 46 (2008) 1061–1078
doi:10.1016/j.rcl.2008.09.004

ambulation. The plantar plate is firm and flexible with an articular-like surface on its dorsal aspect. The plantar plate is composed of fibrocartilage, primarily type I collagen. The collagen bundles are interwoven with fibers oriented longitudinally on its dorsal aspect and transversely on its deep surface to blend with the deep transverse intermetatarsal ligament.[2,3] The reported average length of the plantar plate is 18.8 mm, longer for the second and third toes (20 mm). The plantar plate thickness ranges from 2 to 5 mm and width ranges from 8 to 13 mm. The proximal origin of the plantar plate attaches loosely to the periosteum of the metatarsal shaft to a thin synovial fold, just proximal to the flare of the metatarsal head. Distally the plantar plate inserts firmly and directly into the bone on the plantar surface of the proximal phalanx, just distal to the articular surface.[2]

Other stabilizing structures to the MTP joints include the collateral ligaments, the flexor digitorum longus and brevis tendons, and the extensor hood and sling. The phalangeal collateral ligament is a linear band coursing from the dorsal tubercle of the metatarsal neck to its common insertion with the plantar plate at the plantar base of the proximal phalanx. The accessory collateral ligament fans out from its origin adjacent to the phalangeal collateral ligament to insert broadly along the length of the plantar plate margins.[2] The flexor tendon sheath sits within a shallow central groove on the overlying surface of the plantar plate.[3]

### Mechanism of Injury

The mechanisms that support the longitudinal arch of the foot have been described as the beam mechanism and the truss, or tie-bar mechanism.[4] Hyperextension of the toes at the MTP joint tenses the plantar aponeurosis, raises the longitudinal arch of the foot, inverts the hindfoot, and externally rotates the leg. The hyperextension of the toe winds the plantar aponeurosis around the metatarsal head. This so-called "windlass" mechanism is greatest in the big toe and is seen in gradually lessening degrees in the second, third, and fourth rays, and is almost absent in the fifth.

The transverse arch controls the splay of the forefoot. The stability of the transverse arch is mainly provided by the intercuneiform and intermetatarsal ligaments and the peroneus longus tendon.[5] The five longitudinal processes of the deeper layer of the plantar fascia form a longitudinal arch system. They are inserted into the whole of the transverse arch and are strong.

Although static stabilization of the MTP joint is primarily the function of the plantar plate, dynamic stabilization is provided by the extrinsic and intrinsic musculature of the foot. The ability of the intrinsic and extrinsic foot musculature to stabilize this joint depends largely on the integrity of the plantar plate.[6]

Factors such as hallux valgus deformity, a long second ray, or hypermobile joints all overload the lesser metatarsals leading to synovitis and eventual stretching and rupture of the plantar plate.[7] Acute trauma or chronic microtrauma can cause disruption of the plantar plate.[8] Plantar plate degeneration and rupture is often seen with use of high-heeled shoes and a narrow toe box, but may also occur in athletes. A developmentally short first ray and long second ray predisposes to MTP joint instability and increases stress on the second plantar plate.[7]

### Clinical Examination

Patients may complain that the affected toe "feels as though it is trying to go out of position." They may report that the toe position has changed or that they now walk differently. These are symptoms of MTP joint instability. Excruciating pain on palpation just distal and plantar to the metatarsal head that is disproportionate to any other objective clinical finding is suggestive of intermetatarsal bursitis or acute degeneration of the plantar plate.[6] Generally, patients presenting with pain caused by plantar plate degeneration do not complain of numbness or shooting pains but report focal pain overlying the MTP joint rather than the interspace.

On physical examination, loss of toe purchase with or without medial or lateral deviation may be noted. A submetatarsal callus or a corn over the proximal interphalangeal joint may be seen. Swelling or redness as a result of local edema and warmth may be present. Plantar edema tends to be obvious and can encompass the entire MTP joint area.[6]

Subluxation of the MTP joint may vary from minor to severe. The deformity may be flexible or fixed, depending on the cause. The physical sign is a positive draw test of the MTP joint that reproduces the pain of the patient's complaint.[6] A positive draw test result is present when the proximal phalanx can be translocated 2 mm dorsally above the metatarsal head.

### Imaging

Conventional radiography is important in the assessment of MTP joint instability. Underlying local or systemic pathologies must be excluded. Radiographs are helpful for evaluation of arthropathy, fracture, inflammation, and infection.[9] Shortening, displacement, angulation, rotation, or ablation of a metatarsal thrusts a greater weight-bearing load onto the remaining metatarsal heads. A small displacement of 1 to 3 mm may be sufficient to cause symptoms.[10]

On PD imaging, the normal plantar plate appears as a smooth, low-signal structure abutting the plantar aspect of the metatarsal head, attaching at the proximal phalangeal base adjacent to the joint surface. The plantar plate is difficult to distinguish from the thicker, overlying flexor tendons (**Fig. 1**).[11] High-resolution images may demonstrate a barely visible cleavage plane between the plate and the flexor tendons, more readily seen on coronal short axis images.[3] On gradient-echo (GRE) scans, the plantar plate is slightly higher in signal intensity than the adjacent flexor tendons and thus more easily distinguished from them.[11] Sagittal GRE images demonstrate a narrow zone of high signal intensity hyaline cartilage at the articular surface of the proximal phalanx, with a low signal fibrocartilage of the plantar plate at its distal insertion. This high signal intensity zone is more prominent centrally at the base of the proximal phalanx but should not measure greater than 2.5 mm long. It can appear thinner at the far medial and lateral margins, where the proper collateral ligament blends with the plate to insert directly into bone in a juxta-articular location. Bright signal hyaline cartilage can be distinguished from a tear of the plate by its location adjacent the bone and its focal appearance. Intact collateral ligaments can be demonstrated in the oblique sagittal plane.

Coronal short axis images demonstrate the plantar plate as a thick low signal band centered subjacent to the lesser metatarsal heads, with a shallow groove along its plantar surface housing the flexor tendon sheath. It is thinnest centrally and relatively thick distally, in symmetric fashion, medially to laterally. Proximal to the MTP joint, the accessory collateral ligament is seen as vertically oriented low signal bands to either side of the metatarsal head, which thicken slightly near their attachment to the plantar plate. At the base of the proximal phalanx, the plantar plate and phalangeal collateral ligament attachments appear to blend as a low signal condensation to each side of the flexor tendon. The high signal intensity zone of the hyaline cartilage is not seen in the coronal plane.[3]

Axial images of the forefoot, using T2 fat-suppressed sequences, permit evaluation of marrow signal and can demonstrate hallux valgus and a long second ray, which commonly coexist with and predispose to degeneration and injury of the plantar plate.[3]

On MR imaging, plantar plate tear typically appears as discontinuity and associated increased signal intensity at the plantar plate attachment onto the proximal phalangeal base. The area of plate derangement is isointense with synovium and joint fluid. With degeneration or rupture, the high signal intensity zone at the distal insertion of the plantar plate becomes longer and indistinct (**Figs. 2–4**). As the plantar plate, capsular, and ligamentous structures become insufficient, there is progressive hyperextension of the toe at the MTP joint. Coronal short axis images optimally demonstrate either degenerative thickening or thinning and intrasubstance signal distortion of the plantar plate or collateral ligaments (see **Fig. 3**A, B).[3]

Sonographically, the plantar plate is characterized in the longitudinal plane by a slightly hyperechoic band, with a grainy but homogeneous appearance curving over the metatarsal head to insert into the proximal phalanx (**Fig. 5**A). In the transverse plane, the plantar plate similarly appears as a curved structure overlying the metatarsal head. The short axis view is more heterogeneous because of the undulating nature of the plantar plate, with bundles of echogenic foci (see

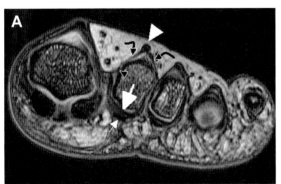
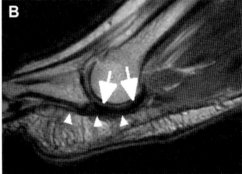

**Fig. 1.** Normal plantar plate anatomy. (*A*) Coronal proton density image of normal plantar plates (*large arrow*) with closely abutting flexor tendons (*small arrow*). Extensor hood (*curved arrows*), extensor digitorum longus (*large arrowhead*), collateral ligaments (*black arrowhead*). (*B*) Sagittal proton density image of the normal plantar plate (*arrows*). Flexor tendon (*arrowheads*).

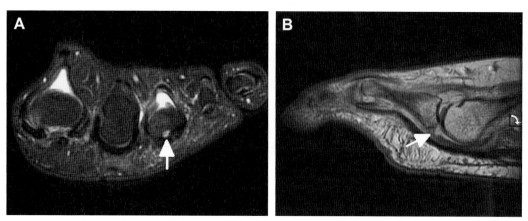

**Fig. 2.** (*A*) Coronal image of a clearly defined central plantar plate tear with focal high signal intensity (*arrow*) and an associated effusion. (*B*) Sagittal image of a full thickness tear (*arrow*).

**Fig. 5**B).[1] This appearance is consistent with histologic reports of the plantar plate collagen bundles appearing interwoven with longitudinally oriented sheets. The distal insertion has multiple interdigitations, longest centrally, shallower dorsally and plantarly.[12] There is a clearly defined margin between the hypoechoic articular cartilage from the hyperechoic fibers of the plantar plate.

Using sonography a tear appears as plantar plate discontinuity and a loss of the normal homogenous, hyperechoic appearance (**Fig. 6**). Most tears occur at the distal insertion onto the

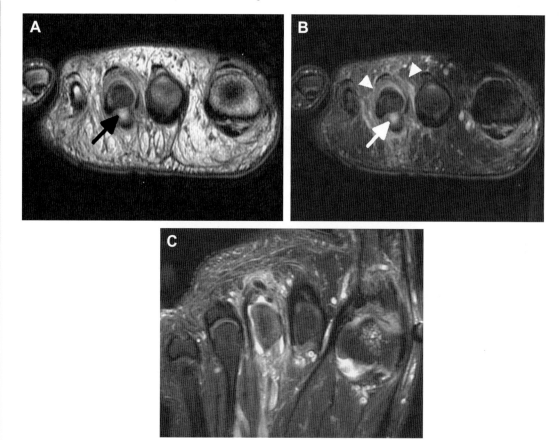

**Fig. 3.** Inflammatory plantar plate tear (*arrow*) with surrounding edema (*arrowheads*). The plantar plate is thickened and the high signal intensity tear is ill defined. (*A*) Proton density coronal, (*B*) T2 fat-suppressed coronal, (*C*) T2 axial.

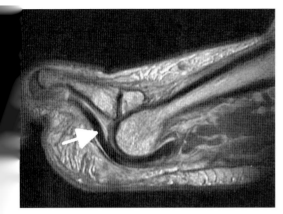

Fig. 4. Dislocated metatarsophalangeal joint. Sagittal proton density image of ruptured capsule and plantar plate.

proximal phalanx. Acute changes include plantar plate thickening, heterogeneity, and hyperemia (see **Fig. 6**B, F).[1] Fibrosis of soft tissues superficial to an abnormal plantar plate can also occur. In the presence of a full-thickness tear of the plantar plate, the flexor tendon may sublux, depending on the location of the tear (see **Fig. 6**E). Osteophyte formation has been reported in the region of derangement in chronic cases of plantar plate disruption (see **Fig. 6**G).[1] Plantar plate tears involve the replacement of normal hyperechoic fibrocartilage with focal hypoechoic defects. These tissues include fat cells, hydropic tubules (watery fluid), blood vessels, loose cellular tissue, and dense irregular tissue (**Fig. 7**A).[12] Direct inspection of plantar plate disruption shows fraying and swelling of fibrocartilage (see **Fig. 7**B).

## Treatment

Initially conservative treatments involve shoe gear modification, including an extra-deep shoe and a toe box with a soft upper portion. Padding and protection of specific callosities or pressure points may be required, which can be combined with taping and strapping of flexible deformities.[13] Painful pressure under the metatarsal heads may be relieved with the use of metatarsal pads or bars.

If symptoms are refractory to conservative therapy surgery is indicated. The general aim is to restore the normal biomechanics of the foot by returning the MTP joint into a neutral position. Tendon transfers, primary plantar plate repair, or combined osseous and soft tissue procedures may be used.[7]

## BONES
### Anatomy

The forefoot includes the five metatarsals, sesamoid bones, and phalanges. The joint between the midfoot and forefoot, the tarsometatarsal joint (Lisfranc joint), is multicompartmental, with variable joint spaces. Multiple sesamoid bones are present in the foot, embedded, partially or totally, in the substance of a corresponding tendon. Sesamoids may be located within the plantar plates of the MTP joints.[14]

### Stress Fractures/Injury

#### History
A stress fracture is an overuse injury. The most common cause of fatigue-type stress fracture is an abrupt increase in the duration, intensity, or frequency of physical activity without adequate periods of rest. Systemic factors, such as hormonal imbalances, nutritional deficiencies, sleep deprivation, and metabolic bone disorders, may contribute to insufficiency-type stress fractures. Stress fractures may be partial or complete.[15] The second metatarsal bone is more prone to

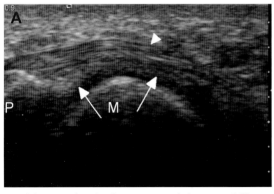

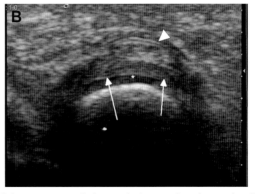

Fig. 5. (A) Normal sagittal sonogram of the central fibers of the metatarsophalangeal plantar plate (*arrows*) as it attaches to the proximal phalanx. Flexor tendon (*arrowhead*). M, metatarsal head; P, proximal phalanx. (B) Transverse sonogram of the normal plantar plate (*arrows*). Articular cartilage (*asterisk*), flexor tendon/sheath (*arrowhead*).

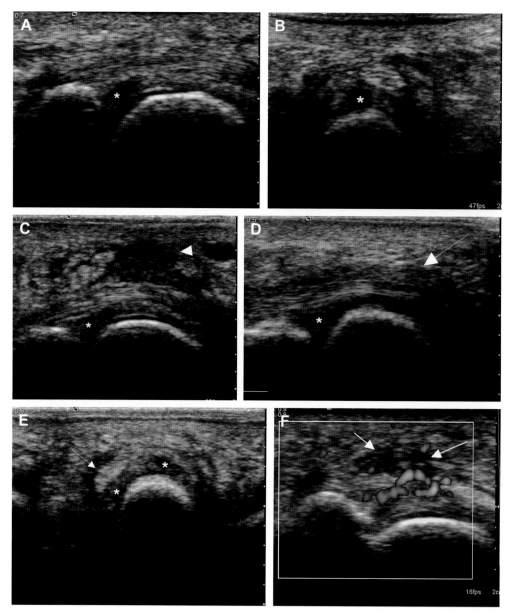

**Fig. 6.** (*A*) Sagittal sonogram of a large partial tear in the plantar plate (*asterisk*). (*B*) Transverse sonogram of a central tear in the plantar plate (*asterisk*). (*C*) Longitudinal image demonstrating moderate adventitial bursitis (*arrowhead*) at the level of the second metatarsophalangeal joint and a full-thickness tear in the plantar plate (*asterisk*). (*D*) Longitudinal sonogram of the fourth metatarsophalangeal joint demonstrating plantar plate rupture (*asterisk*) and associated flexor tenosynovitis. (*E*) Transverse image of plantar plate rupture (*asterisk*), flexor tendon lateral subluxation (*arrow*), and tenosynovitis. (*F*) Hypervascularity of an acute tear of the plantar plate with overlying adventitial bursitis. (*G*) Longitudinal sonogram of the lateral fibers of the second plantar plate with osteophytic change (*arrow*).

stress fracture than the others because of its rigid location where it is countersunk into the cuneiforms at the tarsometatarsal joint.

### Clinical examination

The patient usually complains of pain that is localized to the area of the fracture. On physical examination there is often swelling and warmth over the affected area. Stress of the area causes discomfort.

### Imaging

Initial radiographs may be negative, but subsequent films usually demonstrate abundant callus formation in the area of the stress fracture.[16]

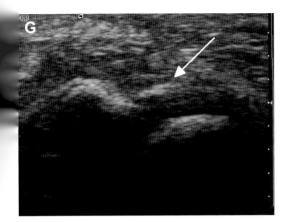

Fig. 6. (*continued*)

MR imaging shows stress fractures as very low signal intensity linear lesions on T1 images, representing the fracture line, surrounded by bone marrow edema, which is low signal on T1 weighting and bright on T2 weighting or short TI inversion recovery images (**Figs. 8, 9**). There may be parosteal soft tissue edema or a small sympathetic effusion in a neighboring joint. Periosteal reaction, if present, appears as a low signal stripe paralleling the cortical bone, occasionally separated from it by high signal edema on fluid-sensitive sequences.[17,18]

Stress fractures can be seen on ultrasound commonly at the metatarsal heads. Ultrasound features include: periosteal reaction appearing as a hyperechoic band along the cortex; periosteal hemorrhage, in which the hyperechoic periosteum is elevated from the cortex by a hypoechoic band; and cortical interruption (see **Fig. 8**C, D).[19] Color Doppler imaging shows perilesional increased flow (see **Fig. 8**D). Local pressure with the transducer is painful and partially reproduces the patient's pain.[20]

### Treatment

Treatment focuses on self-care measures, including rest, ice, and analgesics. Treatment requires off-loading the affected bone. A short-leg walking cast or CAM walker may be used. Fractures at the base of the fifth metatarsal are at risk for nonunion and may require surgical fixation.

## Freiberg Infarction

### History

Freiberg infarction is a disorder affecting the metatarsal head (usually the second or third metatarsal head) characterized by an overload of the subchondral bone plate leading to bone edema, ischemia, and subchondral collapse. There is variable chondral degeneration and osteophyte formation. The cause of Freiberg infarction is not fully understood. Acute or repetitive injury with vascular compromise and subchondral insufficiency is most likely. Freiberg infarction is more common in women and most commonly manifests during adolescence.

### Clinical examination

This condition may mimic synovitis or MTP joint instability. Affected individuals report slowly progressive discomfort in the region of the MTP joint (usually the second) over many years. Physical examination reveals restricted motion.[16]

### Imaging

Early radiographs may be normal. As the subchondral plate collapses, radiographs may demonstrate articular flattening, subarticular sclerosis, and secondary degenerative change, with proliferative bone formation about the involved metatarsal head.[16] Early MR findings include low signal intensity changes in the metatarsal head on T1-weighted images with increased signal intensity

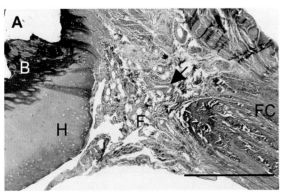

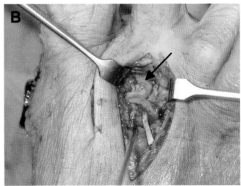

Fig. 7. (*A*) Sagittal histology section demonstrating plantar plate disruption. Normal fibrocartilage (FC) of the plantar plate is replaced with fat cells (F), vessels (*arrow*), disorganized fibrocartilage. This disruption has occurred immediately proximal to the enthesis. B, bone. (Masson trichrome stain, bar = 100 μm). (*B*) Dorsal surgical photograph demonstrates a ruptured plantar plate (*arrow*).

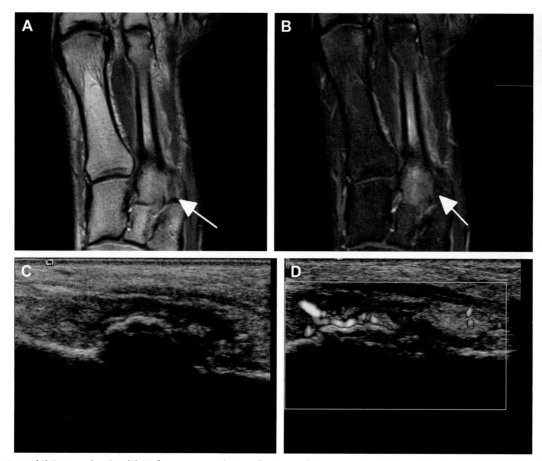

Fig. 8. (*A*) Proton density, (*B*) T2 fat-suppressed stress fracture of the second metatarsal (*arrows*) (*C*) Sonogram of the dorsal aspect of a second metatarsal shaft shows a repairing stress fracture. (*D*) Longitudinal sonogram of the dorsum of the fourth metatarsal base shows a stress fracture with hypervascularity.

on T2-weighted images (**Fig. 10**A, B). A T2 hyperintense stripe usually parallels the subchondral plate at the site of subchondral collapse. The overlying cartilage maybe breached. There is usually a joint effusion. In latter stages, secondary osteoarthritis develops. There may in fact be overlap between these conditions. With disease progression, flattening of the metatarsal head occurs, and low signal intensity changes develop on T2-weighted images as the bone becomes sclerotic (see **Fig. 10**C, D).[17]

### Treatment

In the acute phase, this condition is best treated with a rest, immobilization, and analgesia. An intra-articular injection of corticosteroid may provide some relief. In chronic cases a surgical approach may be indicated. The joint is decompressed with synovectomy and débridement of bone fragments and osteophytes. A shortening osteotomy may be indicated.

## JOINTS
### Anatomy

The lesser MTP joints, second to fifth, are formed by the round metatarsal head that articulates with the concave articular surface of the proximal phalanx. The connections between these bones are the fibrous capsule, the plantar plate, and the intracapsular collateral ligaments.[21] The capsule attaches dorsally just proximal to the dorsal edge of the articular surface of the metatarsal head and extends distally to attach to the base of the proximal phalanx. The capsule itself is thin dorsally. The extensor expansion, however, reinforces the capsule of the MTP joint as the fibers composing the extensor sling are arranged in a transverse manner and encircle the capsule. Plantarly, the joint capsule and extensor expansion blend with the plantar plate and the deep transverse intermetatarsal ligament.[22] The surface of the articulating bones is covered with hyaline cartilage except for a small region at the insertion of the joint

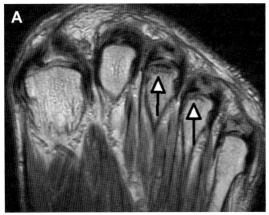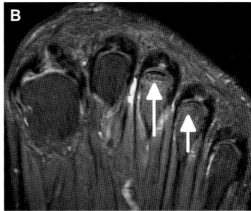

Fig. 9. Subchondral insufficiency fractures of third and fourth metatarsal heads with adjacent plantar plate tears. (A) Proton density, (B) T2 fat-suppressed.

capsule, between the insertion of the fibrous capsule and the hyaline cartilage; here the bone is covered by synovium only and is referred to as the bare area dorsally. On the plantar surface this bare area has been reported to be visible 47% of the time and is referred to as the plantar plate recess.[21] Owing to direct contact with the synovial tissue, without any protecting layer of cartilage, the bone surface in this location is susceptible to synovitis-induced bone destruction.[23]

The periosteum is continuous with the fibrous outer layer of the capsule. The internal synovial layer is arranged in folds and is covered by cells derived from bone marrow and mesenchymal origin. The two layers frequently are separated by fat. The subsynovial tissue is rich in vessels. Synovial fluid is a dialysate of plasma and acts as a lubricant and nutrient.[23]

## Synovitis

### History
Synovitis connotes inflammation of a synovial (joint-lining) membrane. Primary synovitis is characterized by thickening of the synovium, which has become more cellular and engorged with fluid. Synovitis is a major problem in rheumatoid arthritis, juvenile arthritis, lupus, and psoriatic arthritis. Secondary synovitis may occur as a result of rheumatic fever, tuberculosis, trauma (including instability), or gout. Commonly presenting as an effusion, secondary synovitis has an abnormal fluid buildup in a joint that develops in response to synovial inflammation, trauma, anasarca, intra-articular hemorrhage (hemarthrosis), or an adjacent focus of acute inflammation (sympathetic effusion).[24] Most effusions occur as a result of bruising within a joint from acute trauma or

overuse of the joint. Effusions serve to separate, nourish, and lubricate bruised cartilage.[25]

### Clinical examination
Patients note a gradual thickening in the area of the involved joint. They may report feeling as if they are walking on a lump in their shoe. Physical examination reveals generalized thickening and warmth about the involved joint. Synovitis is usually related to overload of the metatarsal as a result of a structural problem, such as a bunion or excessively long metatarsal. Firm palpation of the inflamed synovial tissue causes the patient some degree of discomfort.[16] In an individual who has chronic inflammatory arthritis, the synovial membrane has a doughy or boggy consistency, a feature best appreciated at the joint line or margin.[24]

### Imaging
Conventional radiographs often show hypertrophy of the affected metatarsal shaft from the overload causing the problem.

### Primary synovitis
Proliferative synovitis (pannus) is responsible for bone and cartilage damage in rheumatoid arthritis.[26] It appears as low to intermediate signal on PD sequences. Signal intensity may vary on T2-weighted images. High signal intensity indicates hypervascular pannus. With disease chronicity, fibrous pannus develops and hemosiderin deposition may occur, demonstrating low signal intensity on all imaging sequences.[17]

Ultrasound permits the distinction between joint effusion and synovial proliferation. This distinction is possible because of the difference between the anechoic pattern of fluid collection and the soft echogenicity of synovial proliferation that can

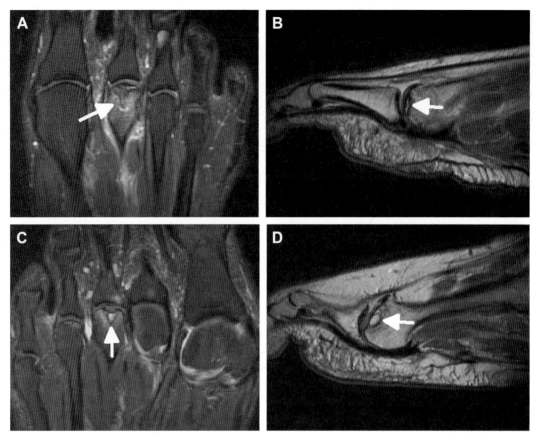

**Fig. 10.** Freiberg disease. (*A*) T2 image shows extensive bone marrow edema and subchondral impaction (*arrow*) and effusion suggesting more acute changes. (*B*) Proton density images show subchondral fracture with impaction of cortex and subchondral bone plate (*arrow*). (*C*) Axial, (*D*) sagittal images of late-stage Freiberg disease with secondary osteoarthritis and subchondral cyst (*arrow*). Collapsed subchondral bone with a low-grade stress response.

appear as a homogeneous thickening of the synovial layer or as irregularly shaped clusters of echoes (bushy and villous appearance) (**Fig. 11A**). Active synovitis is characterized by a marked increase of joint perfusion that can be depicted using power Doppler.[27] When synovitis is present within the joint effusion the synovial lining is thickened. Bone erosions may be present and appear on MR images as sharply marginated areas of trabecular bone loss with a cortical defect. Erosions may be more conspicuous after contrast injection, and appreciated with thin-partition PD sequences.[26] On sonography, bone erosions are observed as loss of sharpness of the outer margins, loss of clarity of the cartilaginous layer, cartilage thinning, and subchondral bone profile irregularities.[19,28] Bone erosions should be visible in two orthogonal planes.[26] Joint cavity widening is the most characteristic feature of acute and chronic synovitis.

### Secondary synovitis

A joint effusion appears on MR imaging as high signal intensity around the affected joint on T2-weighted images, which reflects the presence of fluid or inflammation (see **Fig. 2A**).[29,30] There should be little in the way of contrast enhancement on fat-suppressed T1-weighted sequences.[31]

Sonographically, bone profile and cartilage are the main landmarks when assessing joints, whereas the joint capsule can only be indirectly defined by following the profile of the joint cavity. The bone profile appears as a sharp hyperechoic line and the articular cartilage has a subtle anechoic band with sharp chondrosynovial and osteochondral margins.[32] Joint effusions have a hypoechoic content and increase the distance between the joint capsule and the bone (joint space) (see **Fig. 11B**). The joint effusion is compressible and shows no evidence of flow on Doppler imaging.[26]

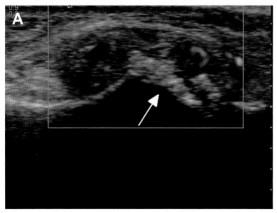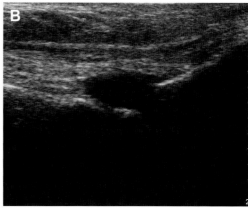

Fig. 11. Synovitis. (A) Longitudinal sonogram of synovial proliferation, bony irregularity (arrow), hyperemia, and mild effusion. (B) Longitudinal sonogram of a moderate effusion and dorsal subluxation of the proximal phalanx.

## Treatment

Primary synovitis is initially treated with nonsteroidal anti-inflammatory medication, whereas secondary synovitis is treated with nonsteroidal anti-inflammatory medication and shoe gear modifications. Wide soft shoes with metatarsal support may improve symptoms, as might insertion of a full-length steel stiffening plate into a sole with an anterior rockerbottom, which immobilizes the forefoot and all MTP joints. If these measures are unsuccessful, an intra-articular corticosteroid injection combined with a steel sole stiffener often helps.[13] Those who have refractory symptoms may progress to surgical synovectomy. The collateral ligaments and extensor digitorum longus tendon may also be divided to provide decompression and reduction of the MTP joint.[13] A metatarsal osteotomy may be performed to unload the distal MTP joint. End-stage joint destruction may require arthroplasty.

## TENDINOPATHY

### Anatomy

Tibialis anterior, extensor hallucis longus, extensor digitorum longus, and peroneus tertius are the muscles of the anterior lower leg that attach to the dorsal aspect of the foot. The four tendons of the extensor digitorum longus lie superficial to the extensor digitorum brevis muscles and tendons. These tendons divide into two lateral slips that insert into the distal phalanx and a central slip that inserts to the middle phalanx. The peroneus tertius tendon inserts into the dorsal surface of the fifth metatarsal. The extensor hallucis longus tendon attaches to the base of the proximal phalanx of the hallux. The tibialis anterior tendon attaches to the medial cuneiform and first metatarsal.[18]

The extensor digitorum brevis and extensor hallucis brevis muscles are intrinsic muscles on the dorsal aspect of the foot. The extensor digitorum muscle belly arises from the calcaneus, with the extensor hallucis brevis muscle lying just medial to it.

The plantar aspect of the foot can be divided into medial, intermediate, and lateral compartments. The medial compartment of the plantar aspect of the foot contains the abductor hallucis muscle, the flexor hallucis brevis muscle, the tendon of the flexor hallucis longus, and the insertions of the posterior tibial tendon and peroneus longus tendon. The flexor hallucis brevis muscle divides into medial and lateral heads, the twin tendons of which are attached to the sides of the base of the proximal phalanx of the hallux. A sesamoid bone usually occurs in each tendon near its attachment. The abductor hallucis attaches with the medial tendon of flexor hallucis brevis to the medial base of the first proximal phalanx. The flexor hallucis longus tendon passes between the two hallucal sesamoids to insert onto the base of the proximal phalanx. Throughout its length it is invested in a synovial sheath.[5]

The intermediate compartment lies deep to the plantar fascia and contains the flexor digitorum brevis muscles, the quadratus plantae muscle, the adductor hallucis muscle, the four lumbrical muscles, and the tendons of the flexor digitorum longus. The tendon of flexor digitorum longus passes forward as four separate tendons, deep to the flexor digitorum brevis, through the fibrous sheaths of the lateral four toes. The adductor hallucis arises by oblique and transverse heads. The medial part of the oblique muscle attaches to the fibular hallucal. The lateral part joins the transverse head and attaches to the fibular sesamoid and directly to the base of the first proximal phalanx.[5]

Deeper, this compartment contains the dorsal and plantar interosseous muscles alongside the metatarsal. The lateral compartment for the fifth digit contains the abductor digiti minimi and flexor digiti minimi muscles.[18]

## Pathology

Chronic trauma and degeneration within a tendon leads to mucoid degeneration, referred to as tendinosis or tendinopathy.[27] Tenosynovitis is inflammation of the tendon sheath and may be caused by synovial inflammatory disease or infection (primary), or mechanical irritation (secondary). Mechanical causes include overuse or plantar plate dysfunction. Acute tenosynovitis is characterized by fluid accumulating in the sheath. Chronic inflammation leads to fibrosis and tendon entrapment.[17]

## Clinical Examination

Tenosynovitis often presents with forefoot tenderness or pain.[33] Palpation of the MTP joint using the pinch test, in which the examining thumb and index finger compress the plantar soft tissues anterior overlying the proximal phalanx, is useful in the diagnosis of tenosynovitis. In the normal case the soft tissue is loose but in the case of tenosynovitis the soft tissue is swollen.[33] Symptoms may be exacerbated by toe flexion with pain fluctuating with altered ankle position.

## Imaging

Tendinosis manifests on MR imaging as fusiform or diffuse tendon thickening and increased intrasubstance signal intensity on PD and T2-weighted images. Bright intrasubstance T2 signal is seen in the context of tendon degeneration.[17] Tenosynovitis is depicted by fluid signal distention of the tendon sheath, and pathologic enhancement of the tendon sheath following intravenous contrast. Stenosing tenosynovitis causes an irregular contour to the tendon sheath. As fibrosis develops within the sheath strands of tissue may be seen extending from the sheath to the tendon. As the pathology progresses the fluid signal in the sheath is replaced by thickened scar giving a lobulated appearance.

On sonography, tendon sheath widening, loss of the normal fibrillar echotexture, and loss of definition of tendon margins are the abnormalities that characterize acute and chronic tendinosis and tenosynovitis (see **Fig. 6**D, E).[32] Transverse scans of tendons in the case of tenosynovitis reveals a synovial sheath filled with fluid, appearing as an hypoechoic or anechoic zone around the tendon. The tendon is often thickened and the contour

may be altered.[33,34] Tendon sheath widening ca... be minimal whereas in others it has an aneu... rysm-like aspect.[27] Chronic inflammatory tenosyn... ovitis may be difficult to differentiate from acut... tenosynovitis but is generally thicker and more complex. Although more commonly affecting the great toe, metatarsalgia and stenosing tenosynovitis of the lesser toes has been reported. Triggering may be elicited with plantar flexion of the toes whereas passive extension may cause pain and a palpable snap along the plantar surface of the metatarsal head.[35]

## Treatment

Avoiding shoes that cause pain may be sufficient. If symptoms persist, shoes with a thick sole and orthotics are prescribed to reduce pressure at the painful site. Local infiltration of a corticosteroid/anesthetic solution helps reduce symptoms.

## INTERMETATARSAL BURSITIS/FIBROSIS
## Anatomy

The intermetatarsal bursae lie between the MTP joints and are located dorsal to the deep transverse intermetatarsal ligament. The bursae in the web spaces between the second and third, and third and fourth digits extend about 1 cm distal to this ligament, but there is no extension of the bursa in the lateral space first and fourth web spaces.

The neurovascular bundle lies beneath the deep transverse intermetatarsal ligament, although distally it veers dorsally, passing around its distal free edge, in close proximity to the bursa.[36] In the plantar aspect of the foot, the posterior tibial vessels and nerves divide into the lateral and medial plantar vessels and nerves, which then run in the medial and central compartments of the foot, respectively.[18]

In its course, the medial branch gives off cutaneous branches that pierce the plantar fascia and supply fine integument and muscles of the sole of the foot, the articulations of the tarsus and metatarsus, and four digital branches. The first of the digital branches supplies the medial border of the great toe, the second bifurcates to supply the adjacent sides of the hallux and second toes, the third digital branch supplies the adjacent sides of the second and third toes, and the fourth supplies the corresponding sides of the third and fourth toes and also receives a communicating branch from the lateral plantar nerve. Each digital nerve gives off cutaneous and articular filaments.

The lateral plantar nerve passes obliquely forward with the lateral plantar artery to the outer side of the foot, dividing into a superficial and deep branch. The superficial branch separates into two digital nerves: one supplies the outer side of the little toe, the other digital branch supplies the adjoining sides of the fourth and fifth toes and communicates with the medial plantar nerve.[5] The first and second lumbrical muscles are innervated by the medial plantar nerve, but the other lumbricals are supplied by the lateral plantar nerve. The lateral plantar nerve innervates the seven interossei and the other small muscles of the foot.[37] These plantar nerves provide a sensory function to the skin of the sole of the foot and foot joints. The plantar nerves provide motor function to the flexor digitorum longus and flexor hallucis longus and to the intrinsic muscles of the foot.

In the dorsal aspect of the foot, the main neurovascular bundle is the dorsalis pedis vessels and deep peroneal nerve, which lie deep to the extensor hallucis longus tendon.[18]

### Pathology

Morton neuromas (also known as interdigital neuromas) are a common cause of ill-defined forefoot pain, most commonly occurring in the second or third interspace between the metatarsal heads, rarely in the first or fourth.[38] Mechanically induced microdamage to the interdigital nerve over a long period of time produces nerve fiber degeneration and excessive intraneural and juxtaneural reparative fibrosis resulting in significant nerve enlargement; this renders the nerve prone to further microtrauma, and thus increasingly symptomatic.[39] In our experience there is a transition from intermetatarsal bursitis to intermetatarsal fibrosis with both entities often coexisting at presentation. Similar to the natural progression from acute to chronic inflammation, there is also progression from bursitis to fibrosis with continued microtrauma. The cause of the insult is controversial; however, instability is a likely contributor. Plantar plate dysfunction leads to MTP joint instability, causing irritation of the intermetatarsal space resulting in acute and chronic inflammation. Excessive weightbearing stress of the forefoot, commonly occurring in women who wear pointed and high-heeled shoes or those who are overweight, predisposes to this condition.

### Clinical Examination

Clinically, the pain of a Morton neuroma can radiate to the two distal involved toes. Pain is often aggravated by tight or high-heeled shoes. The patient can usually point to the specific area of pain. To test for a Morton neuroma a web space compression test can be performed. The metatarsal heads are squeezed together with one hand while simultaneously axially compressing the involved web space beneath the toes with the opposite hand. If a Morton neuroma is present, the web space compression test produces severe pain and often produces a palpable click (Mulder click).

Patients who have bursitis have pain and experience pronounced tenderness at the affected web space. It may mimic Morton neuroma and, in some cases, the bursa becomes entangled around the nerve making the two conditions indistinguishable. The bursa enlarges in a complex manner with fronds of tissue expanding to fill the interspace, potentially enveloping the nerve. Pain may be felt with motion and while at rest. Joint movement may be restricted because of the pain.[40] Pain may be localized to the foot or radiate to the toes.

### Imaging

A Morton neuroma represents perineural fibrosis, which commonly occurs proximal to the metatarsal heads.[41] The perineural mass is usually oriented parallel to the long axis of the metatarsals, deep to the interosseous muscles and distal to the intermetatarsal ligament.[42,43] It appears as a small hypointense mass lesion which is either isointense or slightly hyperintense to skeletal muscle on T1-weighted images and intermediate signal lesion on T2-weighted scans because of the abundant fibrous tissue (**Fig. 12**A, B).[18] Intravenous contrast is not helpful for diagnosis because Morton neuromas show variable enhancement depending on their maturity and associated inflammation.

Morton neuromas have a variable sonographic appearance. A neuroma appears as an ovoid, lobulated, elongated or round hypoechoic mass, with or without a small amount of hyperechoic material (enveloped fat) contained within it (**Fig. 13**A–D). The characteristics of lesions on ultrasound change with time: younger lesions appear hypoechoic and older lesions appear hyperechoic.[44] We found many neuromas to be rounded lesions that were noncompressible; others were elongated along the linear course of the nerve, some with lobulations. The digital nerve may be identified extending to the lesion.[45] The most common location is the third web space, followed by the second web space. Typically, any abnormal web space mass measuring equal to or greater than 3 mm in dorsoplantar thickness (which replaces, displaces, or obscures the neurovascular bundle) is diagnostic of a Morton neuroma.[46,47]

Intermetatarsal bursitis appears as a well-defined fluid collection and demonstrates low

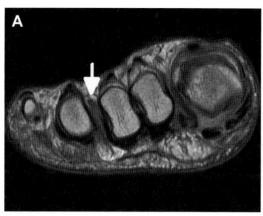
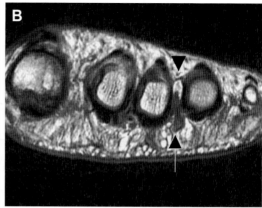

Fig. 12. Intermetatarsal fibrosis. (*A*) Coronal image of intermetatarsal fibrosis (*arrow*). (*B*) Coronal image of third web space intermetatarsal bursitis (*arrowhead*) and fibrosis (*arrow*). Fibrous tissue prolapses to the plantar side of the web space.

signal intensity on T1-weighted images and high signal intensity on T2-weighted images (see **Fig. 12B**). Peripheral enhancement is seen following intravenous administration of contrast, although contrast is not necessary to establish the diagnosis. Small fluid collections with a transverse diameter of 3 mm or less in the first three intermetatarsal bursae may be physiologic.[17]

On sonography, the normal intermetatarsal region contains echogenic areas. Intermetatarsal bursitis is typically depicted as hypoechoic or anechoic zones. These zones may vary from small to large collections, bulging more than 1 mm under the metatarsal head level (see **Fig. 13B, D**).[41] Atypical bursae may be complex with variable compressibility. Significant hyperemia is often seen on Doppler interrogation.[26]

### Treatment

Nonsurgical treatment requires reduction of activity, wearing of a wide shoe with a less constricting toe box, the administration of nonsteroidal anti-inflammatory drugs, and redistribution of weight-bearing with a metatarsal pad placed just proximal to the symptomatic neuroma. Occasionally an injection of corticosteroid in the involved web space relieves symptoms. The use of alcohol ablation in the treatment of Morton neuroma has had promising results.[47] This technique involves injecting ethanol around the nerve, which produces chemical neurolysis through dehydration, necrosis, and precipitation of protoplasm. If conservative treatment fails, surgical excision may be considered (**Fig. 14E, F**).

Intermetatarsal bursitis is similarly treated with wider shoes, a rocker bar (a device added to the soles of the shoes to decrease pressure on the

metatarsals), and local infiltration with a corticosteroid/anesthetic solution. There is occasionally a case for surgical excision, particularly if related to a neuroma.

## ADVENTITIAL BURSITIS
### Anatomy

The aponeurotic fibers of the ball of the foot are arranged in longitudinal, transverse, and vertical bands and tracts. Together with fat bodies encapsulated between the bands and tracts, they form a matrix that ties the skin to the skeleton, allowing longitudinal passage for vessels, nerves, and tendons.[48] The metatarsal fat pad is thick in the region of the MTP joints, which cushions the foot during the toe-off phase of gait.[5]

### Pathology

We are born with multiple bursae to ease friction, especially where tendons lie next to hard surfaces. Adventitial bursae are acquired bursae that form as recurrent stress breaks down the matrix of supporting tissue leading to focal fluid collections. Adventitial submetatarsal bursae develop as a result of excessive friction between soft tissue and underlying bone protuberances of the metatarsal heads. They are not true synovial-lined potential spaces, as are congenital bursae, and are not associated with synovial inflammatory disease.[49]

### Clinical Examination

The fat pad may be warm, with point tenderness and a palpable mass. With chronic inflammation of an adventitial bursa, submetatarsal plantar fibrosis may ensue.

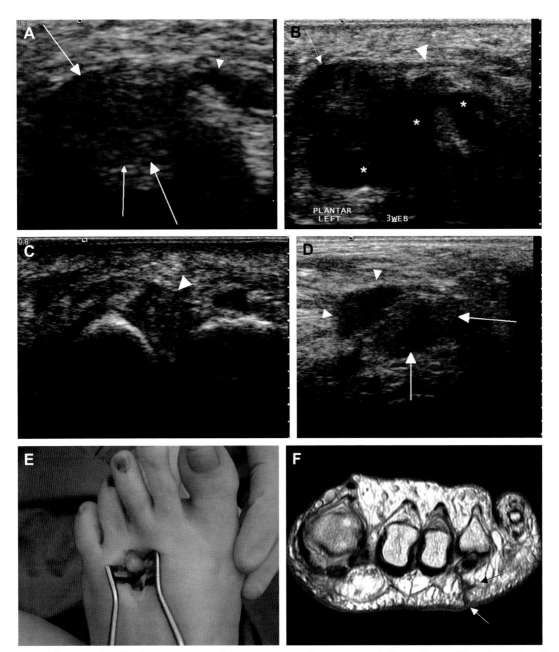

Fig. 13. (A) Plantar longitudinal sonogram of intermetatarsal fibrosis (*arrows*). Normal nerve fibers (*arrowhead*). (B) Plantar sonogram shows intermetatarsal fibrosis (*arrow*) and marked intermetatarsal bursitis (*asterisk*). Normal nerve fibers are seen proximally (*arrowhead*). (C) Transverse sonogram of the plantar aspect of the third web space shows intermetatarsal fibrosis protruding from between the metatarsal heads (*arrowhead*). (D) Dorsal longitudinal sonogram in the third web space shows a superficial intermetatarsal bursitis (*arrowheads*), and deeper intermetatarsal fibrosis (*arrows*). (D) Surgical photograph demonstrating the dorsal excision of a Morton neuroma. (E) A linear scar following surgical resection of third web space intermetatarsal fibrosis/Morton neuroma (*white arrowhead*) is visible (no recurrence of fibrosis).

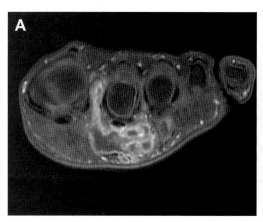
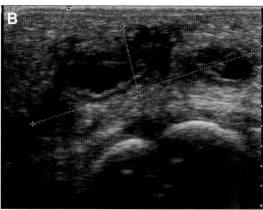

Fig. 14. Adventitial bursitis. (A) Clinically proven adventitial bursitis. Coronal T1 fat-suppressed scans following contrast shows a large cystic lesion with enhancing walls prolapsing from first web space to plantar tissues. (B) A 22-year-old who had rheumatoid arthritis. Longitudinal sonogram of fifth metatarsophalangeal joint shows severe adventitial bursitis.

## Imaging

Submetatarsal bursitis appears as a well-defined fluid collection and demonstrates low signal intensity on PD images and high signal intensity on T2-weighted images (see **Fig. 14A**). Ill-defined signal alterations in the fat pad are common and less likely to be symptomatic than well-defined bursae.[50] Bursae are sometimes continuous from the flexor tendon to the skin or contiguous with the flexor sheath. The bursae can become complex and fibrosis may occur, appearing as bandlike structures of low signal intensity within the submetatarsal fat pad.[50]

On sonography, submetatarsal bursitis may appear as focal or broad areas of ill-defined or well-defined anechoic or heterogenous collections (see **Fig. 14B**). The ill-defined bursitis tends to be totally compressible, and the well-defined collections are less compressible but mobile. Adventitial bursitis is frequently associated with hyperemia on power Doppler (see **Fig. 6G**).

## Treatment

Avoiding painful shoes may be sufficient. If symptoms persist, shoes with a thick sole and orthotics are prescribed and help by reducing pressure at the level of pain. Local infiltration of a corticosteroid/anesthetic solution helps reduce symptoms. There may be a role for excision of an excessively large bursa, or decompression of a bony prominence with a metatarsal osteotomy.

## DISCUSSION

MTP joint instability leads to irritation to the articular cartilage and hastens the progression through effusion, synovitis, tenosynovitis, and arthritic change. Instability typically irritates the intermetatarsal spaces and irritates the intermetatarsal bursae and neurovascular bundles. Many patients who have metatarsalgia commonly have a combination of diagnostic abnormalities. The key is to establish the principal pathology and from there construct an appropriate treatment regimen.

## SUMMARY

Many disorders produce metatarsalgia. MR imaging and, to a lesser extent, sonography permit specific diagnosis. Correlation with the physical examination ensures appropriate treatment.

## REFERENCES

1. Gregg J, Silberstein M, Schneider T, et al. Sonographic and MRI evaluation of the plantar plate: a prospective study. Eur Radiol 2006;16:2661–9.
2. Deland JT, Lee KT, Sobel M, et al. Anatomy of the plantar plate and its attachments in the lesser metatarsal phalangeal joint. Foot Ankle Int 1995;16:480–6.
3. Umans HR, Elsinger E. The plantar plate of the lesser metatarsophalangeal joints. Potential for injury and role of MR imaging. Med Clin North Am 2001;3:659–69.
4. Stainsby G. Pathological anatomy and dynamic effect of the displaced plantar plate and the importance of the integrity of the plantar plate deep transverse metatarsal ligament tie-bar. Ann R Coll Surg Engl 1997;79:58–68.
5. Williams A. Foot and ankle. In: Standring S, editor. Grays anatomy: the anatomical basis of clinical practice. 39th edition. Spain: Elsevier Churchill Livingstone; 2005. p. 1507–49.

6. Yu GV, Judge MS, Hudson JR, et al. Predislocation syndrome. Progressive subluxation/dislocation of the lesser metatarsophalangeal joint. J Am Podiatr Med Assoc 2002;92:182–99.

7. Gregg J, Silberstein M, Clark C, et al. Plantar plate repair and Weil osteotomy for metatarsophalangeal joint instability. J Foot Ankle Surg 2007;13:116–21.

8. Ford LA, Collins KB, Christensen JC. Stabilization of the subluxed second metatarsophalangeal joint: flexor tendon transfer versus primary repair of the plantar plate. J Foot Ankle Surg 1998;37:217–22.

9. Emedicine.com [homepage on the internet] New York: WebMD [updated 21May 2002; cited 8 Feb 2003]. Claw Toe. Available at: http://www.emedicine.com/orthop/topic51.htm. Accessed February 8, 2003.

10. Jahss MH. Fractures and dislocations of the forefoot. In: Radiology, vol. 5. Sydney: JB Lippincott Company; 1986. p. 1–6.

11. Yao L, Do HM, Cracchiolo A, et al. Plantar plate of the foot: findings on conventional arthrography and MRI imaging. AJR 1994;163:641–4.

12. Gregg J, Marks P, Silberstein M, et al. Histologic anatomy of the lesser metatarsophalangeal joint plantar plate. Surg Radiol Anat 2007;29:141–7.

13. Mizel YS, Yodlowski ML. Disorders of the lesser metatarsophalangeal joints. J Am Acad Orthop Surg 1995;3:166–73.

14. Saraffian SK. Anatomy of the foot and ankle—descriptive topographic functional. Philadelphia: JB lippincott company; 1993. p. 452.

15. Reeser JC. Stress fracture. Emedine web site January 21, 2007. Available at: www.emedicine.com/pmr/TOPIC134.HTM. Accessed June 26, 2008.

16. Mann RA, Coughlin MJ. Lesser toe deformities. In American academy of orthopaedic surgeons Instructional Course Lectures. J Bone Joint Surg 1987;36:137–59.

17. Ashman CJ, Klecker RJ, Yu JS. Forefoot pain involving the metatarsal region: differential diagnosis with MR imaging. Radiographics 2001;21:1425–40.

18. Lucas P, Kaplan P, Dussalt R, et al. MRI of the foot and ankle. Curr Probl Diagn Radiol 1997;26:209–66.

19. Marcelis S, Daenen B, Ferrara MA. Peripheral musculoskeletal ultrasound atlas. 1st edition. New York: Thieme Medical Publishers, Inc.; 1996. p. 11–57.

20. Copercini M, Bonvin F, Martinoli C, et al. Sonographic diagnosis of talar lateral process fracture. J Ultrasound Med 2003;22:635–40.

21. Mohana-Borges AV, Theumann NH, Pfirrmann CW, et al. Lesser metatarsophalangeal joints: standard MR imaging, MR arthrography, and MR bursography—initial results in 48 cadaveric joints. Radiology 2003;227:175–82.

22. Powless SH, Elze ME. Metatarsophalangeal joint capsule tears: an analysis by arthrography, a new classification system and surgical management. J Foot Ankle Surg 2001;40:374–89.

23. Sommer OJ, Kladosek A, Weiler V, et al. Rheumatoid arthritis: a practical guide to state-of-the-art imaging, image interpretation, and clinical implications. Radiographics 2005;25:381–98.

24. Baer A. The approach to the painful joint. Emedicine Web site December 6, 2006. Available at: http://www.emedicine.com/med/topic3562.htm. Accessed June 26, 2008.

25. McMorran J. Joint effusion: general practice notebook—a UK medical reference on the world wide web. 2008. Available at:http://www.gpnotebook.co.uk/medwebpage.cfm. Accessed June 22, 2008.

26. Boutry N, Morel M, Flipo RM, et al. Early rheumatoid arthritis: a review of MRI and sonographic findings. AJR 2007;189:1502–9.

27. Grassi W, Filippucci E, Busilacchi P. Musculoskeletal ultrasound. Clin Rheumatol 2004;18:813–26.

28. Koski JM. Ultrasound detection of plantar bursitis of the forefoot in patients with early rheumatoid arthritis. J Rheumatol 1998;25:229–31.

29. Harms SE, Wilk RM, Wolford LM, et al. The temporomandibular joint: magnetic resonance imaging using surface coils. Radiology 1985;157:133–6.

30. Mori S, Kaneda T, Lee K, et al. T2-weighted MRI for the assessment of joint effusion: comparative study of conventional spin-echo and fast spin-echo sequences. Oral Surg Oral Med Oral Pathol Oral Radiol Endod 2004;97:768–74.

31. Wamser G, Bohndorf K, Vollert K, et al. Power Doppler sonography with and without echo-enhancing contrast agent and contrast-enhanced MRI for the evaluation of rheumatoid arthritis of the shoulder joint: differentiation between synovitis and joint effusion. Skeletal Radiol 2004;32:351–9.

32. Grassi W, Filippuci E, Farina A, et al. Sonographic imaging of tendons. Arthritis Rheum 2000;43:969–76.

33. Koski JM. Detection of plantar tenosynovitis of the forefoot by ultrasound in patients with early arthritis. Scand J Rheumatol 1995;24:312–3.

34. Rosenberg ZS, Beltran J, Bencardino JT. From the RSNA refresher courses. Radiological society of North America. MR imaging of the ankle and foot. Radiographics 2000;20:153–79.

35. Martin MG, Masear MG. Triggering of the lesser toes at a previously undescribed distal pulley system. Foot Ankle Int 1998;19:113–7.

36. Bossley CJ, Cairney PC. The intermetatarsophalangeal bursa—its significance in Morton's metatarsalgia. J Bone Joint Surg 1980;62:184–7.

37. Garceau GJ, Brahms MA. A preliminary study of selective plantar-muscle denervation of pes cavus. J Bone Joint Surg Am 1956;38:553–62.

38. Coughlin MJ. Common causes of pain in the forefoot in adults. J Bone Joint Surg 2000;82:781–90.

39. Wu KK. Morton neuroma and metatarsalgia. Curr Opin Rheumatol 2000;12:131–42.
40. Sheon RP. Patient information: bursitis. Uptodate Web site. January 2008. Available at: http://www.uptodate.com/patients/license.html. Accessed June 26, 2008.
41. Ionoggu A, Coari G, Palombi G, et al. Sonography in the study of metatarsalgia. J Rheumatol 2001;28:1338–40.
42. Rockett MS. The use of ultrasound in the foot and ankle. Foot Ankle Clin 2000;5:29–48.
43. Shapiro PP, Shapiro SL. Sonographic evaluation of interidigital neuromas. Foot Ankle Int 1995;16:604–6.
44. Rawool NM, Nazarian LN. Ultrasound of the ankle and foot. Semin Ultrasound CT MR 2000;21:275–84.
45. Lin J, Fessell DP, Jacobson JA, et al. An illustrated tutorial of musculoskeletal sonography: part 3, lower extremity. AJR 2000;175:1313–21.
46. Read JW, Noakes JB, Kerr D, et al. Morton's metatarsalgia: sonographic findings and correlated histopathology. Foot Ankle Int 1999;20:153–61.
47. Hughes RJ, Ali K, Jones H, et al. Treatment of Morton's neuroma with alcohol injection under sonographic guidance: follow-up of 101 cases. AJR 2007;188:1535–9.
48. Bojsen-Moller F, Flagstade KE. Plantar aponeurosis and internal architecture of the ball of the foot. J Anat 1976;121:599–611.
49. Brown RR, Rosenberg S, Schweitzer Z, et al. MRI of medial malleolar bursa. AJR 2005;184:979–83.
50. Studler U, Mengiardi B, Bode B, et al. Fibrosis and adventitious bursae in plantar fat pad of forefoot: MR imaging findings in asymptomatic volunteers and MR imaging—histologic comparison. Radiology 2008;246:863–70.

# Imaging of Painful Conditions of the Hallucal Sesamoid Complex and Plantar Capsular Structures of the First Metatarsophalangeal Joint

Timothy G. Sanders, MD[a,b,]*, Sharik Kabir Rathur, MD[c]

**KEYWORDS**
- Ankle • Foot • Sesamoid ossicles • Turf toe
- Magnetic resonance • Computed tomography

## ANATOMY OF THE FIRST METATARSOPHALANGEAL JOINT

The first metatarsophalangeal (MTP) joint is a condyloid articulation with the proximal articular surface of the proximal phalanx demonstrating a shallow elliptical cavity that articulates with the rounded articular surface of the first metatarsal head. Normal motion is highly variable but typically ranges between 30 degrees of flexion and 50 degrees of extension with very little medial–lateral motion and no axial rotation.[1,2] The joint capsule is lax along the plantar aspect of the joint with a strong distal attachment to the base of the proximal phalanx and a weaker proximal attachment along the plantar aspect of the first metatarsal neck. The joint is stabilized both medially and laterally by collateral ligaments and along the dorsal aspect of the joint by an expansion of the extensor tendon mechanism.[3,4] The soft tissue anatomy along the plantar aspect of the joint is complex. Discussion is divided into two separate sections entitled the "hallucal sesamoid complex" and "plantar plate" anatomy.

### Hallucal Sesamoid Complex Anatomy

A sesamoid bone is defined as a bone that is embedded within a tendon and typically occurs in a location where a tendon passes over a joint.[1] Sesamoid bones are so named because they are similar in shape and appearance to a sesame seed. The patella is the largest and best-known sesamoid bone in the body, but sesamoids also occur in several other locations including numerous sites within the hands and feet. The patella acts as a nice anatomic model for other sesamoid bones in the body, which all have a very similar anatomic configuration. Although sesamoids are embedded within a tendon, one side of the bone is typically covered with hyaline cartilage and

[a] National Musculoskeletal Imaging, 1930 N. Commerce Parkway, Suite #5, Weston, FL 33326, USA
[b] Department of Diagnostic Radiology, College of Medicine, University of Kentucky, Lexington, KY 40536–0298, USA
[c] Department of Diagnostic Radiology, University of Miami, Jackson Memorial Hospital, 1611NW 12th Ave, Miami, FL 33136, USA
* Corresponding author.
*E-mail address:* radmantgs@cs.com (T.G. Sanders).

Radiol Clin N Am 46 (2008) 1079–1092
doi:10.1016/j.rcl.2008.09.001
0033-8389/08/$ – see front matter © 2008 Elsevier Inc. All rights reserved.

articulates with the underlying joint.[1,5] This anatomic configuration places the tendon at a slightly increased distance from the joint, thus decreasing the force applied to the tendon during motion of the joint and improving the mechanical advantage of the tendon. The presence of a sesamoid bone also helps to prevent flattening and fraying of the tendon as tension increases on the tendon during motion of the joint.

The hallucal sesamoid complex is composed of two separate sesamoids, the medial (tibial) and lateral (fibular) sesamoids (**Fig. 1**). Their ossification is complete between 9 and 14 years-of-age.[6] The tibial sesamoid is the larger and longer of the two and it is embedded within the medial head of the flexor hallucis brevis tendon. The lateral sesamoid is the smaller and rounder and it lies embedded within the lateral head of the flexor hallucis brevis tendon.[3,4] The dorsal surface of the hallucal sesamoids are covered with hyaline cartilage that articulate with the plantar aspect of the first metatarsal head. Unique to the hallucal sesamoids is the fact that in addition to protecting the surrounding tendons, they also serve a vital function in weight bearing. The hallucal sesamoid complex normally transmits up to 50% of the body weight and during the push-off stage of gait and may transmit as much as 300% of the body weight.[3] The hallucal sesamoids disperse the body weight at the level of the first metatarsophalangeal joint and thus act to protect the tendons that are located along the plantar aspect of the joint as well as to provide a cushioning effect for the first metatarsal head.

Although the two sesamoids lie primarily within the medial and lateral heads of the flexor hallucis tendon, the adjacent soft tissue anatomy is quite complex. The tibial sesamoid also serves as the distal attachment site of the abductor hallucis tendon. The fibular sesamoid serves as the distal attachment site of the adductor hallucis tendon and receives fibers from the transverse intermetatarsal ligament. The sesamoids are also embedded within a thickened portion of the plantar aspect of the joint capsule referred to as the plantar plate. The central portion of the plantar plate located between the two sesamoids is also referred to as the intersesamoid ligament. There is a small gap between the fibular and tibial sesamoids that allows passage of flexor hallucis longus tendon beneath the first metatarsophalangeal joint (**Fig. 2A**). This configuration also provides protection to the flexor hallucis tendon as it courses along the plantar aspect of the joint. Portions of the capsule also attach to the sesamoids. Along the medial aspect of the joint, the tibial sesamoid attaches to the phalanx via a thickening of the capsule sometimes referred to as the medial sesamoid phalangeal ligament, and to the metatarsal via a capsular thickening referred to as the medial metatarsosesamoid ligament (**Fig. 2B**). The fibular or lateral sesamoid attaches via the lateral sesamoid phalangeal and the lateral metatarsosesamoid ligaments (**Fig. 2C**).[7]

Faulty ossification may lead to a bipartite or rarely a multipartite configuration of the hallucal sesamoids (**Fig. 3**). The tibial sesamoid may demonstrate a bipartite configuration in up to 30% of individuals while a bipartite configuration of the fibular sesamoid is rather uncommon.[3,5,8] The hallucal sesamoid complex receives the

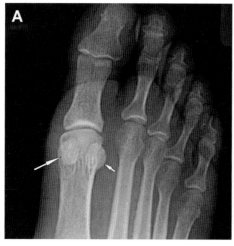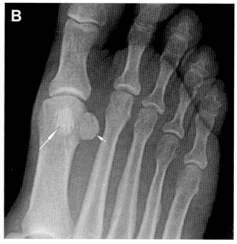

**Fig. 1.** Normal sesamoids. AP radiograph (*A*) of the forefoot shows the tibial (medial) sesamoid (*long arrow*) and the fibular (lateral) sesamoid (*short arrow*). Note that on an AP view of the forefoot, the sesamoids overlap the first metatarsal head. Lateral oblique radiograph (*B*) of the forefoot allows better visualization of the fibular sesamoid (*short arrow*), which is now projected off of the first metatarsal head. Tibial sesamoid (*long arrow*) overlaps the metatarsal head on this projection.

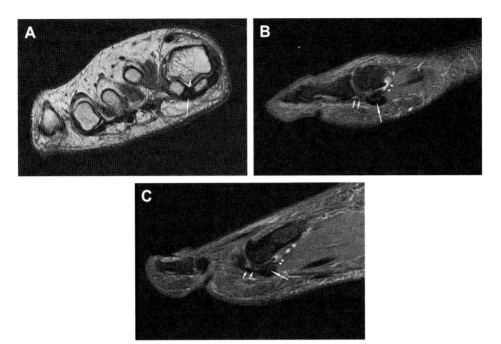

Fig. 2. Normal plantar plate anatomy. Short axis proton density image (A) shows the intersesamoid ligament (*short arrow*) between the two sesamoids. The flexor hallucis longus tendon (*long arrow*) is protected at the level of the first metatarsophalangeal joint sitting within the gap between the two sesamoids. Sagittal image (B) through the tibial sesamoid (*long arrow*) shows the medial sesamoidal phalangeal ligament (*short arrows*) and the metatarsosesamoid ligament (*arrow heads*). (C) Sagittal image through the fibular sesamoid (*long arrow*) shows the lateral sesamoidal phalangeal ligament (*short arrows*). The lateral metatarsosesamoid ligament (*arrow heads*) is only seen in part on this image.

majority of its blood supply from either the plantar arch or from the medial plantar artery with each sesamoid typically supplied by a single artery that enters the sesamoid from a proximal and plantar direction.[4,9] There is very little collateral blood supply and little to no recurrent supply. This configuration of the blood supply may play an important role in certain pathologic conditions such as avascular necrosis, poor healing, and nonunion of fractures.[10,11]

## Plantar Plate Anatomy

The plantar plate, sometimes referred to as the volar accessory ligament is a fibrocartilaginous thickening of the plantar aspect of the capsule of the first MTP joint. The plantar plate actually represents a reinforced thickened portion of the volar aspect of the joint capsule with a very strong distal attachment along the plantar aspect of the base of the proximal phalanx and a weaker attachment proximally through the capsule to the plantar aspect of the first metatarsal neck.[12–14] The plantar plate extends both medially and laterally to contain the tibial and fibular sesamoids; the segment of the plantar plate located between the two sesamoids has been referred to as the intersesamoid ligament (**Fig. 2**). The plantar

plate, in conjunction with the hallucal sesamoid complex and the adjacent tendinous attachments, plays a vital role in providing support and stability to the first metatarsophalangeal joint.

## THE PAINFUL HALLUCAL SESAMOID COMPLEX

The sesamoids provide a significant cushioning effect for the first metatarsophalangeal joint and they are also important with regard to weight-bearing with up to three times the body weight transferred across the sesamoids during the push-off phase of normal gait. Sesamoid pathology can be varied and is often difficult to differentiate clinically from other forms of pathology at level of the first MTP joint. When abnormalities are isolated to the sesamoids, the patient usually presents with limited and painful dorsiflexion of the joint. Physical examination may reveal swelling and synovitis along the plantar aspect of the joint. Pain is usually elicited with direct palpation or when the examiner pushes the affected sesamoid distally.[1,3,4]

## Sesamoiditis

The definition of sesamoiditis varies throughout the literature, but sesamoiditis is most often used

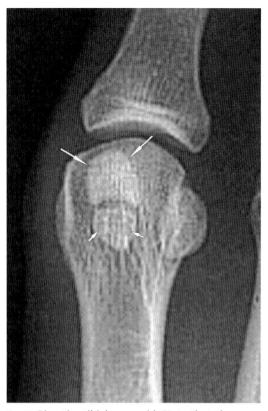

Fig. 3. Bipartite tibial sesamoid. Note that there are two separate fragments of the tibial sesamoid: the distal fragment *(long arrows)* and the proximal fragment *(short arrows)*. The fragments are rounded with sclerotic margins completely surrounding both ossification centers.

sesamoiditis can be considered equivalent to a focal tendinosis; indeed, it is sometimes associated with inflammatory changes of the surrounding tendon and adjacent soft tissue structures.[1,4,15]

Sesamoiditis often occurs in the young athlete in the setting of repetitive trauma to the plantar aspect of the forefoot and it may be associated with stress related marrow edema, stress fracture or even an acute fracture of one or both of the sesamoids. Alternatively, sesamoiditis may occur in the context of osteoarthritis, inflammatory arthropathy, avascular necrosis, or infection.

Radiography can play an important role in the initial evaluation of the painful sesamoidal complex. Depending upon the precise etiology of pain, radiographs may be normal or may demonstrate sclerosis or fragmentation of the involved sesamoid. Radiographs can also provide a more specific diagnosis including fracture or osteoarthritis as the source pain. Radiographic evaluation should include AP and lateral radiographs. The medial oblique view can be helpful in assessment of the tibial sesamoid, while the lateral oblique view may be of help in assessing the fibular sesamoid.[16] When an isolated sesamoid abnormality is suspected clinically, a special sesamoid view can be obtained as an oblique coronal radiograph in which the beam is directed tangential to the metatarso-sesamoid articulation, allowing direct visualization of the joint without osseous overlap.[15] Nuclear medicine bone scan will demonstrate increased uptake within the affected sesamoid bone, while MR imaging will show diffuse marrow edema (decreased T1 and increased T2-weighted signal) replacing the normal fat signal within the affected sesamoid (**Fig. 4**). Historically, nuclear medicine bone scan has been used to detect abnormalities of the sesamoids. Bone scan is sensitive, demonstrating radiotracer uptake in the context of abnormality, but does not clarify

as a nonspecific descriptive term referring to any painful inflammatory condition of the sesamoid bones. As previously described, the sesamoid bones of the first metatarsophalangeal joint are embedded within the medial and lateral heads of the flexor hallucis brevis tendon and as such,

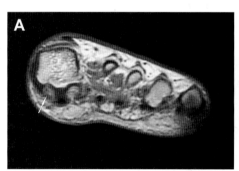
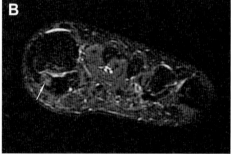

Fig. 4. Sesamoiditis. Proton density (*A*) and STIR (*B*) short axis images through the first metatarsophalangeal joint reveals diffuse marrow edema with the tibial sesamoid in this patient who has metatarsalgia indicating sesamoiditis.

he nature of the pathology and as such, plays little ole in evaluation of sesamoiditis. MR imaging typically permits more specific diagnosis of fracture, stress fracture, avascular necrosis or underlying pathology, and as such is considered as the imaging modality of choice for assessment of sesamoiditis.

## Sesamoid Trauma

Traumatic injuries of the sesamoids may occur as a result of high or low impact injury including direct trauma, forced dorsiflexion of the great toe, or repetitive stress. Various traumatic injuries of the hallucal sesamoids have been described and include acute fracture, avulsion fracture, subluxation or dislocation, stress fracture, or diastasis of a bipartite/multipartite sesamoid.[16–20]

Most acute sesamoidal fractures involve the tibial sesamoid, as this sesamoid sits more directly under the first metatarsal head and is more directly involved in weight-bearing, placing this sesamoid at increased risk for injury. Furthermore, the position of the fibular sesamoid allows it to slip into the first metatarsal interspace between the first and second metatarsal heads, thus providing some protection from direct trauma. Clinically suspected sesamoid fractures should be initially evaluated with conventional radiographs. Radiographic signs that have been described in association with a sesamoid fracture include irregular margins with unequal separation of sesamoidal fragments, absence of similar radiographic findings on the contralateral side, or evidence of attempted healing (periosteal new bone). Visualization of a fracture or diastasis of sesamoidal fragments that represents a change from pre-injury radiographs is a definitive sign of fracture, but pre-injury radiographs are rarely available.[20] It is often difficult to differentiate a bipartite or multipartite sesamoid from an acute fracture on the basis

of radiographs alone and more advanced imaging is often required.

Nuclear medicine bone scan is nonspecific but will demonstrate focal increased uptake within the fractured sesamoid.[19] CT and MRI are both very helpful in evaluating for acute fracture of a hallucal sesamoid. The sagittal and coronal (long axis) imaging planes using CT are most useful in detecting fractures and separation of fracture fragments.[17] On MR imaging, the fracture will be seen as a low signal intensity line on T1-, and as a high or low signal intensity line on T2-weighted imaging (Fig. 5). MRI has the added benefit of demonstrating diffuse marrow edema (bright signal on STIR or T2-weighted imaging with fat saturation and diffuse low T1 signal abnormality). When evaluating the sesamoids with either CT or MR imaging, differentiation of a bipartite sesamoid from an acute fracture often requires evaluation of the morphology of the sesamoid, including the margins and shape of the fragments. A bipartite sesamoid is usually larger than a nonpartite sesamoid and usually demonstrates rounded fragments with smooth sclerotic margins, while a fracture fragment will often reveal irregular nonsclerotic margin often with some degree of separation of the fragments.[21]

Athletes exposed to excessive running, jumping, or forced dorsiflexion of the first MTP joint are at increased risk for stress fractures of the hallucal sesamoids, and although either sesamoid may suffer from stress fracture, the medial sesamoid is more commonly affected.[17,18] Individuals present clinically with tenderness to palpation over the affected sesamoid with worsening of pain during participation in the offending activity.

Radiographs of the foot are often normal in individuals with hallucal sesamoidal stress fracture. Possible findings however include a complete or incomplete fracture, sclerosis, or a bipartite or multipartite configuration. Nuclear medicine bone

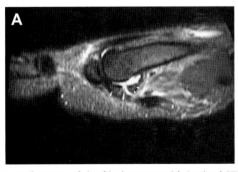
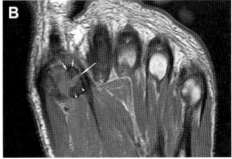

Fig. 5. Acute fracture of the fibular sesamoid. Sagittal STIR (A) and long axis T1 (B) images through the first metatarsophalangeal joint demonstrate an acute vertical fracture (long arrows) through the fibular sesamoid. Note that there is bright T2 signal within the fracture on the STIR image with low T1 signal on the coronal image. There is slight distraction of the proximal fragment (arrow heads) and the distal fragment (short arrows).

scan, as previously mentioned, is nonspecific but will reveal increased uptake in the affected sesamoid. CT imaging maybe normal but usually reveals a complete or incomplete fracture, with or without separation of fragments. In the early stages of stress response, MR imaging is nonspecific demonstrating diffuse marrow edema within the sesamoid. With persistent activity, a fracture develops and MR imaging will demonstrate a vertical low signal intensity line best seen on sagittal or long axis images through the involved sesamoid (**Fig. 6**). If the offending activity persists, the fracture can go on to completion and in the later stages, flattening and fragmentation of the sesamoid may occur.[22]

Traumatic dislocation or subluxation of the sesamoids usually occur as a result of significant trauma to the great toe and are most often seen in conjunction with plantar capsular injury or disruption. These injuries have also been reported in ballet dancers and soccer players. Radiographs are usually sufficient to establish the diagnosis, but MR imaging can be useful in fully delineating the associated soft tissue injuries.

Delayed union and nonunion are common complications of sesamoid fracture, in part due to the tenuous blood supply of the sesamoids and possibly also related to the tremendous force applied across the sesamoids during normal weight-bearing.[4] Over time, nonunion fracture fragments will develop sclerotic margins, which are nicely depicted on CT or MR imaging. Marrow edema may persist within the fracture fragments of a symptomatic nonunion (**Fig. 7**).

Initial treatment of sesamoidal fractures is usually conservative with rest, partial weight-bearing, avoidance of aggravating activity, and possible short leg casting. High level athletes or those who fail conservative treatment may undergo surgical resection of the proximal fragment. However, due to the crucial role of the sesamoids in distribution of force during weight-bearing, complete sesamoidal resection is ill advised as it may lead to serious complications including hallux valgus or cock-up deformity of the hallux.[16]

### Avascular Necrosis

Avascular necrosis of the hallucal sesamoids represents an uncommon cause of metatarsalgia. Patients typically present with insidious onset of pain overlying the affected sesamoid. Although numerous etiologies have been suggested, it is repetitive trauma that is most often cited as the probable etiology in the majority of cases.[9–11,23,24] The tibial and fibular sesamoids appear to be involved with near equal frequency and females are affected slightly more often than men.[6,23] The condition is most often reported in adolescents or young adults who participate in athletic activity.

Radiographs are usually normal during the first 6 months following onset of symptoms, but eventually radiographic abnormalities develop, which include fragmentation, a stippled appearance, and increased density.[6,9] Fragmentation into several fragments is classic and usually excludes other etiologies such as acute fracture or stress fracture. Nuclear medicine bone scan is nonspecific but will demonstrate increased uptake within the affected sesamoid. CT imaging will show findings similar to radiographs but typically demonstrates the abnormalities of fragmentation and increased density earlier and with increased precision (**Fig. 8**). MR imaging will show abnormality of the involved sesamoid very early with marrow edema present at the time of initial symptoms. This is manifest as

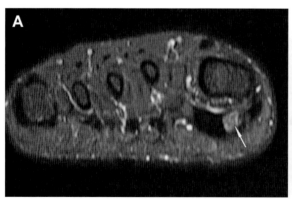
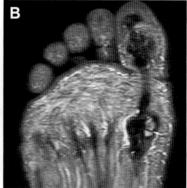

**Fig. 6.** Stress fracture of the tibial sesamoid. This long distance runner developed insidious onset pain of at the level of her first metatarsophalangeal joint, exacerbated by running. Short axis (*A*) and long axis (*B*) T2-weighted images reveal diffuse marrow edema within the tibial sesamoid (*long arrow*) and an incomplete stress fracture (*short arrow*) noted on the long axis image.

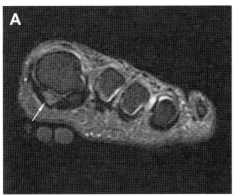
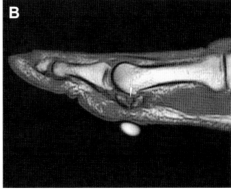

Fig. 7. Nonunion of a tibial sesamoid fracture. Short axis T2-weighted image with fat saturation (A) shows marrow edema (arrow) within the tibial sesamoid in a patient with chronic pain in this region. Sagittal T1-weighted image (B) shows a vertical fracture (arrow) with sclerotic margins of both fracture fragments indicating nonunion.

low T1 and bright T2-signal throughout the marrow space of the involved sesamoid (Fig. 8). This is also a nonspecific finding and is similar to the appearance of a nonspecific sesamoiditis and early stress related changes. Late MR findings include fragmentation and areas of mixed T1 and T2 signal representing areas of sclerosis intermixed with marrow edema (Figs. 9 and 10). The presence of extensive fragmentation is nearly diagnostic of avascular necrosis and usually excludes acute or stress related fractures.

Avascular necrosis does not usually respond well to conservative treatment and often requires surgical excision of the involved sesamoid, although excision of both sesamoids is not generally recommended.[6,25] A limited excision of the necrotic portion of the sesamoid may be an acceptable surgical alternative to complete excision of the involved sesamoid.

## Arthritis

The first metatarsophalangeal joint is a true synovial joint composed of three separate articulations including the metatarsophalangeal and two metatarsosesamoidal articulations. Osteoarthritis, gout, and inflammatory arthropathies commonly involve this joint and can lead to various changes of the sesamoids including chondral loss with joint space narrowing of the metatarsosesamoidal joints, subchondral sclerosis, marrow edema, erosions, and subchondral cysts. Advanced arthritis often leads to progressive hallux valgus deformity and metatarsosesamoidal subluxation or dislocation (Fig. 11).[21,26]

## Infection

Osteomyelitis of the sesamoids most often occurs from contiguous spread either from the underlying soft tissue infection or from septic arthritis of the first MTP joint. Sesamoidal osteomyelitis is often seen in the diabetic foot and may be associated with overlying skin ulcers, cellulites, and draining sinus tracks. MR imaging is the most sensitive imaging modality for evaluation of osteomyelitis and usually demonstrates marrow edema throughout the involved sesamoid. There may also be

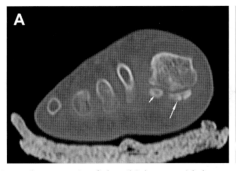
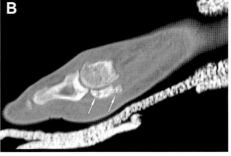

Fig. 8. Avascular necrosis of the tibial sesamoid demonstrated on CT imaging. Short axis (A) and sagittal (B) CT images through the tibial sesamoid (long arrows) reveals mixed sclerosis and fragmentation of the tibial sesamoid in this patient with avascular necrosis of the tibial sesamoid. The fibular sesamoid (short arrow) is normal in appearance.

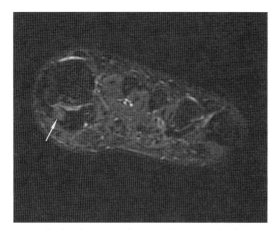

Fig. 9. Early changes of avascular necrosis demonstrated on MR imaging. Short axis STIR image shows diffuse nonspecific marrow edema *(arrow)* within the tibial sesamoid. MR shows no fracture or fragmentation in this early case of avascular necrosis.

associated cortical destruction.[21,26] The presence of an overlying skin defect, adjacent soft tissue abscess, or sinus track increases the specificity of MR imaging with regard to the diagnosis of osteomyelitis.

### Nerve Impingement

Occasionally, the tibial sesamoid can result in impingement on the medial branch of the plantar digital nerve along the medial aspect of the hallux. Symptoms typically include decreased sensation and radiating pain. No specific imaging findings are associated with impingement of the medial plantar digital nerve and treatment is supportive with resection of the tibial sesamoid reserved for refractory cases of pain.[27]

### Absent Sesamoid

As previously described, the sesamoids play a key role in cushioning of the metatarsal head and in appropriate weight distribution across the first MTP joint. An absence of one of the sesamoids is a known cause of metatarsalgia. The most common reason for an absent sesamoid is previous surgical resection (**Fig. 12**). There are also case reports of congenitally absent tibial sesamoids that result in MTP joint pain.[28] Total resorption of the tibial sesamoid resulting from infection has been reported as a mimic of a congenitally absent sesamoid and may present with MTP joint pain as a result of altered biomechanics of the joint.[26] Radiographs, CT and MR imaging will all demonstrate the absence of the tibial sesamoid. MR imaging may also reveal soft tissue changes such as tendinitis or capsular injury associated with the altered anatomy.

### PLANTAR PLATE INJURIES (TURF TOE)

The term "turf toe" has been used loosely to describe various soft tissue injuries about the first MTP joint; however, turf toe is strictly defined as a plantar capsular ligament injury of the first MTP joint.[15,29] Turf toe is a common injury that may lead to significant morbidity and prolonged recovery times if not identified and treated promptly. Turf toe was first described in athletes playing American football on artificial turf.[29] The incidence of injury has increased with the widespread use of new artificial playing surfaces introduced in the late 1960s combined with lighter more flexible footwear designed for these surfaces, which typically provide less support to the MTP joints. Artificial surfaces have been found to become harder with aging and wear.[30] This harder surface

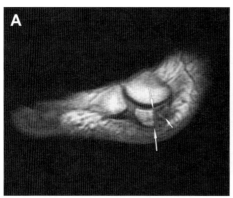
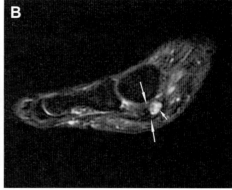

Fig. 10. Late avascular necrosis of the tibial sesamoid demonstrated on MR imaging. Sagittal T1 (*A*) and STIR (*B*) images in a patient who has a previous vertical fracture *(long arrows)* through the tibial sesamoid demonstrate mixed T1 and bright T2 signal abnormality *(short arrow)* within the proximal fragment indicating avascular necrosis complicating the fracture. The missed signal on T1 indicates a combination of sclerosis and marrow edema.

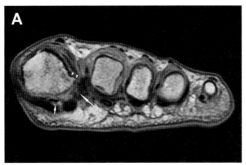
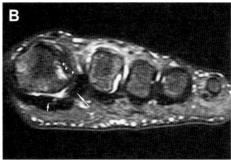

Fig. 11. Osteoarthritis of the first metatarsophalangeal joint. Short axis T1 (A) and T2 (B) images through the first metatarsophalangeal joint shows changes of osteoarthritis. The arrows' heads point to a small lateral osteophyte and subchondral marrow edema of the metatarsal head. Long arrow points to the fibular sesamoid, which shows subchondral sclerosis and lateral subluxation. The tibial sesamoid (short arrows) is also laterally subluxed but with no significant sclerosis or marrow edema.

combined with the higher coefficient of friction of artificial turf as compared to natural grass has been implicated in turf toe.[15,29,30] The footwear initially designed for artificial turf was lighter and more flexible allowing increased dorsiflexion of the first metatarsal phalangeal joint than traditional cleats, thus increasing the risk of hyperextension injury. The development of more modern shoes with stiffened forefoot has been shown to reduce injury rate.[31]

### Mechanism of Injury

Turf toe is a hyperextension injury most commonly seen in American football athletes playing on artificial turf; however, injuries have been reported in many other sports. The most common mechanism is forced hyperextension of the first MTP joint during a football pile-up. The injury occurs in players lying in the prone position with the first toe planted on the playing surface with the heel elevated, when another player falls across the back of his leg. This forces the MTP joint into hyperextension, injuring the plantar capsuloligamentous structures.[32] Another less common mechanism is seen in lineman, where valgus and hyperextension forces are introduced as the player repeatedly pushes off from the down position. This is believed to lead to a chronic repetitive-type injury of the plantar plate, and individuals with this mechanism of injury often describe a more insidious onset of symptoms.[32,33] This type of injury may also be associated with an underlying pes planus deformity.[33] Other predisposing factors for turf toe include hypermobility of the ankle joint, prior injury to the first MTP joint, and increasing age of the athlete.[2] There has been recent description of hyperextension injuries at the MTP joints of skimboarders, referred to as "skimboarder's

toe". This should be differentiated from turf toe because skimboarder's toe results in dorsal MTJ pain and disruption of the extensor expansion instead of the plantar plate.[34]

Hyperflexion injuries have also been reported as a mechanism of turf toe; however, hyperflexion of the MTP joints typically results in dorsal capsular injuries, which do not meet the strict definition of turf toe.[13,32] A separate entity has been described in beach volleyball players, referred to as "sand toe".[35] This is a hyperflexion injury involving the first and lesser MTP joints resulting in dorsal capsular injuries that lead to significant disability and prolonged recovery times.[35]

Turf toe injury is described as a sprain or tear of the plantar capsule–ligament complex of the first MTP joint, the most important component being the plantar plate. The detailed anatomy of the plantar plate and hallucal sesamoid complex is described in an earlier section. Hyperextension results in stretching or tearing of the opposing plantar plate, with the injury most often occurring at its weakest point near the proximal attachment to the metatarsal head neck junction. The injury is usually located just distal to the sesamoids and may allow sesamoid retraction or proximal migration.[31] Sesamoid fracture or diastasis of a bipartite sesamoid have also been described in association with plantar plate injury.[15,36] In extreme dorsiflexion, the proximal phalanx may compress the dorsal metatarsal head resulting in a focal osteochondral impaction injury.[15,33] Dorsal dislocation of the great toe has also been associated with turf toe.[13,15]

### Clinical Presentation of Turf Toe Injuries

Individuals with turf toe most commonly present after an acute injury and typically describe worsening pain and disability over the subsequent

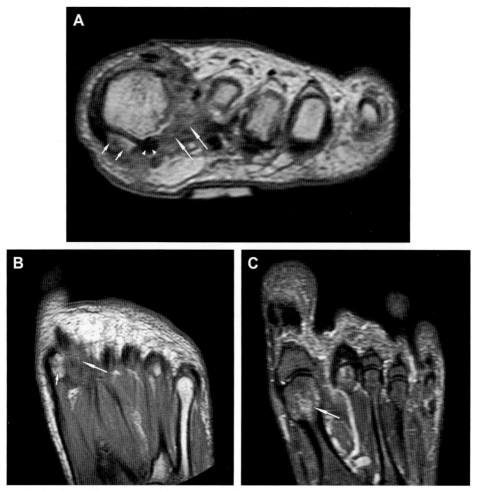

Fig. 12. Surgically absent fibular sesamoid as a cause of metatarsalgia associated with altered weight bearing. Proton density short axis image (A) shows a normal tibial sesamoid *(short arrows)*, normal flexor hallucis longus tendon *(arrow heads)*, and a surgically absent fibular *(long arrows)* sesamoid. Long axis T1 image (B) shows the normal tibial sesamoid *(short arrow)* and the absence of the fibular sesamoid *(long arrow)*. Long axis T2 image (C) shows marrow edema within the first metatarsal head in this patient who has continued foot pain associated with altered biomechanics of walking following a complete resection of the fibular sesamoid.

24 hours.[15,29] Clinical presentation and extent of disability varies depending on the severity of the injury. Physical examination reveals swelling, hyperemia, and point tenderness over the plantar surface first MTP joint.[29] Pain and guarding limits active range of motion, but passive range of motion may be increased due to plantar plate disruption.[15] Functional disability is a result of impaired push-off, and football players may complain of difficulty assuming the "down" position.[29] The duration of impairment depends upon the severity of injury and may persist from a few days to many weeks.[29]

Treatment and recovery time varies significantly depending on the severity of injury. Turf toe injuries

are categorized based on severity.[31] Grade 1 injury is defined as a stretching type injury (sprain) of the plantar capsular–ligamentous complex without loss of functional integrity. Individuals presenting with a Grade I sprain typically complain of mild tenderness and swelling along the plantar aspect of the MTP joint but without ecchymosis. Athletes are able to bear weight and are usually able to continue playing. Treatment is symptomatic with rest, ice, compression, and elevation (RICE), taping or a stiff insole.[13,14,31,33] A Grade 2 injury is defined as a partial tear of the plantar capsular–ligamentous complex. This manifests clinically as mild to moderate tenderness, edema, and ecchymosis. Athletes are usually limp with weight bearing and are unable to compete. Recovery time can be as long as 2 weeks. Treatment includes RICE and immobilization with or without crutches.[13,14,31,33] Grade 3 injury is defined as a complete tear of the plantar plate, and it may have associated injuries including: osteochondral impaction of the dorsal metatarsal head, sesamoid fracture, diastasis of a bipartite sesamoid, sesamoid retraction/proximal migration, or MTP joint dislocation.[13,31,33] Athletes present with severe tenderness, swelling, and ecchymosis, and may be out of play for 4–6 weeks or longer. These individuals require long term immobilization in a cast or boot; they may require surgery depending upon their response to conservative management and the presence associated injuries.[13,31,33,36]

## Imaging of Turf Toe Injuries

Evaluation with radiographs and MR imaging plays an important role in confirming the presence of and grading the extent of plantar plate injury, evaluating for associated injuries, and in guiding appropriate clinical management.[14] Initial evaluation of turf toe injury usually begins with radiographs which may demonstrate soft tissue swelling, avulsion fractures, sesamoid fractures, diastasis of bipartite sesamoids, proximal migration of the sesamoids (Fig. 13) due to plantar plate disruption, or MTP joint dislocation.[13,15,29] Stress views may be useful in demonstrating ligamentous laxity or disruption.[13] Comparison views of the unaffected hallux may also be of benefit.[13] Follow-up

radiographs may demonstrate interval proximal migration on the sesamoids, indicating complete disruption of the plantar plate.[14] Chronic turf toe injuries may result in hallux rigidus, which manifests as dorsal spurring at the MTP joint.[7] Arthrograms to evaluate for capsular injury have been performed historically; however, MR imaging is more useful in directly assessing the plantar soft tissues.

MR imaging is ideal for grading the extent of plantar plate injury, which is usually best depicted on sagittal and short axis axial T2-weighted images through the first MTP joint. Grade I injury demonstrates soft tissue edema and swelling along the plantar aspect of the first MTP joint. There may be mild thickening and edema within the plantar capsular structures, but no partial or full thickness tear will be present (Fig. 14). Grade II injury reveals a partial thickness tear/disruption of the plantar capsule (Fig. 15), and a Grade III injury manifests as a complete disruption of the plantar capsular structures and may demonstrate associated sesamoid pathology, such as edema or fracture, diastasis, or proximal migration (Fig. 16). Associated osteochondral lesions of the dorsal metatarsal head may also be demonstrated and a thorough evaluation of the adjacent musculotendinous structures should be performed.[7] Coronal (long axis) images are best suited for evaluation of the collateral ligaments; sagittal and short axis images are useful in evaluation of the surrounding tendons and sesamoid bones.[12,13,15,37] Disruption of the plantar plate

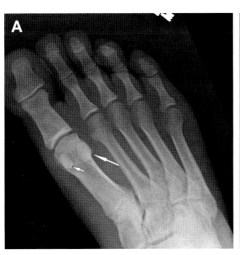 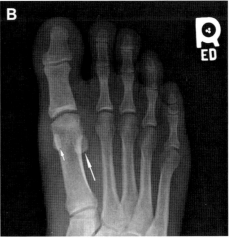

Fig. 13. Complete disruption of the plantar plate resulting in proximal migration of the sesamoids. (A) AP radiograph in the immediate post-injury period shows normal position of the tibial (short arrow) and fibular (long arrow) sesamoids. (B) AP radiograph approximately one month after injury shows proximal migration of the tibial (short arrow) and fibular (long arrow) sesamoids, indicating a complete disruption of the plantar plate distal to the sesamoids.

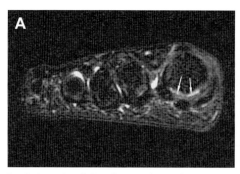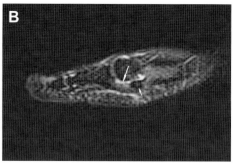

**Fig. 14.** Grade I sprain of the plantar plate. Short axis (*A*) and sagittal (*B*) images through the first metatarsopha-langeal joint reveal soft tissue edema *(long arrows)* within the plantar plate and superficial to the plantar plate. There is no capsular disruption with no evidence of a partial or full thickness tear of the capsular structures. Fibular sesamoid *(short arrow)*.

intersesamoid ligament may allow interposition of the flexor hallucis longus tendon between the sesamoids resulting in divergence of the medial and lateral sesamoids on axial images.[14]

### Treatment of Turf Toe

Turf toe was initially thought to have low morbidity but is now known to result in significant short and long term morbidity and disability.[33] One study showed that while ankle inversion injury is a much more common injury amongst American football players, turf toe actually results in more lost game time, which indicates the importance of this injury.[2] Turf toe is usually treated success-fully with conservative management, and surgery is reserved for refractory or complicated cases.[36] Conservative therapy usually includes RICE. Rest is very important to allow the injury to heal; however, the implications of a turf toe injury are often underestimated and noncompliance is fre-quently encountered.[33] Support or immobilization

with tape, orthotics, walking boot, or casting may be required depending on the severity of injury.[29,36] Physical therapy with early mobilization is beneficial to preserve range of motion, however, returning to practice too early results in prolonged recovery.[33]

Surgery is rarely indicated, but it may be required if there is poor response to conservative management or other associated injuries are present. Surgical indications include: sesamoid fracture, diastasis of a bipartite sesamoid, proxi-mal migration of sesamoids, loose body, chondral flap, or failure to respond to conservative manage-ment.[13,32,36] Capsular-ligamentous repair and resection of the distal fragment of a sesamoid frac-ture/diastasis may be performed.[33]

### SUMMARY

Numerous distinct pathologic entities involving the hallucal sesamoidal complex and capsular struc-tures of the first MTP joint can result in

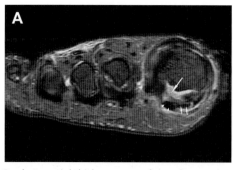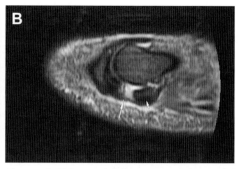

**Fig. 15.** Grade II partial thickness tear of the plantar plate. Short axis T2 image (*A*) shows a partial tear of the plan-tar plate *(long arrow)* between the fibular sesamoid and flexor hallucis longus tendon *(arrow heads)*. The medial aspect of the plantar plate *(short arrows)* demonstrates soft tissue edema and a stretching type injury but remains intact. Sagittal T2 image (*B*) shows partial thickness disruption of the lateral sesamoidal phalangeal ligament *(long arrow)* with adjacent soft tissue edema, but some fibers remain intact. The fibular sesamoid *(short arrow)* is partially retracted.

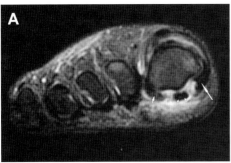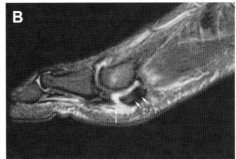

Fig.16. Grade III full thickness tear of the plantar plate. Short axis T2 image (A) shows a complete tear of the plantar plate. The Flexor hallucis longus tendon (arrow heads) is interposed between the tibial (long arrow) and fibular (short arrow) sesamoids, which demonstrate medial and lateral displacement. Sagittal T2 image (B) shows a complete disruption (long arrow) of the plantar plate with a fluid filled gap at the expected location of the plantar capsule. The tibial sesamoid (short arrow) is proximally retracted.

metatarsalgia of the first MTP joint. Although history and clinical presentation are very important in establishing a working differential for the etiology of pain, there is often significant overlap with regard to clinical presentation and physical findings. Targeted imaging to include radiographs, nuclear medicine bone scan, CT and MR imaging can play a pivotal role in accurately diagnosing the source of pain.

## REFERENCES

1. Grace DL. Sesamoid problems. Foot Ankle Clin 2000;5(3):609–27.

2. Rodeo SA, O'Brien S, Warren RF, et al. Turf-toe: an analysis of metatarsophalangeal joint sprains in professional football players. Am J Sports Med 1990; 18(3):280–5.

3. McBryde AM, Anderson RB. Sesamoid foot problems in the athlete. Clin Sports Med 1988;7:41–60.

4. Dedmond BT, Cory JW, McBryde A Jr. The hallucal sesamoid complex. J Am Acad Orthop Surg 2006; 14(13):745–53.

5. Mellado JM, Ramos A, Salvado E, et al. Accessory ossicles and sesamoid bones of the ankle and foot: imaging findings, clinical significance and differential diagnosis. Eur Radiol 2003;13(Suppl 4): L164–77.

6. Toussirot E, Jeunet L, Michel F, et al. Avascular necrosis of the hallucal sesamoids update with reference to two case-reports. Joint Bone Spine 2003; 70(4):307–9.

7. Crain JM, Phancao JP, Stidham K. MR imaging of turf toe. Magn Reson Imaging Clin N Am 2008; 16(1):93–103.

8. Munuera PV, Dominguez G, Reina M, et al. Bipartite hallucal sesamoid bones: relationship with hallux valgus and metatarsal index. Skeletal Radiol 2007; 36(11):1043–50.

9. DiGiovannis CW, Patel A, Calfree R, et al. Osteonecrosis in the foot. J Am Acad Orthop Surg 2007;15(4):208–17.

10. Fleischli J, Cheleuitte E. Avascular necrosis of the hallucal sesamoids. J Foot Ankle Surg 1995;34(4): 358–65.

11. Julsrud ME. Osteonecrosis of the tibial and fibular sesamoids in an aerobics instructor. J Foot Ankle Surg 1997;36:31–5.

12. Wilson L, Dimeff R, Miniaci A, et al. Radiologic case study. First metarsophalangeal plantar plate injury (turf toe). Orthopedics 2005;28(4). 344, 417–9.

13. Watson TS, Anderson RB, Davis WH. Periarticular injuries to the hallux metatarsophalangeal joint in athletes. Foot Ankle Clin 2000;5(3):687–713.

14. Allen LR, Flemming D, Sanders TG. Turf toe: ligamentous injury of the first metatarsophalangeal joint. Mil Med 2004;169:xix–xxiv.

15. Umans HR. Imaging sports medicine injuries of the foot and toes. Clin Sports Med 2006;25(4):763–80.

16. Mittlmeier T, Haar P. Sesamoid and toe fractures. Injury 2004;35(Suppl 2):SB87–97.

17. Biedert R. Which investigations are required in stress fracture of the great toe sesamoids? Arch Orthop Trauma Surg 1993;112(2):94–5.

18. Wall J, Feller JF. Imaging of stress fractures in runners. Clin Sports Med 2006;25(4):781–802.

19. Georgoulias P, Georgiadis I, Dimakopoulos N, et al. Scintigraphy of stress fractures of the sesamoid bones. Clin Nucl Med 2001;26(11):944–5.

20. Brown TI. Avulsion fracture of the fibular sesamoid in association with dorsal dislocation of the metatarsophalangeal joint of the hallux: report of a case and review of the literature. Clin Orthop Relat Res 1980;(149):229–31.

21. Karasick D, Schweitzer ME. Disorders of the hallux sesamoid complex: MR features. Skeletal Radiol 1998;27(8):411–8.

22. Burton EM, Amaker BH. Stress fracture of the great toe sesamoid in a ballerina: MRI appearance. Pediatr Radiol 1994;24(1):37–8.

23. Ozkoc G, Akpinar S, Ozalav M, et al. Hallucal sesamoid osteonecrosis: an overlooked cause of forefoot pain. J Am Podiatr Med Assoc 2005; 95(3):277–80.

24. Velkes S, Pritsch M, Horoszowski K. Osteochondritis of the first metatarsal sesamoids. Arch Orthop Trauma Surg 1988;107(6):369–71.

25. Waizy H, Jager M, Abbara-Czardybon M, et al. Surgical treatment of AVN of the fibular (lateral) sesamoid. Foot Ankle Int 2008;29(2):231–6.

26. Potter HG, Pavlov H, Abrahams TG. The hallux sesamoids revisited. Skeletal Radiol 1992;21(7): 437–44.

27. Richardson EG. Hallucal sesamoid pain: causes and surgical treatment. J Am Acad Orthop Surg 1999;7(4):270–8.

28. Kanatli U, Ozturk AM, Ercan NG, et al. Absence of the medial sesamoid bone associated with metatarsophalangeal pain. Clin Anat 2006;19(7):634–9.

29. Bowers KD Jr, Martin RB. Turf-toe: a shoe-surface related football injury. Med Sci Sports 1974;8(2): 81–3.

30. Bowers KD Jr, Martin RB. Impact absorption, new and old Astroturf at West Virginia University. Med Sci Sports 1974;6(3):217–21.

31. Clanton TO, Butler JE, Eggert A. Injuries to the metatarsophalangeal joints in athletes. Foot Ankle 1986; 7(3):162–76.

32. Coker TP, Arnold JA, Weber DL. Traumatic lesions of the metatarsophalangeal joint of the great toe in athletes. Am J Sports Med 1978;6(6):326–34.

33. Clanton TO, Ford JJ. Turf toe injury. Clin Sports Med 1994;13(4):731–41.

34. Donnelly LF, Betts JB, Fricke BL. Skimboarder's toe: findings on high-field MRI. AJR Am J Roentgenol 2005;184(5):1481–5.

35. DeLee & Drez's orthopaedic sports medicine. 2nd Edition. Philadelphia: Saunders; 2003. Turf Toe.

36. Browner: skeletal trauma: basic science, management, and reconstruction. 3rd Edition. Philadelphia: Saunders; 2003. Turf Toe.

37. Tewes DP, Fischer DA, Fritts HM, et al. MRI findings of acute turf toe. A case report and review of anatomy. Clin Orthop Relat Res 1994;(304):200–3.

# Imaging of Soft Tissue Lesions of the Foot and Ankle

Laura W. Bancroft, MD[a,b,*], Jeffrey J. Peterson, MD[c],
Mark J. Kransdorf, MD[c]

**KEYWORDS**

• Foot • Ankle • Tumor-like conditions • Tumor • MRI

The differential diagnosis of soft tissue lesions of the foot can be narrowed significantly with the aid of imaging. The cystic nature of ganglia, synovial cysts, and bursitis can be confirmed with MR imaging or sonography. Location and signal characteristics of noncystic lesions of the foot can suggest a diagnosis of Morton's neuroma, giant cell tumor of tendon sheath, and plantar fibromatosis. Synovial-based lesions of the foot and ankle can be differentiated with a variety of imaging modalities, based on the presence or absence of mineralization, lesion density, signal intensity, and enhancement pattern. Finally, knowledge of the incidence of specific neoplasms of the foot and ankle based on patient age aids radiologists in providing a limited differential diagnosis.

## TUMOR-LIKE LESIONS
### Cystic Tumor–Like Lesions

#### Ganglia

Ganglia are the most common soft tissue masses in the foot and ankle, representing more than 40% of suspected soft tissue masses.[1] Ganglia are myxoid lesions that occur around joints or tendon sheaths and often are multiloculated. They likely are caused by the coalescence of small cysts formed by myxomatous degeneration of periarticular connective tissue.[2] Ganglia often are diagnosed clinically and never imaged; however, MR imaging can be helpful if the ganglion is palpable or symptomatic because of extension along a nerve

or tendon or into the tarsal tunnel.[3] Palpable lesions in the foot and ankle are most common around the tarsometatarsal joint, and clinicallyoccult ganglia are most common in the sinus tarsi and tarsal canal.[1] Classic MR imaging features include a well-defined, cystic structure that is hyperintense on fluid-sensitive sequences (**Fig. 1**). Ganglia are well defined on sonography, and can be variable in appearance, ranging from anechoic to hypoechoic, often with multiple internal septations.[4]

#### Synovial cysts

Synovial cysts are synovial-lined, juxta-articular fluid collections that can form in response to effusions associated with internal joint derangement or arthritis.[2] MR imaging of uncomplicated synovial cysts in the foot and ankle delineate fluid signal intensity foci communicating with an abnormal joint (**Fig. 2**). Complicated cysts resulting from prior hemorrhage or infection have more complex signal intensities.

#### Adventitial bursa

Adventitial bursae form when abnormal friction develops between opposing rigid structures. Adventital bursae are not uncommon in the foot and, when inflamed, the resulting adventitial bursitis may simulate a painful mass. In a study of 24 patients who had hallux valgus and hallux rigidus, Schweitzer and colleagues found a 70% incidence of adventitial bursitis subjacent to the first metatarsophalangeal joint, likely related to altered stress on the submetatarsal soft tissue.[5] MR imaging

---

[a] Department of Radiology, University of Central Florida, Florida Hospital, 601 East Rollins Street, Orlando, FL 32803, USA
[b] Mayo Clinic College of Medicine, Rochester, MN, USA
[c] Mayo Clinic, 4500 San Pablo Boulevard, Jacksonville, FL 32224, USA
* Corresponding author. Department of Radiology, University of Central Florida, Florida Hospital, 601 East Rollins Street, Orlando, FL 32803.
E-mail address: laura.bancroft@flhosp.org (L.W. Bancroft).

Radiol Clin N Am 46 (2008) 1093–1103
doi:10.1016/j.rcl.2008.08.007

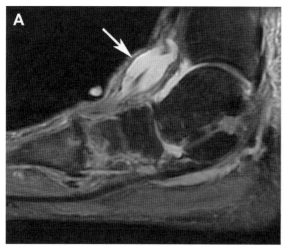
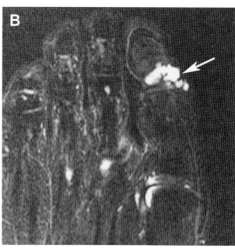

Fig. 1. Ganglion. (*A*) Sagittal FSE T2-weighted, fat-suppressed image through the foot demonstrates a well-circumscribed cystic focus (*arrow*) along the extensor hallucis longus tendon sheath, consistent with ganglion. Overlying soft tissue marker indicates that this was palpable. (*B*) Long-axis STIR image through the forefoot shows a multiloculated ganglion (*arrow*) adjacent to the first interphalangeal joint.

reflects the degree of active inflammation. Inactive bursitis shows little fluid and enhancement interrupting the subcutaneous fat, whereas active inflammation shows greater degrees of fluid and peripheral enhancement (**Fig. 3**).

## Noncystic Tumor–Like Lesions

### Morton's neuroma
Morton's neuroma, also known as interdigital neuroma, is a benign nontumorous lesion associated with neural degeneration and perineural fibrosis, most often located within the second and third interspaces.[6] Patients typically complain of pain radiating to the toes and numbness, although approximately a third of patients are asymptomatic.[7] MR imaging is accurate in diagnosing Morton's neuromas, and coronal short-axis T1-weighted imaging through the level of the metatarsophalangeal joints is the most important imaging plane.[6] MR imaging typically demonstrates a rounded intermediate soft tissue nodule in the affected interspace outlined by the adjacent fat. The relatively low signal intensity of Morton's neuroma is because this is reactive fibrosis and not a true neuroma (**Fig. 4**).[6]

### Rheumatoid nodules
Rheumatoid nodules occur in approximately 20% to 30% of rheumatoid patients, more commonly affecting women who have advanced disease.[8] Histologically, these are granulomatous foci with areas of central necrosis.[9] Nodules occur along the superficial subcutaneous tissues overlying areas susceptible to trauma, bursae, joints, tendons, or ligaments.[8] Although rheumatoid nodules are most common along the extensor surface of the upper extremity, they also can occur in the foot. MR imaging features include a nonspecific, ill-defined mass with prolonged T1 and T2 relaxation times (**Fig. 5**).[9] Diagnostic confidence can be improved if there is a clinical history of rheumatoid arthritis and active inflammatory marrow signal changes, joint effusion, and synovitis.

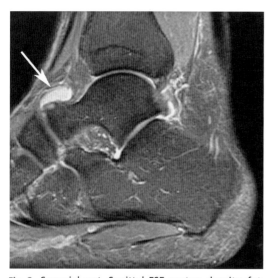

Fig. 2. Synovial cyst. Sagittal FSE proton density, fat-suppressed image shows a synovial cyst (*arrow*) extending dorsally from the degenerative talonavicular joint.

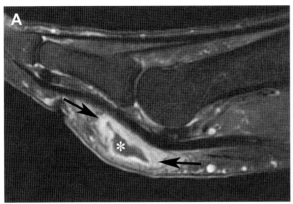
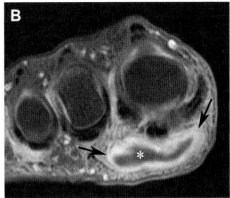

Fig. 3. Adventital bursitis. (*A*) Sagittal and (*B*) coronal, short-axis, enhanced, T1-weighted, fat-suppressed images through the forefoot show a peripherally enhancing (*arrows*) fluid collection (*asterisk*) in the superficial plantar soft tissues adjacent to the first metatarsal head, consistent with adventitial bursitis.

### Callus

Soft tissue callus is a superficial soft tissue thickening overlying pressure points that forms in response to mechanical pressure. Calluses typically are seen within the submetatarsal soft tissues of the forefoot. Although benign and relatively common in the average adult population, calluses potentially can ulcerate and lead to deeper infection in diabetic patients. MR imaging can define the extent of the intermediate to low signal intensity calluses (**Fig. 6**), which should not be confused with more ominous pathology.[10]

### Synovial-Based Processes

#### Synovial chondromatosis

Primary synovial chondromatosis is an uncommon, benign disorder in which multiple hyaline cartilage nodules are formed within a joint, tendon sheath, or bursa (**Fig. 7**).[11] Although historically believed to be metaplastic transformation of synovium into cartilage, chromosome 6 aberrations have been identified in cases of synovial chondromatosis, strongly suggesting a neoplastic process.[12,13] The knee is the most commonly involved joint (more than 50% of cases), followed by the elbow, hip, and shoulder; the foot and ankle are uncommonly involved.[2] Patients typically are in the third through fifth decades and men are affected two to four times more often than women.[2,14]

Radiographs may be unremarkable or show a synovial-based mass with or without erosions; calcifications occur in approximately 70% to 95% of cases.[11] MR imaging or MR arthrography usually shows many similar-sized bodies within the joint, tendon sheath, or bursa. The signal characteristics of the bodies depend on whether or not they are mineralized. Unmineralized bodies closely parallel imaging characteristics of hyaline

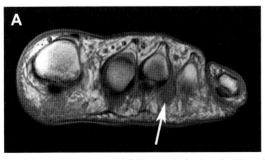
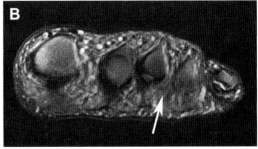

Fig. 4. Morton's neuroma. (*A*) Coronal, short-axis, T1-weighted image through the level of the metatarsophalangeal joints demonstrates a rounded intermediate signal soft tissue nodule (*arrow*) in the third intermetatarsal space, plantar to the transverse ligament. The subcutaneous fat serves as effective contrast to this Morton's neuroma. (*B*) This nodule (*arrow*) is less conspicuous on FSE T2-weighted image. The relatively low signal intensity of Morton's neuroma is because this is reactive fibrosis and not a true neuroma.

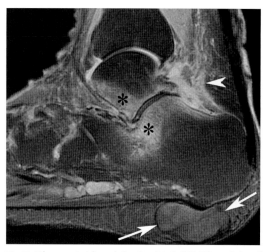

Fig. 5. Rheumatoid nodule. Sagittal, FSE T2-weighted fat-suppressed image shows a well-circumscribed rheumatoid nodule (*arrows*) in the plantar soft tissues of this patient who had rheumatoid arthritis. Notice the active inflammatory marrow signal changes (*asterisks*), joint effusion, and synovitis (*arrowhead*) about the subtalar joint.

cartilage, with hyperintense, lobulated signal on fluid-sensitive sequences. Mineralized osteochondral bodies can appear as signal voids resulting from dense mineralization or they may approximate fatty marrow signal intensity.[2,11]

### Pigmented villonodular synovitis

Pigmented villonodular synovitis (PVNS) is a commonly used synonym for what the World

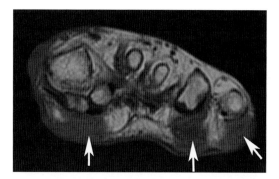

Fig. 6. Callus. Coronal, short-axis, T1-weighted image through the forefoot shows three foci of intermediate signal intensity (*arrows*) that replace the plantar fat pad deep to the metatarsal heads. These calluses form at pressure points in response to mechanical pressure. Notice the intrinsic muscular atrophy in this diabetic patient.

Health Organization officially terms, *diffuse-type giant cell tumor* (**Fig. 8**).[15] PVNS is a proliferation of synovium that grossly resembles a shaggy red beard and may be located intra-articularly, extra-articularly, or both. In a review of 14 cases of PVNS in the foot and ankle from the Scottish Bone Tumor Registry, the mean age of affected individuals was 26 years old with a slight female predominance.[16] Pathology involved the hindfoot in the majority of cases, followed by the mid- and forefoot.[16]

Lesions are not mineralized; however, joint effusions can be dense on conventional radiography. PVNS can result in erosions on both sides of a joint. MR imaging of PVNS commonly demonstrates hemosiderin deposition within the inflamed synovium. T1-weighted imaging typically shows mixed intermediate to low signal intensity soft tissue throughout the involved joint, persistent low signal intensity on fluid-sensitive sequences, and characteristic "blooming" (further signal loss) on gradient-echo imaging. Complete excision is the treatment of choice; however, a 14% recurrence rate has been reported.[16]

### Gout

The tophaceous form of gout is a tumor-like process that occurs most commonly as a late manifestation of the disease. Radiographic changes develop only after repeated attacks and develop in approximately 40% of patients. Focal urate deposits typically are dense on radiographs and often are associated with well-marginated erosions of the adjacent bone. Tophi are denser than skeletal muscle but not as dense as bone, with rare calcification on CT (**Fig. 9**). On CT, tophi have a mean attenuation of 160 to 170 Hounsfield units. Although lesions typically involve the metatarsophalangeal or interphalangeal joint of the great toe, tophaceous gout can result in extensive, multiple, soft tissue masses with destruction of multiple bones of the foot (**Fig. 10**).[17] Gouty tophi typically are isointense to muscle on T1-weighted sequences but can display variable signal intensity on fluid-sensitive sequences.[18] Tophi typically demonstrate variable, heterogeneous, predominantly peripheral gadolinium enhancement.

## TUMORS

In an evaluation of more than 39,000 tumor cases compiled from a referral database, Kransdorf reported the most common benign soft tissue tumors of the foot and ankle based on patient age.[19,20] In the pediatric subset, fibromatosis and granuloma annulare proved the most common benign tumors sent

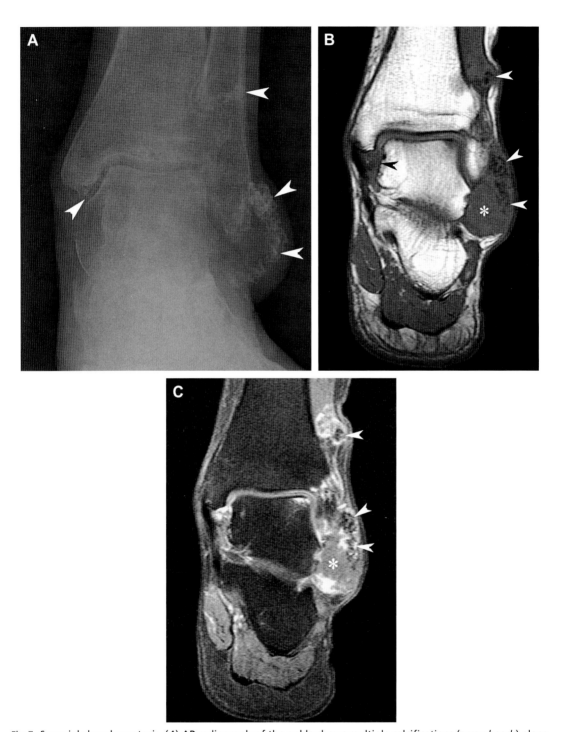

Fig. 7. Synovial chondromatosis. (*A*) AP radiograph of the ankle shows multiple calcifications (*arrowheads*) along the lateral malleolus, fibula and medial ankle joint. Coronal T1-weighted images (*B*) pre- and (*C*) post contrast delineate the corresponding signal voids (*arrowheads*) that represent multiple osteochondral bodies in the peroneal tendon sheath and ankle joint. Intermediate signal intensity soft tissue (*asterisks*) in the tendon sheath is due to unmineralized, neoplastic chondral bodies.

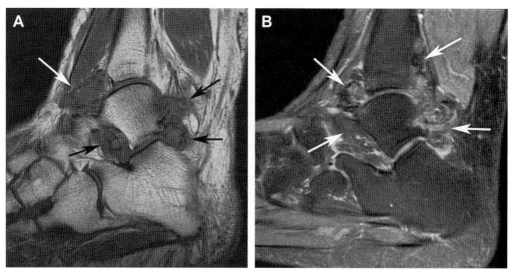

**Fig. 8.** PVNS. (*A*) Sagittal T1-weighted image through the ankle shows extensive, mixed intermediate to low signal intensity soft tissue (*arrows*) throughout the ankle joint, subtalar joint, and sinus tarsi. (*B*) FSE T2-weighted, fat-suppressed image shows persistent low signal intensity resulting from hemosiderin deposition within the extensive synovitis. Gradient-echo imaging characteristically results in further signal loss, termed blooming.

for referral; synovial sarcoma, dermatofibrosarcoma protuberans, and rhabdomyosarcoma were the most common malignant tumors of the foot and ankle. In the adult foot and ankle, fibromatosis and giant cell tumor of tendon sheath were the most common benign tumors; synovial sarcoma, malignant fibrous histiocytoma (undifferentiated pleomophic sarcoma), and

leiomyosarcoma were the most common malignant tumors.

## Plantar Fibromatosis

Plantar fibromatosis is a type of superficial fibromatosis categorized under "fibroblastic/myofibroblastic tumors" by the World Health

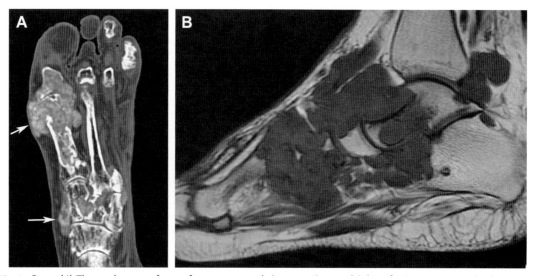

**Fig. 9.** Gout. (*A*) The tophaceous form of gout can result in extensive, multiple soft tissue masses. This long-axis, reformatted, CT image shows mineralized tophi (*arrows*) destroying the first metatarsal and the midfoot. (*B*) Sagittal T1-weighted image of multifocal gout in a different patient presents with extensive intermediate signal soft tissue masses throughout the synovial joints of the hind- and midfoot.

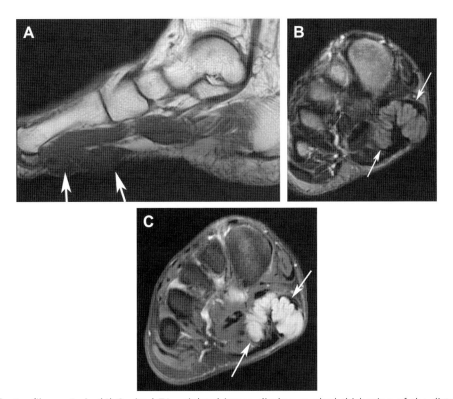

Fig. 10. Plantar fibromatosis. (A) Sagittal T1-weighted image displays marked thickening of the distal plantar fascia (arrows), which is isointense to skeletal muscle. Coronal, short-axis (B), FSE T2-weighted, and (C) enhanced, T1-weighted, fat-suppressed images show an accordion-like arrangement (arrows) of redundant fibromatosis along the plantar fascia.

Organization.[21] Plantar fibromatosis is a nodular fibrous proliferation arising from the plantar aponeurosis, often in non–weight-bearing regions.[22] Lesions occur more often in men, are bilateral in 20% to 50% of cases, and are more common in epileptics, diabetics, and alcoholics who have liver disease.[22,23] On sonography, plantar fibromatosis typically is a fusiform, hypoechoic, or heterogeneous mass located in the middle or distal plantar fascia.[4] On MR imaging, these infiltrative masses grow along the aponoreuosis; most are heterogeneous, isointense to slightly hyperintense to skeletal muscle on fluid-sensitive sequences, and exhibit variable enhancement (Fig. 11).[24]

## Giant Cell Tumor of Tendon Sheath

Giant cell tumor of tendon sheath is one of the so-called fibrohistiocytic tumors designated by the World Health Organization, in which a circumscribed proliferation of synovial-like tissue arises from the synovium of tendon sheaths.[25] This is the localized form of giant cell tumors, occurring most often in patients between ages 30 and 50 and more often in

women. On sonography, lesions typically are solid, homogeneous, hypoechoic masses with internal vascularity.[26] Giant cell tumors of tendon sheath are focal soft tissue nodules located along tendon sheaths, demonstrating decreased signal on T1- and T2-weighted sequences (similar to pigmented villondular synovitis) as a result of hemosiderin content[27] (see Fig. 9). Local excision is the treatment, and recurrence rates in the literature range from 0 to 30%.[25,28]

## Lipoma

Lipoma is a benign tumor comprised of mature adipocytes and is the most common mesenchymal soft tissue tumor in adults.[29] Tumors are most common in patients between ages 40 and 60, are more common in obese patients, and can be multiple in approximately 5% of patients.[29] Cytogenetic markers have been found in the majority of lipomas, including aberrations of 12q13–15.[30]

Lipomas are common benign tumors that usually are never imaged. Because of their fatty composition, lipomas are less dense than surrounding

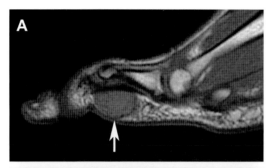

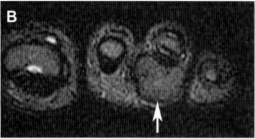

Fig. 11. Giant cell tumor of tendon sheath. (*A*) Sagittal T1-weighted image shows a well-circumscribed nodule (*arrow*) along the third flexor tendon sheath that is slightly hyperintense to skeletal muscle. (*B*) Coronal, short axis, conventional T2-weighted image shows a rim of low signal intensity around the intermediate to low signal nodule (*arrow*). Signal characteristics are in keeping with pathologically proved giant cell tumor of tendon sheath.

soft tissue on radiographs. On sonography, lipomas are variable in their echogenicity but often are elliptic, well circumscribed, and have their longest dimension paralleling the skin.[4] MR imaging is diagnostic, demonstrating a soft tissue mass that is isointense to subcutaneous fat on all sequences (**Fig. 12**). A few thin septations may be present, but

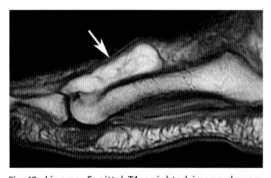

Fig. 12. Lipoma. Sagittal T1-weighted image demonstrates a fatty mass (*arrow*) paralleling the metatarsal shaft contains a few thin septae, consistent with lipoma. Notice there are fewer septae in the lipoma relative to the plantar subcutaneous fat. Lipomas are common benign tumors that usually are never imaged.

they should be fewer in number relative to the adjacent subcutaneous fat. Displacement of muscle fibers in intramuscular lipomas could be mistaken for septations if not fully evaluated on several imaging planes.

## Soft Tissue Chondroma

Soft tissue chondroma is one of two "chondro-osseous tumors" designated by the World Health Organization.[31] Chondromas are benign extraosseous and extrasynovial soft tissue tumors composed primarily of mature hyaline cartilage, occurring in a variety of age ranges, with a slight male predominance.[31] Although most lesions occur around the fingers, soft tissue chondromas can occur around the foot and ankle. Mineralization is invariably present on radiographs. MR imaging demonstrates a soft tissue mass approximating cartilage signal intensity. If mineralization is present, this is evident by corresponding signal voids (**Fig. 13**). Lesions can become large and may be mistaken for chondrosarcoma.[32] Surgical excision typically is curative; however, up to 20% recur and malignant transformation to chondrosarcoma has been reported in rare instances.[31]

## Synovial Sarcoma

Synovial sarcoma is classified under "tumors of uncertain differentiation" by the World Health Organization.[33] These are mesenchymal, spindle-cell tumors that display epithelial differentiation and biphasic morphology, histologically resemble synovial cells (but are not actually derived from them), and have a cytogenic hallmark of t(X;18)(p11;q11).[33] Synovial sarcoma can occur in any age group but most occur in young adults and there is a male predominance.[33] Most cases of synovial sarcoma arise in the deep soft tissues around the knee; synovial sarcoma occurs less commonly in the foot and ankle. Lesions typically are lobulated soft tissue masses that can invade multiple compartments of the foot and erode into the bones (**Fig. 14**). Approximately a third of cases demonstrate mineralization on radiographs.[2] MR imaging shows fluid-fluid levels in approximately 10% to 25% of cases due to prior hemorrhage, and MR imaging also may show "triple" signal intensity resulting from a combination of cystic and solid components.[2,34] Surgical resection is the treatment. Approximately half of synovial sarcomas recur and approximately 40% metastasize to the lungs, bones, or regional lymph nodes.[33]

## Undifferentiated Pleomorphic Sarcoma

Undifferentiated high grade pleomorphic sarcoma (UPS) is categorized as a "so-called fibrohistiocytic

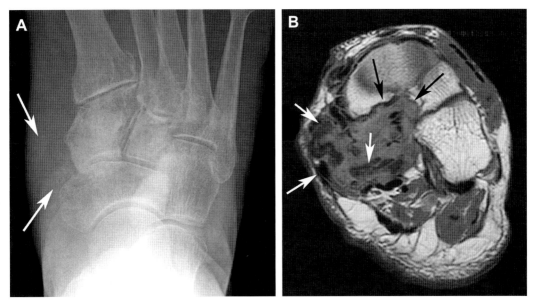

Fig. 13. Soft tissue chondroma. (*A*) AP radiograph of the midfoot shows multiple coarse calcifications (*arrows*) within a medially located soft tissue mass. (*B*) Coronal, short-axis, T1-weighted image through the mass shows signal voids (*white arrows*) corresponding to the regions of radiographically visible mineralization. Subtle scalloping (*black arrows*) of the cuneiforms, as opposed to cortical destruction, reflects the nonaggressive nature of this tumor.

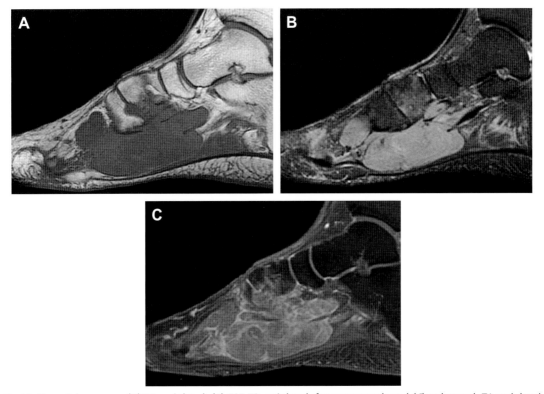

Fig. 14. Synovial sarcoma. (*A*) T1-weighted; (*B*) FSE T2-weighted, fat-suppressed; and (*C*) enhanced, T1-weighted images show a large, lobulated soft tissue mass along the plantar aspect of the foot, which invades multiple compartments of the foot and erodes into the bones. The mass proved to be a synovial sarcoma at resection.

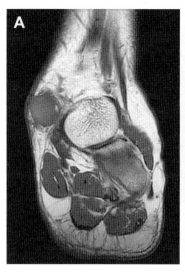 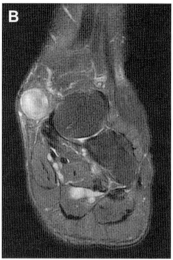

**Fig. 15.** Leiomyosarcoma. Corona (A) T1-weighted and (B) FSE T2 weighted fat suppressed image through the hindfoot demonstrate a well-circumscribed, nonspecific superficial nodule medial to the ta lus. Resection was performed, with pathologic diagnosis of leiomyosarcoma. Patient underwent tumor resection with sural artery fasciocutaneous flap, preoperative and intraoperative adjuvant radiation therapy.

tumour" by the World Health Organization, and was previously termed malignant fibrous histiocytoma (MFH).[35] Pleomorphic (MFH-like) sarcoma represents the most common type of sarcoma in patients older than 40 years of age, and there is a slight male predominance.[35] Although approximately half of these tumors occur in the lower extremity, undifferentiated pleomorphic sarcoma is more common in the thigh than in the foot and ankle.[36] Imaging reveals nonspecific solid soft tissue masses, with the majority of tumors occurring in the deep intramuscular compartments.[36] MR imaging characteristics depend upon the variable amount of collagen, myxoid tissue, necrosis and hemorrhage.[36] Fluid-sensitive sequences often reveal hyperintense signal within the mass, although signal is variable and masses can also be hypointense to skeletal muscle. High grade pleomorphic sarcomas have a poor prognosis, with an overall 5-year survival of 50–60%.[37]

## Leiomyosarcoma

Leiomyosarcoma is a malignant smooth muscle tumor that usually occurs in middle-aged or old patients, and most often in the retroperitoneum.[38] Tumors can originate from the major blood vessels, soft tissue or dermis. Leiomyosarcomas only account for approximately 10–15% of limb sarcomas, and can occasionally be seen in the foot and ankle.[38] Radiographic mineralization is reported in approximately 15% of soft tissue lesions, and magnetic resonance imaging features are nonspecific (**Fig. 15**) with large lesions demonstrating hemorrhage, necrosis and cystic change.[39] Subcutaneous lesions are generally larger and associated with a less favorable prognosis than dermal lesions.[39] Leiomyosarcoma is

capable of both local recurrence and distant metastases, although regional lymph node involvement is rare.[38]

## REFERENCES

1. Weishaupt D, Schweitzer MR, Morrison WB, et al. MRI of the foot and ankle: prevalence and distribution of occult and probable ganglia. J Magn Reson Imaging 2001;14:464–71.
2. Kransdorf MJ, Murphey MD. Synovial tumors. In: Kransdorf MJ, Murphey MD, editors. Imaging of soft tissue tumors. 2nd edition. Philadelphia: Lippincott Williams & Wilkins; 2006. p. 381–436.
3. Costa CR, Morrison WB, Carrino JA, et al. MRI of an intratendinous ganglion cyst of the peroneus brevis tendon. AJR Am J Roentgenol 2003;181:890–1.
4. Pham H, Fessell DP, Femino JE, et al. Sonography and MR imaging of selected benign masses in the ankle and foot. AKR Am J Roentgenol 2003;180: 99–107.
5. Schweitzer ME, Maheshwari S, Shabshin N. Hallux valgus and hallux rigidus: MRI findings. Clin Imaging 1999;23:397–402.
6. Zanetti M, Ledermann T, Zollinger H, et al. Efficacy of MR imaging in patients suspected of having Morton's neuroma. AJR Am J Roentgenol 1997; 168:529–32.
7. Bencardino J, Rosenberg ZS, Beltran X, et al. Morton's neuroma: is it always symptomatic? AJR Am J Roentgenol 2000;175:649–53.
8. Boutry N, Flipo RM, Cotten A. MR imaging appearance of rheumatoid arthritis in the foot. Semin Musculoskelet Radiol 2005;9:199–209.
9. Sanders TG, Linares R, Su A. Rheumatoid nodule of the foot: MRI appearances mimicking an

indeterminate soft tissue mass. Skeletal Radiol 1998; 27:457–60.

0. Schweitzer ME, Morrison WB. MR imaging of the diabetic foot. Radiol Clin North Am 2004;42:61–71.

11. Murphey MD, Vidal JA, Fanburg-Smith JC, et al. Imaging of synovial chondromatosis with radiologic-pathologic correlation. RadioGraphics 2007; 27:1465–88.

12. Weiss SW, Goldblum JR. Cartilaginous soft tissue tumors. In: Enzinger and weiss's soft tissue tumors. 4th edition. St Louis: Mosby; 2001. p. 1361–88.

13. Buddingh EP, Krallman P, Neff JR, et al. Chromosome 6 abnormalities are recurrent in synovial chondromatosis. Cancer Genet Cytogenet 2003;140:18–22.

14. Unni KK, Inwards CY, Bridge JA, et al. Synovial tumors. In: Tumors of the bone and joints. 4th edition. Silver Spring, MD: ARP Press; 2005. p. 386–432.

15. de St. Aubain Somerhause N, Dal Cin P. Diffuse-type giant cell tumour. In: Fletcher CDM, Unni JJ, Mertens F, editors. World Health Organization classification of tumours: tumours of soft tissue and bone. Lyon FR: IARC Press; 2000. p. 112–4.

16. Sharma H, Jane MJ, Reid R. Pigmented villonodular synovitis of the foot and ankle: forty years of experience from the Scottish bone tumor registry. J Foot Ankle Surg 2006;45:329–36.

17. Johnson PT, Fayad LM, Fishman EK. CT of the foot: selected inflammatory arthritides. J Comput Assist Tomogr 2007;31:961–9.

18. Yu JS, Chung C, Recht M, et al. MR imaging of tophaceous gout. AJR Am J Roentgenol 1997;168: 523–7.

19. Kransdorf MJ. Benign soft-tissue tumors in a large referral population: distribution of specific diagnoses by age, sex, and location. AJR Am J Roentgenol 1995; 164:395–402.

20. Kransdorf MJ. Malignant soft-tissue tumors in a large referral population: distribution of diagnoses by age, sex, and location. AJR Am J Roentgenol 1995;164: 129–34.

21. Goldblum JR, Fletcher JA. Superficial fibromatoses. In: Fletcher CDM, Unni JJ, Mertens F, editors. World Health Organization classification of tumours: tumours of soft tissue and bone. Lyon FR: IARC Press; 2000. p. 81–2.

22. Weiss SW, Goldblum JR. Fibromatoses. In: Enzinger and weiss's soft tissue tumors. 4th edition. St. Louis: Mosby; 2001. p. 309–46.

23. Robbin MR, Murphey MD, Temple T, et al. Imaging of musculoskeletal fibromatosis. RadioGraphics 2001;21:585–600.

24. Morrison WB, Schweitzer ME, Wapner KL, et al. Plantar fibromatosis. Radiology 1994;193:841–5.

25. De St. Aubain Somerhausen N, Dal Cin P. Giant cell tumour of tendon sheath. In: Fletcher CDM, Unni JJ, Mertens F, editors. World Health Organization classification of tumours: tumours of soft tissue and bone. Lyon FR: IARC Press; 2000. p. 110–1.

26. Middleton WD, Patel V, Teefey SA, et al. Giant cell tumors of the tendon sheath: analysis of sonographic findings. AJR Am J Roentgenol 2004;183:337–9.

27. Jelinek JS, Kransdorf MJ, Shmookler BM, et al. Giant cell tumor of the tendon sheath: MR findings in nine cases. AJR Am J Roentgenol 1994;162:919–22.

28. Gholve PA, Hosalkar HS, Kreiger PA, et al. Giant cell tumor of tendon sheath: largest single series in children. J Pediatr Orthop 2007;27:67–74.

29. Nielsen GP, Mandahi N. Lipoma. In: Fletcher CDM, Unni JJ, Mertens F, editors. World Health Organization classification of tumours: tumours of soft tissue and bone. Lyon FR: IARC Press; 2000. p. 20–2.

30. Mandahl N, Hoglund M, Mertens F, et al. Cytogenetic aberrations in 188 benign and borderline adipose tissue tumors. Genes Chromosomes Cancer 1994;9:207–15.

31. Nayler S, Heim S. Soft tissue chondroma. In: Fletcher CDM, Unni JJ, Mertens F, editors. World Health Organization classification of tumours: tumours of soft tissue and bone. Lyon FR: IARC Press; 2000. p. 180–1.

32. Papagelopoulos PJ, Savvidou OD, Mavrogenis AF, et al. Extraskeletal chondroma of the foot. Joint Bone Spine 2007;74:285–8.

33. Fisher C, de Bruijn DHR, Geurts van kessel A. Synovial sarcoma. In: Fletcher CDM, Unni JJ, Mertens F, editors. World Health Organization classification of tumours: tumours of soft tissue and bone. Lyon FR: IARC Press; 2000. p. 200–4.

34. Nakanishi H, Araki N, Sawai Y, et al. Cystic synovial sarcomas: imaging features with clinical and histopathologic correlation. Skeletal Radiol 2003;32:701–7.

35. Fletcher CDM, van den Berg E, Molenaar WM, et al. Pleomorphic malignant fibrous histiocytoma/undifferentiated high grade pleomorphic sarcoma. In: Fletcher CDM, Unni JJ, Mertens F, editors. World Health Organization classification of tumours: tumours of soft tissue and bone. Lyon FR: IARC Press; 2000. p. 120–2.

36. Kransdorf MJ, Murphey MD, et al. Malignant fibrous and fibrohistiocytic tumors. In: Kransdorf MJ, Murphey MD, editors. Imaging of soft tissue tumors. 2nd edition. Philadelphia: Lippincott Williams & Wilkins; 2006. p. 257–97.

37. Gustafson P. Soft tissue sarcoma. Epidemiology and prognosis in 508 patients. Acta Orthop Scand Suppl 1994;259:1–31.

38. Evans HL, Shipley J. Leiomyosarcoma. In: Fletcher CDM, Unni JJ, Mertens F, editors. World Health Organization classification of tumours: tumours of soft tissue and bone. Lyon FR: IARC Press; 2000. p. 131–4.

39. Kransdorf MJ, Murphey MD, et al. Muscle tumors. In: Kransdorf MJ, Murphey MD, editors. Imaging of soft tissue tumors. 2nd edition. Philadelphia: Lippincott Williams & Wilkins; 2006. p. 298–327.

# Current Concepts in Imaging Diabetic Pedal Osteomyelitis

Andrea Donovan, MD[a],*, Mark E. Schweitzer, MD[b]

**KEYWORDS**

- Diabetes • Foot • Osteomyelitis
- Neuropathic arthritis • Imaging

The prevalence of diabetes mellitus in the United States estimated at 7%. Diabetes-related foot ulceration and infection are associated with considerable morbidity and health care expense.[1,2] The lifetime risk for foot ulceration in diabetic patients is as high as 25%.[3] More than one-half of foot ulcers become infected,[4–7] which may necessitate hospital admission.[8] The health care cost associated with diabetic foot ulceration and infection was estimated at $10.9 billion in 2001 in the United States alone.[2] Although many diabetic foot infections are limited to soft tissue, osseous involvement occurs in 20% to 65% of cases.[9,10]

The diagnosis and management of diabetes-related osteomyelitis is challenging and requires a multidisciplinary team approach.[10] Radiologists have an important role to confirm diagnosis and evaluate the extent of infection. This may help reduce the incidence of infection-related morbidities, the need for and duration of hospitalization, and the incidence of major limb amputation.[11] Diabetes-related foot infection is the most common cause of nontraumatic amputation of the lower extremity.[9,12,13] It is estimated that one amputation is performed every 30 seconds somewhere in the world as a consequence of diabetes. Amputation is a major risk for future contralateral limb amputation secondary to altered weight bearing.[10,14] Early diagnosis of infection is important to reduce the risk for amputation.[15] The current approach to treatment of pedal infection includes early and aggressive orthodic use for altered weight bearing,

wound care, appropriate antibiotics,[16] and medical and surgical revascularization procedures to limit or obviate amputation.[17,18] If amputation becomes necessary, however, imaging may help limit the extent of resection by mapping the preoperative extent of infection.[19,20]

## PATHOGENESIS OF DIABETIC PEDAL OSTEOMYELITIS

Nearly all diabetes-related foot infections result from contiguous spread from a skin ulcer.[21] The risk factors for the development of a foot ulcer are strongly related to vascular disease and resultant neuropathy. These factors act in combination with other factors, such as unrecognized trauma, to accelerate superimposed infection and impede healing.[22,23] Micro- and macroangiopathy are recognized as initiating events in the cascade of foot ulceration and infection.[24] The current diagnosis of vascular insufficiency is based primarily on evaluation of macroangiopathy[25–27] and this may guide revascularization with grafting, angioplasty, or stenting procedures.[28] Microangiopathy in diabetic patients, however, is a major contributor to peripheral vascular disease and subsequent end-organ ischemia. Microvascular basement membrane alterations related to longstanding hyperglycemia are a hallmark of diabetes, and result in impaired capillary vascular dilation and permeability. The result is a decrease in end-organ perfusion reserve,[29] which contributes to impaired

[a] Department of Medical Imaging, Sunnybrook Health Sciences Centre, Room AG 278, 2075 Bayview Avenue, Toronto, Ontario M4N 3M5, Canada
[b] Department of Radiology, The Ottawa Hospital, General Campus, 501 Smyth Road, Module S-1, Ottawa, Ontario K1H 8L6, Canada
* Corresponding author.
*E-mail address:* andrea.donovan@sunnybrook.ca (A. Donovan).

Radiol Clin N Am 46 (2008) 1105–1124
doi:10.1016/j.rcl.2008.08.004

wound healing despite revascularization.[22] Furthermore, a lack of adequate stress-induced capillary vasodilation contributes to neuroarthropathy after minor trauma and to osteomyelitis after soft tissue infection. The later is to some degree related to the limited ability to respond to and localize early infection.

Peripheral neuropathy plays an important role in ulcer development and may be attributed to disturbances in sensory, motor, or autonomic function.[23,30] Motor neuropathy leads to atrophy of the intrinsic foot musculature and, to a lesser degree, the calf musculature. The resultant abnormal foot anatomy and biomechanics lead to excess pressure, callus formation, and ulcers. Loss of protective sensation related to sensory neuropathy leads to repetitive unattended injury and inadequate ulcer healing. Autonomic dysfunction leads to hypohydrosis and to dry, cracked skin, which accelerates skin ulceration.[10,31] Ulcer healing is impaired further by arterial vascular insufficiency and immunodeficiency in longstanding diabetes. A nonhealing ulcer can progress to a soft tissue infection, such as an abscess, or develop into a sinus tract extending to adjacent bone and subsequent osteomyelitis.

The microbiology of pedal osteomyelitis parallels that of the contiguous soft tissue infection and, therefore, usually is polymicrobial.[9] The most common pathogen cultured from infected bone samples is *Staphylococcus aureus*, followed by *S epidermidis*. Extension of infection into vascular channels impairs blood flow and may result in bone necrosis and sequestration of devitalized bone in chronic infection.

## EVALUATION OF DIABETIC PATIENTS WHO HAVE SUSPECTED OSTEOMYELITIS

The clinical diagnosis of diabetes-related osteomyelitis relies on identification and characterization of an associated foot ulcer. An ulcer that measures more than 2 cm$^2$ has an increased likelihood of underlying osteomyelitis.[9] Although a probe-to-bone test frequently is used clinically, it is not reliable in many cases.[32,33] An elevated erythrocyte sedimentation rate (greater than 70 mm/h) is 100% sensitive but absent in 70% of patients who have osteomyelitis.[34] The gold standard test for diagnosing osteomyelitis remains microbiologic diagnosis with a bone biopsy.[10] Superficial cultures are not sufficient as results do not correlate with those of bone biopsies.[35]

Imaging of the diabetic foot plays an important role in the diagnosis of osteomyelitis and evaluation of the extent of infection. One of the greatest challenges to radiologists is differentiating neuroarthropathy from superimposed infection. Until recently, guidelines for appropriate imaging of diabetes-related pedal osteomyelitis were unavailable. In August 2008, however, the American College of Radiology (ACR) released ACR Appropriateness Criteria to guide selection of appropriate imaging modality in diabetic patients who have suspected osteomyelitis.[36] ACR recommendations are based on several clinical scenarios, including early neuropathy, soft tissue swelling, skin ulcer, and suspected osteomyelitis. The appropriateness rating scale ranges from 1 to 9, with a rating of 1 the least appropriate and a rating of 9 the most appropriate. Radiography is recommended as the initial screening examination and MR imaging with or without contrast is recommended as the examination of choice. In patients who have contraindications to MR imaging, bone scintigraphy with $^{111}$In-labeled white blood cell scanning may be used. For detection of radiographically occult neuropathy, three-phase bone scan or CT may be used.

## RADIOGRAPHY EVALUATION OF PEDAL OSTEOMYELITIS

Radiographs are recommended as the initial imaging test to evaluate pedal osteomyelitis (ACR Appropriateness Criteria, rating 9).[36] The earliest radiographic changes of osteomyelitis include soft tissue swelling and blurring of adjacent fat planes. The classic findings include the triad of osteolysis, periosteal reaction, and bone destruction, although these usually are not apparent until 10 to 20 days after infection.[37] Radiographs have a sensitivity of 60% and specificity of 80% in diagnosing acute osteomyelitis.[38–40] Characteristic progressive changes, however, can be seen on serial radiographs. When a diagnosis of osteomyelitis is uncertain, the current Infectious Diseases Society of America guidelines recommend repeat radiographs after treatment in 2 to 4 weeks, rather than proceeding to advanced imaging modalities.[10] Important information can be obtained from radiographs, including evidence of prior amputation, foreign body, or abnormal alignment related to neuropathic disease. These may not be readily apparent on MR imaging, especially with nonerect imaging. Radiographic findings may aid in the selection and interpretation of subsequent imaging tests.

## NUCLEAR MEDICINE EVALUATION OF PEDAL OSTEOMYELITIS

Nuclear medicine plays a limited role in evaluation of diabetic pedal osteomyelitis.[41,42] It may help to dentify patients, however, in early, preradiographic stages of neuropathic osteoarthropathy. Technetium ($^{99m}$Tc) three-phase bone scan of the foot is recommended to evaluate soft tissue swelling in the absence of an ulcer (ACR Appropriateness Criteria, rating 5).[36] Bone scintigraphy is more sensitive than radiography or MR imaging in detecting neuroarthropathy.[43] Combined bone $^{99m}$Tc-methylene diphosphonate and $^{111}$In-labeled white blood cell scintigraphy is highly sensitive (90%) for detecting osteomyelitis, but specificity (70%–80%) may be hampered by coexisting pathologic processes, such as neuroarthropathy, trauma, or cellulitis.[44–46] It may be used, however, to image patients who have contraindication to MR imaging (ACR Appropriateness Criteria, rating 4). $^{67}$Ga is a marker of infection and inflammation, but uptake in areas with osteoblastic activity may give false-positive results (sensitivity 80% and specificity 69%).[47] Although $^{99m}$Tc-hexamethylpropyleneamine oxime white blood cell scintigraphy is highly sensitive (88%) and specific (96%), it is limited by being time consuming and requiring special equipment and trained personnel.[48] Immunoscintigraphy with $^{99m}$Tc-labeled antigranulocyte monoclonal antibody fragment has shown varied results (sensitivity 67%–90% and specificity 75%–85%).[49,50]

$^{18}$F-fluorodeoxy-D-2-glucose (FDG) is an indicator of cellular glucose metabolism and accumulates at sites of infection.[51] FDG–positron emission tomography (FDG-PET) offers the advantage of shorter study time, higher resolution, and higher target-to-background ratio than other metabolic procedures.[52] Increased uptake, however, also may be present in other disease processes with accelerated metabolic activity, such as a fracture or neoplasm.[53] Recent evaluation of PET/CT in diabetic patients who have clinically suspected osteomyelitis showed accurate differentiation between osteomyelitis and soft tissue infection.[54] Furthermore, FDG-PET may have use in the setting of diabetes to differentiate neuropathic disease from osteomyelitis.[55,56] A low-degree periarticular FDG uptake was observed in patients who have Charcot arthropathy osteoarthropathy, with maximum standardized uptake value (SUV$_{max}$) ranging from 0.7 to 2.4 (mean, 1.3 ± 0.4). The SUV$_{max}$ at sites of diabetic osteomyelitis in the absence of neuropathic disease measured 2.9 to 6.2 (mean 4.38 ± 0.39), compared with SUV$_{max}$ of 6.5 in one patient who had Charcot arthropathy and superimposed infection.[56] Further studies are needed to evaluate the role of FDG-PET in the evaluation of neuropathic osteoarthropathy with superimposed osteomyelitis. Currently, the ACR does not recommend PET/CT in evaluation of diabetes-related pedal osteomyelitis (ACR Appropriateness Criteria, rating 1). In the future, PET/MR also may have an important role by providing metabolic and soft tissue information. The associated costs, however, may not be insignificant.

## CT EVALUATION OF PEDAL OSTEOMYELITIS

CT may be useful to evaluate soft tissue swelling without an apparent ulcer[36] (ACR Appropriateness Criteria, rating 5). The diagnostic considerations in this setting include early neuroarthropathy or soft tissue infection. CT may detect neuroarthropathy that is not radiographically apparent. In patients who have an ulcer, CT is not recommended to evaluate osteomyelitis (ACR Appropriateness Criteria, rating 1).[36] It may be useful, however, in patients who have a contraindication to MR imaging (ACR Appropriateness Criteria, rating 5).[36] CT changes in acute osteomyelitis are not common but, when present, include replacement of normal intramedullary fat, periosteal reaction, and cortical destruction.[57] The soft tissues often demonstrate fat stranding or, occasionally, a focal collection.[58]

## ULTRASONOGRAPHY EVALUATION OF PEDAL OSTEOMYELITIS

Ultrasound currently is not recommended to evaluate the diabetic foot[36] (ACR Appropriateness Criteria, rating 1). In countries where ultrasound is more readily available than MR imaging, however, it represents the next imaging modality after radiography for evaluation of pedal infection. The presence of a subperiosteal abscess is the most common sonographic manifestation of pedal osteomyelitis. This is not present, however, in all cases. Care must be given to avoid misinterpreting a soft tissue abscess as a periosteal abscess and osteomyelitis.[59] The ultrasound criteria for infection are based primarily on long bone infection, and data on the usefulness of ultrasound to diagnose pedal osteomyelitis are limited.[36]

## MR IMAGING EVALUATION OF PEDAL OSTEOMYELITIS

MR imaging is the modality of choice for evaluation of pedal osteomyelitis and soft tissue infection (ACR Appropriateness Criteria rating 9). A recent meta-analysis evaluating the usefulness of MR imaging in diagnosing diabetic pedal osteomyelitis demonstrated a sensitivity of 90% and a specificity of 83%.[60] Unlike other imaging modalities (discussed previously), MR imaging has the advantage of providing exquisite anatomic detail of soft tissue and osseous structures. Clinical decision making in patients who have pedal infection is guided by the extent of infection and vascular perfusion.[61] Resection of infected and necrotic tissue is required to heal a chronic wound.[62] Accurate delineation of the extent of infection and associated soft tissue complications by MR imaging facilitates tissue sparing surgical resection, making MR imaging clinically useful and cost effective.[11]

### MR Imaging Protocol

The study should be tailored to individual patients and specific clinical questions by selecting the appropriate coil and protocol. Whenever possible, the foot should be examined without bandages to identify the ulcer. The authors recommend placing markers over shallow ulcers, which may not be apparent on imaging. The field of view is selected to include the area of clinical concern, usually tailored to forefoot, midfoot, or hindfoot. Use of a large field of view, such as that of the entire foot, should be avoided. Furthermore, both feet should not be imaged simultaneously.

For optimal visualization of toe ulcers, a forefoot protocol is recommended. The ideal coil is a small, 3- or 5-in surface coil; a wrist coil also can be used if the forefoot is small and not significantly deformed. A field of view of 10 to 14 cm is recommended. Forefoot anatomy is unique and imaging planes are distinct from those of the hindfoot. It is important for radiologists and technologists to use the same terminology to minimize the potential for confusion. A plane perpendicular to the toes may be termed, the short-axis view, and a plane parallel to the toes, the long-axis view. A minimum of two planes should be obtained to best visualize the area of interest. The most useful plane for imaging the toes is the short-axis view, as it provides excellent visualization of the ulcer and relationship to the underlying osseous structures. The corresponding longitudinal plane should be tangential to the ulcer (eg, sagittal view for a plantar ulcer and long-axis view for a medial ulcer). T1-weighted and T2-weighted, fat-suppressed, short-axis images are recommended to evaluate for marrow changes and adjacent soft tissue abnormalities. For flexed or deformed toes, a sagittal plane is most useful. Sagittal images also are helpful for evaluating septic arthritis and osteomyelitis associated with plantar or dorsal ulceration. T1-weighted and short tau inversion recovery (STIR) sequences are recommended in the sagittal plane. Fat suppression is more uniform with STIR than chemically fat-saturated T2-weighted images because of curvature of the foot surface. A long-axis view is best for depicting anatomic relationships and the extent of infection.

A T2-weighted fat-suppressed sequence may be used.

The midfoot and hindfoot are best imaged with an extremity chimney-type knee coil and a 14- to 16-cm field of view. The use of a sagittal plane is essential and T1- and STIR-weighted sequences should be used. Midfoot neuropathic disease and hindfoot calcaneal ulcers are best evaluated in the sagittal plane. Axial and coronal planes are useful for evaluating the adjacent soft tissues, especially in the presence of medial or lateral ulceration.

Contrast-enhanced images are useful for evaluating soft tissue complications, such as sinus tracts, abscesses, or areas of necrosis. This information is invaluable in the preoperative planning of limited limb resection. Pre- and post-contrast, T1-weighted, fat-suppressed sequences should be obtained to differentiate enhancement from inadequate fat suppression. Faster, gradient-echo sequences are used as an alternative to conventional T1-weighted sequences when limited time is available for the examination. The authors have found a pre- and postcontrast volumetric interpolated breath-hold examination useful, as diabetic patients often cannot tolerate long examinations.

A special mention is warranted regarding gadolinium use in imaging diabetic patients and potential complications related to nephrogenic systemic fibrosis (NSF). A link was reported between gadolinium-containing contrast agents and NSF in patients who have renal failure.[63–65] In 2006, the Food and Drug Administration issued a warning concerning gadolinium-based contrast agents.[66] Current ACR guidelines for the administration of gadolinium are based on the calculated glomerular filtration rate (GFR), patient age, and presence of diabetes or hypertension.[67] The ACR does not recommend routine laboratory evaluation in all patients before MR imaging because 90% of patients who have NSF are already on dialysis and the remainder have known, advanced renal failure. Individual radiology department guidelines, however, for the administration of gadolinium may be more rigorous, especially in patients who have diabetes. At the authors' institution, all patients who have diabetes undergo prescreening with calculation of GFR. Patients who have a moderately reduced GFR (30–60 mL/min/1.73 m$^2$) are considered for alternative imaging but still can receive gadolinium after a risk/benefit assessment. Consistent with current ACR guidelines,[36] gadolinium usually is not administered to patients who have severely reduced GFR (<30 mL/min/1.73 m$^2$).

## Skin Callus

Foot deformity in diabetic patients is common and results primarily from ligament disorders, tendon disorders, muscle atrophy, and joint disease.[68,69] Altered biomechanics and friction from ill-fitting footwear lead to callus formation at pressure points. The sites of callus formation occur at predictable weight-bearing sites, such as the forefoot beneath the first or fifth metatarsal heads and the tip of the great toe. One-fifth of calluses are seen in the hindfoot at the heel.[70] In the neuropathic foot, callus location is different: hallux valgus predisposes to callus formation medial to the first metatarsal, and rocker-bottom deformity related to midfoot-dominant neuropathic disease is associated with callus formation underneath the cuboid.[71] On MR imaging, callus appears as a focal prominence within the subcutaneous fat, usually characterized by low signal intensity on T1-weighted sequences and low to intermediate signal intensity on T2-weighted sequences (**Fig. 1**). Occasionally, callus enhancement post contrast may be mistaken for soft tissue infection, but atypical location and lack of adjacent soft tissue changes should aid in correct diagnosis.

In addition to callus formation, chronic friction may result in adventitial bursa formation at common pressure points. A thin, flattened fluid focus is situated over an osseous prominence and adjacent to a callus (**Fig. 2**). The absence of adjacent soft tissue inflammation should be confirmed on postcontrast images, as preservation of the adjacent subcutaneous fat may be a reliable sign to distinguish adventitial bursa from an abscess.

## Ulceration and Sinus Tract

Several factors contribute to callus breakdown, including dry skin related to autonomic dysfunction, altered weight bearing related to motor neuropathy, and persistent friction at pressure points.[72] Recognition of callus is important as prompt callus removal may reduce the likelihood of skin ulceration.[73]

Ulcer distribution is influenced by cumulative mechanical trauma as a result of an individual patient's gait characteristics, type of foot wear, and level of activity. Ulcer location generally parallels that of the callus distribution (listed previously), including the surface adjacent to the first and fifth metatarsal heads (**Fig. 3**), the plantar surface of the second and third metatarsal heads, and the dorsal surface of the toes in the setting of claw toe deformities.[70,74] In patients who have Charcot osteoarthropathy and rocker-bottom deformity, midfoot ulceration may occur superficial to the cuboid. Forefoot and midfoot ulcers typically are superficial and occur in ambulatory patients. In contrast, broad, deeper ulcers are more typical in nonambulatory patients, whereby chronic pressure on an externally rotated foot results in hindfoot ulceration predominantly at the calcaneus and the lateral malleolus.[70]

Ulceration can be differentiated from simple callus on MR imaging. A typical ulcer appears as a focal skin interruption with "heaped-up" margins and an associated soft tissue defect (see **Figs. 3** and **4**). Unlike a callus, ulcers are bright on T2-weighted sequences and demonstrate intense peripheral enhancement related to granulation tissue at the ulcer base. Occasionally, there may be deep extension of the ulcer to the level of the adjacent osseous prominence via a sinus tract. Contrast administration is useful to delineate sinus tracts identified by "tramtrack" enhancement (see **Fig. 4**).[75,76] A sinus tract should be evaluated in all imaging planes; a tract may appear round on a tangential cut and potentially be mistaken for

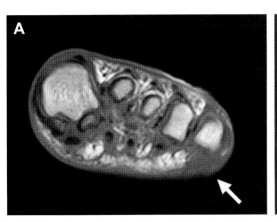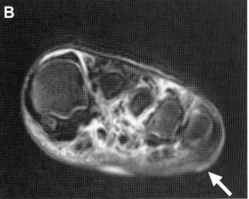

**Fig. 1.** Callus signal characteristics. (*A*) Short-axis T1-weighted and (*B*) short-axis, T2-weighted, fat-suppressed images show low T1 and low T2 signal intensity soft tissue underneath the fifth metatarsal base without skin disruption (*arrows*). The marrow signal adjacent to the callus is normal.

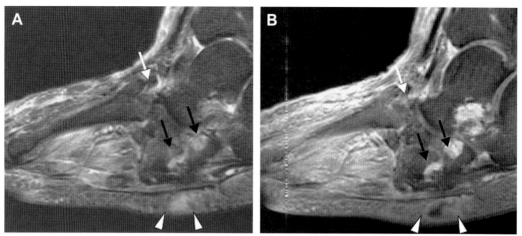

Fig. 2. Adventitial bursitis. (*A*) Sagittal, T2-weighted, fat-suppressed and (*B*) sagittal, T1-weighted, gadolinium-enhanced, fat-suppressed images show neuropathic changes in the midfoot with collapse and fragmentation (*white arrow*) and rocker-bottom deformity. There is evidence of bursa formation underneath the cuboid (*arrowheads*) characterized by high T2 signal intensity and peripheral rim enhancement. Note that subcutaneous fat superficial to the bursa is maintained. Subchondral cysts (*black arrows*) at the calcaneocuboid joint mitigate against the presence of infection.

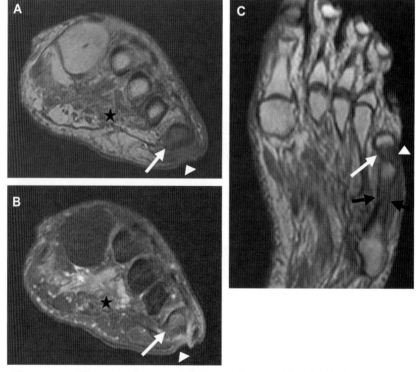

Fig. 3. Ulcer with osteomyelitis and a fracture. (*A*) Short-axis T1-weighted; (*B*) short-axis, T2-weighted, fat-suppressed; and (*C*) long-axis T1-weighted images show a skin ulcer underneath the fifth metatarsal base (*arrowheads*). The ulcer is hypointense on T1- and hyperintense on T2-weighted sequences with focal skin discontinuity. The adjacent fifth metatarsal base demonstrates marrow edema characterized by a hypointense T1 and hyperintense T2 signal compatible with osteomyelitis (*white arrows*). Also note fatty atrophy of the intrinsic foot musculature (*star*) (*A*, *B*) related to diabetic neuropathy. In (*C*), a low signal intensity fracture line at the fifth metatarsal shaft (*black arrows*) is situated away from the skin ulcer. Low marrow signal intensity surrounds the fracture. This case illustrates the importance of using marrow morphology in addition to signal change to make the correct diagnosis.

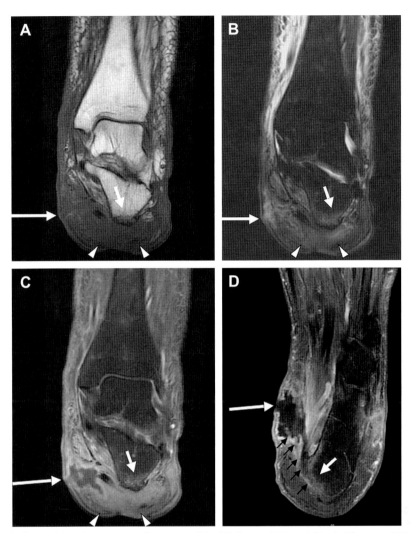

Fig. 4. Calcaneal ulcers with a sinus tract and osteomyelitis. (*A*) Coronal T1-weighted; (*B*) coronal T2-weighted fat-suppressed; (*C*) coronal T1-weighted, gadolinium-enhanced, fat-suppressed; and (*D*) axial T1-weighted, gadolinium-enhanced, fat-suppressed images show two heel ulcers: one at the plantar surface (*arrowheads*) depicted by skin discontinuity and the other medially (*long white arrow*) depicted by a heaped-up margin, best appreciated with contrast administration. Phlegmonous enhancing soft tissue is seen deep to the plantar ulcer. A medial sinus tract is only apparent after contrast administration with a peripheral rim of enhancement extending to the calcaneus (*black arrows*) (*D*). There is associated marrow edema with enhancement in the calcaneus compatible with osteomyelitis (*short white arrow*).

an abscess. Familiarity with typical ulcer location and the ability to identify a sinus tract are necessary to evaluate for osteomyelitis by MR imaging.

## Soft Tissue Swelling, Cellulitis, and Abscess

Ulcers can progress to more advanced soft tissue infections, including cellulitis, phlegmon, and abscess. Clinically, cellulitis presents with a warm, red, and swollen leg. Diffuse soft tissue swelling also is common in the acute stage of neuropathic disease, and in diabetic patients in general.[23] Osteomyelitis is an unlikely diagnosis in diabetic

patients who have soft tissue swelling but lack an ulcer. Therefore, the role of imaging in soft tissue swelling is to diagnose neuropathic disease and to identify soft tissue infection.[77–79] If radiographs are normal and the clinical suspicion for infection is low, the next most appropriate test is a three-phase bone scan. If clinical suspicion for infection is high, however, MR imaging may be indicated. On MR imaging, soft tissue edema and cellulitis demonstrate fat reticulation characterized by intermediate T1- and high T2-weighted signal intensity.[80] The distinguishing feature is enhancement post contrast seen with cellulitis and not with edema related to diabetes or neuropathic disease.[77]

Soft tissue mass effect or phlegmon is an indicator of possible osteomyelitis. Phlegmonous soft tissue replaces the subcutaneous fat and is characterized by an ill-defined, low T1- and intermediate to hyperintense T2-weighted signal intensity, which is not as bright as fluid (see **Fig. 4**). Vague enhancement post contrast does not demonstrate a discrete rim of enhancement, which otherwise is of an abscess.

Abscesses are uncommon in diabetic patients but when present demonstrate characteristic fluid signal intensity with peripheral rim enhancement after contrast administration (**Fig. 5**). The majority of abscesses are small and obscured by adjacent soft tissue edema unless contrast is administered.

The vast majority of pedal abscesses represent areas of contiguous skin infection. The majority of abscesses occur in the forefoot, where they are situated close to adjacent skin ulcer, whereas midfoot and hindfoot abscesses may be several centimeters away from the ulcer.[77] Abscesses are significantly more frequent in patients who have osteomyelitis and after foot surgery.[77] The presence of an abscess precludes nonsurgical management, which otherwise may be possible in uncomplicated osteomyelitis. Routine use of contrast is recommended as it aids in abscess identification and enables optimal assessment of the extent of soft tissue infection. MR imaging mapping of soft tissue involvement helps surgeons plan targeted and limited surgical intervention and avoid unnecessary empiric exploration.[19]

Foreign bodies are seen commonly in diabetic patients who have sensory neuropathy or after surgery. A careful search for a foreign body should be performed in patients who have soft tissue infection and no adjacent ulcer. A foreign body usually has a low signal intensity on T1- and T2-weighted sequences and may be associated with blooming.[81] The surrounding rim of enhancement is related to a foreign body granulomatous reaction and should not be mistaken for an abscess.[78] T2 signal intensity is helpful in distinguishing a foreign body from an abscess. Contrary to an abscess, a foreign body is not of fluid signal intensity (see **Fig. 5**).

## Gangrene

End-organ ischemia in diabetic patients may lead to gangrene. Noninfected devitalized tissue is termed, "dry gangrene," whereas the term, "wet gangrene," is reserved for cases of superimposed infection. Contrast-enhanced MR imaging is useful to delineate areas of soft tissue devascularization. On imaging, gangrene is characterized by a nonenhancing area that is sharply demarcated from the

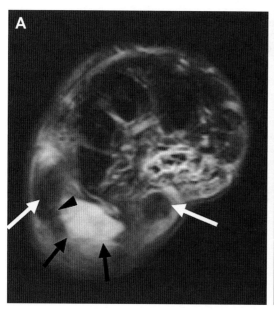 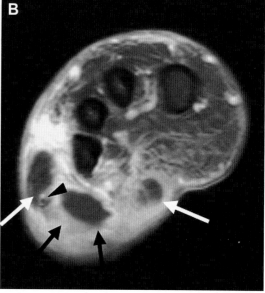

**Fig. 5.** Abscess versus foreign body granuloma. (*A*) Short-axis, T2-weighted, fat-suppressed and (*B*) short-axis, T1-weighted, gadolinium-enhanced, fat-suppressed images show a plantar fluid collection with peripheral rim enhancement (*black arrows*). Medial and lateral to this collection are round T2 hypointense areas with extensive surrounding enhancement (*white arrows*) compatible with foreign bodies and adjacent reactive hyperemia. There is a small focus of susceptibility artifact related to the lateral foreign body (*arrowhead*).

surrounding viable tissue. The periphery of the devitalized tissue may demonstrate reactive hyperemia and enhancement.[82] Although necrotic tissue should be resected completely, viable tissue should be preserved to promote successful wound healing. Current clinical MR imaging protocols may not be able to identify ischemic, but viable, tissue at risk. Future use of dynamic contrast-enhanced (DCE) MR imaging with quantitative analysis of tissue enhancement may be used to map the extent of ischemic but viable tissue before surgical resection.[83] Most cases of gangrene are diagnosed clinically do not, and should not, proceed to advanced imaging.

Soft tissue infection in a critically ischemic foot is more likely to proceed to gangrene because of increased metabolic demands; the metabolic requirements for healing outweigh those necessary to maintain tissue viability.[82] Wet gangrene may demonstrate soft tissue gas on imaging. Gradient-echo sequences are most sensitive in identifying small foci of blooming artifact related to air (**Fig. 6**). Care should be taken to distinguish soft tissue gas related to gangrene from that related to a skin ulcer serving as a portal of air entry into soft tissues. Gangrene usually is associated with nonenhancing devitalized tissue and

demonstrates more extensive soft tissue gas than that seen surrounding an ulcer.[84]

## Osteomyelitis

The sensitivity and specificity of MR imaging for diagnosing osteomyelitis exceeds 90% in the absence of neuropathic disease.[60] Marrow replacement by a low signal intensity on T1-weighted images and a corresponding high signal intensity on T2-weighted images is characteristic for osteomyelitis,[75] with or without notable cortical disruption. In addition, these findings are diagnostic for osteomyelitis in the presence of an adjacent ulcer and absence of underlying neuropathic disease or alternate etiology for marrow abnormality, such as a fracture or marrow necrosis (see **Fig. 3**). The simplest MR imaging method is to follow the ulcer or sinus tract down to bone and evaluate the T1 signal of the marrow. A noticeably decreased T1 signal is indicative of osteomyelitis.

Although T2 hyperintensity is highly sensitive for osteomyelitis, T1-weighted sequences should be used to confirm the diagnosis. Attention must be given to cases where the marrow appears hyperintense on T2-weighted sequences but has no corresponding low signal intensity on T1-weighted

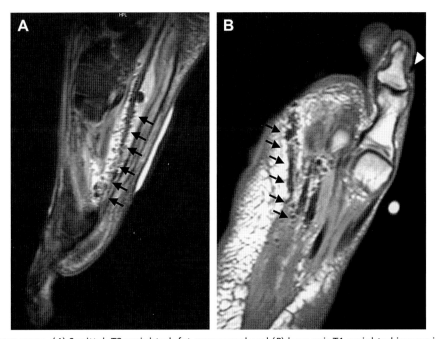

**Fig. 6.** Gas gangrene. (*A*) Sagittal, T2-weighted, fat-suppressed and (*B*) long axis T1-weighted images in a patient who had foot crepitus and an ulcer over the great toe (*arrowhead*) (*B*). There are multiple low- signal intensity foci with evidence of blooming artifact (*arrows*) along the flexor tendon sheath. The tendon sheath distension with fluid is best seen in (*A*). This extensive soft tissue gas is unlikely secondary to air dissecting from the skin ulcer. The patient had clinical signs of infection, and the imaging findings are compatible with infected, wet gangrene.

sequences. Even in the presence of enhancement, this marrow is not involved with osteomyelitis. Rather, it represents a reactive change, such as that related to adjacent soft tissue infection (**Fig. 7**), or osteitis related to cortical, but not to medullary, infection.

The postoperative imaging of diabetic foot is increasingly common. The criteria for diagnosing osteomyelitis at the amputation stump are the same as described previously, and there should be no marrow abnormality on imaging even in the immediate postoperative period. Marrow hypointensity on T1-weighted images indicates osteomyelitis,

and isolated hyperintensity on T2-weighted images is compatible with reactive marrow change (see **Fig. 7**). A less abrupt surgical "cut" is associated with more postoperative edema. Therefore, interpretations should be made with care in patients treated by débridement rather than amputation.

Several secondary signs may help confirm the diagnosis of osteomyelitis. Periosteal reaction is a helpful sign that favors the diagnosis of osteomyelitis and may manifest as circumferential high signal on T2-weighted sequences with associated enhancement. The diagnosis of osteomyelitis

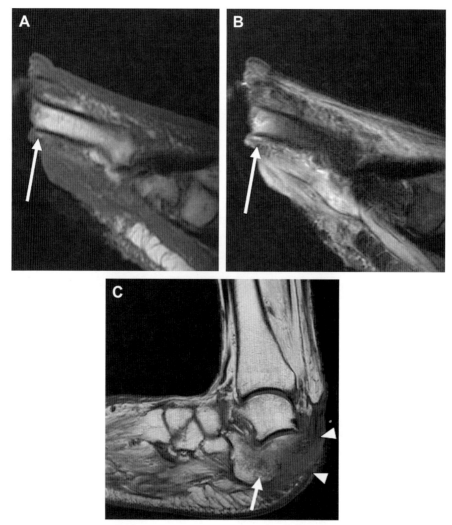

**Fig. 7.** Osteitis versus osteomyelitis after amputation. (*A*) Sagittal T1-weighted and (*B*) sagittal T2-weighted, fat-suppressed images through the great toe demonstrate evidence of transmetatarsal amputation. There is a large soft tissue defect at the amputation stump with T2 marrow hyperintensity and no corresponding marrow abnormality on the T1-weighted image (*arrow*). The imaging findings are compatible with reactive marrow edema and osteitis with no evidence of osteomyelitis. (*C*) Sagittal T1-weighted image in another patient after partial calcaneal resection shows a large soft tissue ulcer (*arrowheads*) with extensive calcaneal marrow hypointensity deep to the ulcer (*arrow*) compatible with osteomyelitis.

also is more likely in the presence of soft tissue findings (discussed previously), including a sub-tending skin ulcer, sinus tract, cellulitis, soft tissue abscess, or a foreign body.[70,76]

## Septic Arthritis

Most cases of septic arthritis in diabetic feet are secondary to contiguous spread from an adjacent soft tissue infection.[70,85] The most common joints involved are those adjacent to a callus or ulcer. Septic arthritis is common at the interphalangeal joints related to dorsal ulceration; at the metatar-sophalangeal joints related to lateral ulceration; at the first and fifth MTP joints; at the midfoot in neuropathic feet; and at the talocrural and subtalar joints related to ulceration at the malleoli or the calcaneus.

By MR imaging, the involved joint demonstrates a complex joint effusion with intense, usually thick, synovial enhancement (**Fig. 8**). Direct communication of joint fluid with an adjacent sinus tract may be present. In those cases, the joint effusion may decompress and appear reduced in size on follow-up imaging despite ongoing septic arthritis. The adjacent soft tissues may show perisynovial edema, and the subchondral marrow may show a thin rim of reactive marrow edema with marginal erosions.[86] It is important to distinguish reactive marrow changes secondary to septic arthritis from the changes of superimposed osteomyelitis. Proximal extension of subchondral edema beyond the subchondral bone, and diffuse, fairly overt, T1 hypointensity in the adjacent marrow has a high likelihood of being associated with osteomyelitis.[87]

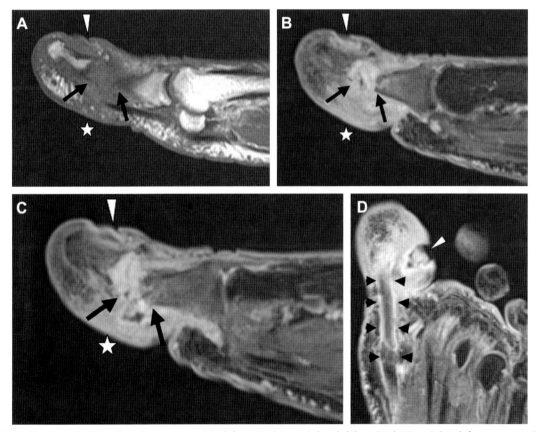

**Fig. 8.** Septic arthritis and septic tenosynovitis. (A) Sagittal T1-weighted; (B) sagittal, T2-weighted, fat-suppressed; and (C) sagittal, T1-weighted, gadolinium-enhanced, fat-suppressed images through the forefoot demonstrate a dorsal ulcer (*white arrowhead*) with plantar cellulitis (*star*). The interphalangeal joint demonstrates a joint effusion with thick enhancement (*arrows*) and erosions, compatible with septic arthritis. The marrow abnormality is localized to the subarticular bone rather than diffuse. Therefore, there is no associated osteomyelitis. (D) Axial T1-weighted, gadolinium-enhanced, fat-suppressed image shows a plantar ulcer (*white arrowhead*) with enhancement surrounding the flexor hallucis longus tendon sheath (*black arrowheads*) in keeping with septic tenosynovitis.

## Spread of Infection

Soft tissue infection in diabetic feet often is aggressive and does not respect the usual fascial planes and compartments of the foot. The foot is divided into several compartments: plantar compartment (medial, central, and lateral), interosseous, and dorsal.[88] An infection may spread centripetally from an ulcer and violate these anatomic boundaries. The extension of infection into adjacent compartments is observed most commonly with ulcers and infection originating in the lateral compartment. A study by Ledermann and colleagues[89] showed that only 20% of infections in the lateral compartment did not spread into adjacent compartments. Proximal spread of infection in the foot, unlike in the hand, is unusual but tends to spread along the Achilles and peroneal tendons.

Septic tenosynovitis may result from spread of infection from adjacent pressure ulceration. Tendons are situated over osseous prominences where they are separated from the skin only by a thin layer of subcutaneous fat tissue. The tendons most commonly involved in septic tenosynovitis are the peroneals related to a lateral malleolus ulcer and the Achilles related to a calcaneal ulcer. In the forefoot, nearly two thirds of tendon infections involve the flexor tendons and are related to plantar location of forefoot ulceration. In rare cases, progression of soft tissue infection may lead to tendon destruction.[21] On MR imaging, circular peritendinous enhancement of a tendon coursing through an area of cellulitis and adjacent to infected pedal ulcer may be a specific sign of tendon infection (see **Fig. 8**).[90] In a study by Ledermann and colleagues, tendon thickening, tendon hyperintensity on T2-weighted images, and tendon enhancement were not shown to be specific for infection and may be seen with other inflammatory, neoplastic, or post-traumatic conditions.[89] A positive correlation was reported between the presence of tendon infection and osteomyelitis, presumably because these entities are related to extension of advanced infection.[89]

## OSTEOMYELITIS VERSUS NEUROPATHIC ARTHROPATHY

Neuropathic arthropathy may mimic osteomyelitis clinically and by imaging. This is especially true in the acute stage of neuropathic disease when patients present with a warm, swollen, and erythematous foot.[91] In patients who have soft tissue swelling, scintigraphy is very sensitive for detecting neuroarthropathy, and MR imaging is useful for diagnosing soft tissue infection. In early stages of neuroarthropathy, MR imaging shows soft tissue edema, fluid collections, effusions, and marrow abnormalities[92,93] with periarticular soft tissue and marrow enhancement postcontrast administration.[94] It is important to detect neuropathic disease as early as possible (before radiographic changes), to place patients in orthodics, and slow the progression of foot deformity.

Patients in the coalescence or subacute stage of neuroarthropathy demonstrate bone resorption. The chronic, consolidation stage is associated with a return to a stable, yet deformed foot and is characterized by the familiar pattern of debris, destruction, dislocation, and density radiographically.[95,96] MR imaging may show deformity, osseous fragmentation, and joint effusions (**Fig. 9**). This quiescent, advanced stage of neuroarthropathy should not mimic infection clinically, and any signs or symptoms of infection in these patients strongly suggest the true presence of infection.

Distinction between neuropathic arthropathy and osteomyelitis on foot MR imaging may be facilitated by an appreciation that osteomyelitis almost exclusively develops by contiguous spread of infection from skin ulceration at predictable sites[70] whereas neuropathic arthropathy primarily is an articular disease. Thus, the imaging finding of a marrow abnormality without an adjacent ulcer along with the presence of periarticular disease favors neuropathic disease over infection.

As discussed previously, the location of osteomyelitis parallels the location of most common sites of ulceration, such as those at the metatarsal heads, toes, calcaneus and malleoli.[70] Therefore, the most useful distinguishing feature of osteomyelitis is location. Neuropathic arthropathy most commonly affects Lisfranc's and the metatarsophalangeal joints, whereas osteomyelitis is seen distal to Lisfranc's joint, at the calcaneus and the malleoli. Evaluation for osteomyelitis at the midfoot is most challenging, and secondary signs of infection, including visualization of direct spread from an ulcer over a rocker-bottom deformity and a sinus tract, should be used.

## SUPERIMPOSED INFECTION IN NEUROPATHIC ARTHROPATHY

The presence of neuropathic disease may limit the specificity of MR imaging for detecting superimposed infection. The likelihood of osteomyelitis in neuropathic patients who have an ulcer that extends to bone is higher than that in patients who have no preceding neuroarthropathy (**Fig. 10**). Therefore, the role of imaging in these patients is

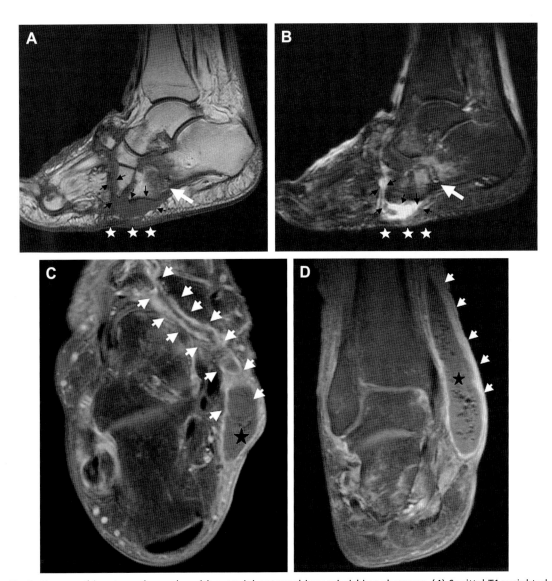

**Fig. 9.** Neuropathic osteoarthropathy with synovial outpouchings mimicking abscesses. (A) Sagittal T1-weighted and (B) sagittal T2-weighted fat-suppressed images show a rocker-bottom deformity and midfoot fragmentation. There is a joint effusion extending from Lisfranc's joint to the plantar soft tissues (*black arrows*) (A, B). Note that the subcutaneous fat is maintained superficial to the joint effusion (*stars*) (A, B). Subchondral marrow edema at the calcaneocuboid joint (*white arrow*) (A, B) is related to neuropathic osteoarthropathy. The effusion can be followed on the corresponding (C) axial and (D) coronal T1-weighted, gadolinium-enhanced, fat suppressed images. The effusion extends from Lisfranc's joint (*white arrows*) (C, D) into the soft tissues superficial to the medial malleolus, communicating with a large collection (*black star*). Low-signal intensity foci within the medial collection represent gas related to a recent diagnostic aspiration. This appearance is typical for synovial outpouchings and effusions in neuropathic osteoarthropathy. The absence of a skin ulcer and typical location should aid in distinguishing them from abscess and infection.

to evaluate the extent of the disease rather than to make a diagnosis.[89] Radiographs and MR imaging are recommended. MR imaging with the use of contrast is recommended to assess the extent of disease and to evaluate tissue perfusion.[36] Several imaging features were shown to be useful in distinguishing neuropathic disease with or without

superimposed infection. In a recent study by Ahmadi and colleagues,[97] several imaging features were shown to be useful in distinguishing neuropathic disease with or without superimposed infection. The soft tissue features commonly associated with superimposed joint infection included replacement of adjacent subcutaneous fat signal

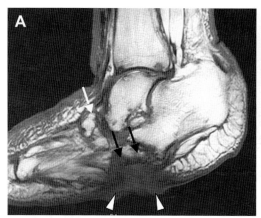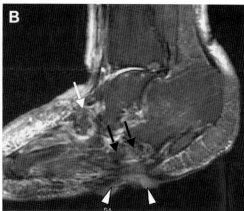

Fig. 10. Plantar ulcer and osteomyelitis in neuropathic osteoarthropathy. (*A*) Sagittal T1-weighted and (*B*) sagittal, T2-weighted, fat-suppressed images show a large plantar ulcer under the cuboid (*arrowheads*) with replacement of the subcutaneous fat to the level of the cuboid. There is associated cuboid marrow edema characterized by low T1 and high T2 signal intensity (*black arrows*) compatible with osteomyelitis. Note rocker-bottom deformity and midfoot fragmentation and disorganization (*white arrow*).

intensity and the presence of adjacent soft tissue collection. These soft tissue collections were larger when adjacent to neuropathic joints with superimposed infection. Sinus tracts were more common in infected cases and often resulted in a paradoxic decrease in the size of fluid collections on follow-up imaging after the development of superimposed infection. Soft tissue abnormalities that did not help distinguish neuropathic disease with from those without superimposed infection included skin ulceration, soft tissue enhancement, and rim enhancement of fluid collections adjacent to joints. Two potentially helpful signs for excluding infection in neuropathic patients are the presence of subchondral cysts (see **Fig. 2**) and intra-articular bodies. The disappearance of these findings on follow-up studies indicates superinfection.[98]

Marrow changes associated with superimposed osteomyelitis more commonly show diffuse involvement. In contrast, limited periarticular involvement is seen with neuropathic disease, where the pathologic process is joint centered. The authors have found the use of a ghost sign to be helpful in distinguishing acute neuropathy from superimposed infection. A positive ghost sign indicates a superimposed infection, and a negative ghost sign excludes infection in neuropathic foot. Bones that "disappear" on T1-weighted sequence but "appear" and become morphologically more distinct on T2-weighted sequences or after contrast administration (ie, positive ghost sign) are likely to be superinfected (**Fig. 11**). To contrast these findings to the neuropathic foot, a ghost sign is absent as the bones are truly "dissolved" and destroyed.

## SUMMARY OF AMERICAN COLLEGE OF RADIOLOGY APPROPRIATENESS CRITERIA ON IMAGING DIABETES-RELATED OSTEOMYELITIS

In the presence of an ulcer extending to bone, osteomyelitis likely is present.[36] Radiographs and MR imaging should be performed concurrently. MR imaging is the imaging test of choice to confirm the diagnosis and to evaluate the extent of infection. If there is no ulcer, but clinical suspicion for infection is high, radiographs and MR imaging are recommended. If the results of MR imaging are indeterminate, a bone biopsy may be performed.

In the presence of soft tissue swelling but no ulcer, osteomyelitis is unlikely to be present. The goal of imaging in this scenario is to distinguish between neuroarthropathy and soft tissue infection. Radiographs should be the initial imaging test. If radiographs are negative for neuroarthropathy, patients should have additional imaging: a three-phase bone scan if the clinical suspicion for infection is low and MR imaging if the suspicion for infection is high.

## FUTURE DIRECTIONS IN IMAGING PEDAL OSTEOMYELITIS
### High Field Imaging

Increased spatial resolution and higher contrast with high field imaging on 3T MR imaging systems may enable the identification of more subtle marrow abnormalities and facilitate an earlier diagnosis of osteomyelitis.[99] High field imaging offers the advantage of reduced acquisition time and consequently may reduce motion-related artifact,

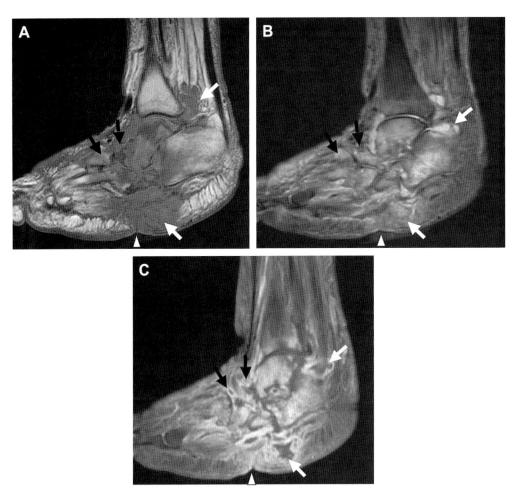

Fig. 11. Neuroarthropathy with superimposed osteomyelitis: ghost sign. (A) Sagittal T1-weighted; (B) sagittal, T2-weighted, fat-suppressed; and (C) sagittal, T1-weighted, gadolinium-enhanced, fat-suppressed images show fragmentation and subluxation at the midfoot (black arrows) with a rocker-bottom deformity and a plantar ulcer (arrowhead). There is an appearance of "dissolved" midfoot osseous structures in (A) with extensive, diffuse T1 hypointensity. On a T2-weighted image in (B), the midfoot osseous structures take on a more regular, well-defined appearance with marrow hyperintensity. This phenomenon represents a positive ghost sign and is consistent with the diagnosis of osteomyelitis superimposed on underlying neuroarthropathy. Diffuse marrow enhancement is seen in (C). There are multiple fluid collections about the foot, most arising from midfoot articulations and from the talocrural joint with thick synovial enhancement (white arrows).

which often is present when imaging patients who have foot ulcers. An additional advantage is the ability to achieve large volume coverage while maintaining high spatial resolution and high temporal resolution. This has proved useful in 3T magnetic resonance angiography of the foot in diabetic patients[100] where good temporal resolution allows discrimination of arteries from veins. High spatial resolution provides valuable information on the vascular status of the foot, including the presence and degree of collateral pathway, and accurate depiction of target vessels suitable for surgical bypass.[101]

Ultra–high field, 7T MR imaging provides additional signal-to-noise gain, which may be used for multinuclear applications with low gamma sodium and phosphorus nuclei.[102] Current clinical scanners are limited by low signal-to-noise ratio, low spatial resolution, and long acquisition times. High field sodium imaging in a cartilage model is shown to have a diagnostic advantage compared with proton MR imaging.[103–105] In the future, functional imaging with phosphorous on 7T may be used to evaluate muscle and bone metabolism. This may facilitate an earlier detection of pedal osteomyelitis and may aid in detection of superimposed infection in patients who have underlying neuroarthropathy.

## Tissue Perfusion and Viability

There is increasing interest in developing an accurate diagnostic tool to assess soft tissue microvascularity and perfusion. Precise mapping of viable tissue with functional imaging may aid surgeons in planning limited resection and deciding whether or not to proceed to revascularization.

Muscle perfusion has been evaluated in nuclear medicine using scintigraphy methods and PET.[106,107] Because of limited availability and spatial resolution, however, these modalities have not gained wide clinical acceptance. Although CT perfusion offers good spatial resolution, there remains a risk for contrast agent–related adverse reactions and considerable radiation exposure.[108] Contrast-enhanced ultrasound has shown good reproducibility but is operator dependent and not widely available.[109] Functional MR imaging techniques offer the advantage of good spatial resolution, wide availability, and no associated radiation.[83] There are two broad functional MR imaging technique categories to assess skeletal muscle perfusion—those with and without intravenous contrast administration. DCE MR imaging has been shown to be accurate in measuring skeletal muscle perfusion.[110,111] Noncontrast techniques include arterial spin labeling, where blood is magnetically labeled and serves as an intrinsic contrast agent to measure microvascular blood flow,[112] and blood oxygen level–dependent MR imaging.[113] These functional MR imaging techniques have been used in combination with rest/exercise or postischemic hyperemia paradigms to evaluate muscle perfusion reserve.[113] Evaluation of tissue at risk in the feet of diabetic patients would be facilitated greatly by these techniques.[114] In the future, muscle perfusion quantification could be used as an endpoint in clinical trials for novel angiogenic therapeutic agents for treatment of peripheral vascular disease.[115]

## SUMMARY

Diabetic pedal osteomyelitis is primarily a manifestation of vascular insufficiency with resultant tissue ischemia, neuropathy, and infection. Nearly all cases of pedal osteomyelitis arise from a contiguous ulcer and soft tissue infection. MR imaging is the modality of choice to assess for the presence of osteomyelitis and associated soft tissue complications, to guide patient management, and to aid in limited limb resection.

## REFERENCES

1. Reiber GE, Lipsky BA, Gibbons GW. The burden of diabetic foot ulcers. Am J Surg 1998;176(2A Suppl):5S–10S.
2. Gordois A, Scuffham P, Shearer A, et al. The health care costs of diabetic peripheral neuropathy in the US. Diabetes Care 2003;26(6):1790–5.
3. Singh N, Armstrong DG, Lipsky BA. Preventing foot ulcers in patients with diabetes. JAMA 2005;293(2):217–28.
4. Lavery LA, Armstrong DG, Wunderlich RP, et al. Diabetic foot syndrome: evaluating the prevalence and incidence of foot pathology in Mexican Americans and non-Hispanic whites from a diabetes disease management cohort. Diabetes Care 2003;26(5):1435–8.
5. Armstrong DG, Lipsky BA. Advances in the treatment of diabetic foot infections. Diabetes Technol Ther 2004;6(2):167–77.
6. Armstrong DG, Lipsky BA. Diabetic foot infections: stepwise medical and surgical management. Int Wound J 2004;1(2):123–32.
7. Lavery LA, Armstrong DG, Wunderlich RP, et al. Risk factors for foot infections in individuals with diabetes. Diabetes Care 2006;29(6):1288–93.
8. Reiber GE. The epidemiology of diabetic foot problems. Diabet Med 1996;13(Suppl 1):S6–11.
9. Lipsky BA. Osteomyelitis of the foot in diabetic patients. Clin Infect Dis 1997;25(6):1318–26.
10. Lipsky BA, Berendt AR, Deery HG, et al. Diagnosis and treatment of diabetic foot infections. Clin Infect Dis 2004;39(7):885–910.
11. Morrison WB, Schweitzer ME, Wapner KL, et al. Osteomyelitis in feet of diabetics: clinical accuracy, surgical utility, and cost-effectiveness of MR imaging. Radiology 1995;196(2):557–64.
12. Trautner C, Haastert B, Giani G, et al. Incidence of lower limb amputations and diabetes. Diabetes Care 1996;19(9):1006–9.
13. Jeffcoate WJ, Harding KG. Diabetic foot ulcers. Lancet 2003;361(9368):1545–51.
14. Berendt AR, Peters EJ, Bakker K, et al. Specific guidelines for treatment of diabetic foot osteomyelitis. Diabetes Metab Res Rev 2008;24(Suppl 1):S190–1.
15. Bamberger DM, Daus GP, Gerding DN. Osteomyelitis in the feet of diabetic patients. Long-term results, prognostic factors, and the role of antimicrobial and surgical therapy. Am J Med 1987;83(4):653–60.
16. Senneville E, Lombart A, Beltrand E, et al. Outcome of diabetic foot osteomyelitis treated nonsurgically: a retrospective cohort study. Diabetes Care 2008;31(4):637–42.
17. Yasuhara H, Hattori T, Shigeta O. Significance of phlebosclerosis in non-healing Ischaemic foot

ulcers of end-stage renal disease. Eur J Vasc Endovasc Surg 2008;36(3):346–52.

18. Faglia E, Mantero M, Caminiti M, et al. Extensive use of peripheral angioplasty, particularly infrapopliteal, in the treatment of ischaemic diabetic foot ulcers: clinical results of a multicentric study of 221 consecutive diabetic subjects. J Intern Med 2002;252(3):225–32.

19. Durham JR, Lukens ML, Campanini DS, et al. Impact of magnetic resonance imaging on the management of diabetic foot infections. Am J Surg 1991;162(2):150–3 [discussion: 153–4].

20. Horowitz JD, Durham JR, Nease DB, et al. Prospective evaluation of magnetic resonance imaging in the management of acute diabetic foot infections. Ann Vasc Surg 1993;7(1):44–50.

21. Lipsky BA, Pecoraro RE, Wheat LJ. The diabetic foot. Soft tissue and bone infection. Infect Dis Clin North Am 1990;4(3):409–32.

22. Stadelmann WK, Digenis AG, Tobin GR. Impediments to wound healing. Am J Surg 1998;176(2A Suppl):39S–47S.

23. Rathur HM, Boulton AJ. The neuropathic diabetic foot. Nat Clin Pract Endocrinol Metab 2007;3(1): 14–25.

24. Ierardi RP, Shuman CR. Control of vascular disease in patients with diabetes mellitus. Surg Clin North Am 1998;78(3):385–92.

25. Andreisek G, Pfammatter T, Goepfert K, et al. Peripheral arteries in diabetic patients: standard bolus-chase and time-resolved MR angiography. Radiology 2007;242(2):610–20.

26. Lapeyre M, Kobeiter H, Desgranges P, et al. Assessment of critical limb ischemia in patients with diabetes: comparison of MR angiography and digital subtraction angiography. AJR Am J Roentgenol 2005;185(6):1641–50.

27. Kreitner KF, Schmitt R. MultiHance-enhanced MR angiography of the peripheral run-off vessels in patients with diabetes. Eur Radiol 2007;17(Suppl 6): F63–68.

28. Faglia E, Dalla Paola L, Clerici G, et al. Peripheral angioplasty as the first-choice revascularization procedure in diabetic patients with critical limb ischemia: prospective study of 993 consecutive patients hospitalized and followed between 1999 and 2003. Eur J Vasc Endovasc Surg 2005;29(6): 620–7.

29. Edmonds ME, Roberts VC, Watkins PJ. Blood flow in the diabetic neuropathic foot. Diabetologia 1982; 22(1):9–15.

30. Younger DS, Bronfin L. Overview of diabetic neuropathy. Semin Neurol 1996;16(2):107–13.

31. Reiber GE, Vileikyte L, Boyko EJ, et al. Causal pathways for incident lower-extremity ulcers in patients with diabetes from two settings. Diabetes Care 1999;22(1):157–62.

32. Shone A, Burnside J, Chipchase S, et al. Probing the validity of the probe-to-bone test in the diagnosis of osteomyelitis of the foot in diabetes. Diabetes Care 2006;29(4):945.

33. Lavery LA, Armstrong DG, Peters EJ, et al. Probe-to-bone test for diagnosing diabetic foot osteomyelitis: reliable or relic? Diabetes Care 2007;30(2):270–4.

34. Bridges RM Jr, Deitch EA. Diabetic foot infections. Pathophysiology and treatment. Surg Clin North Am 1994;74(3):537–55.

35. Wheat LJ, Allen SD, Henry M, et al. Diabetic foot infections. Bacteriologic analysis. Arch Intern Med 1986;146(10):1935–40.

36. Schweitzer ME, Daffner RH, Weissman BN, et al. ACR appropriateness criteria on suspected osteomyelitis in patients with diabetes mellitus. J Am Coll Radiol 2008;5(8):881–6.

37. Caputo GM, Cavanagh PR, Ulbrecht JS, et al. Assessment and management of foot disease in patients with diabetes. N Engl J Med 1994; 331(13):854–60.

38. Levine SE, Neagle CE, Esterhai JL, et al. Magnetic resonance imaging for the diagnosis of osteomyelitis in the diabetic patient with a foot ulcer. Foot Ankle Int 1994;15(3):151–6.

39. Shults DW, Hunter GC, McIntyre KE, et al. Value of radiographs and bone scans in determining the need for therapy in diabetic patients with foot ulcers. Am J Surg 1989;158(6):525–9 [discussion: 529–30].

40. Enderle MD, Coerper S, Schweizer HP, et al. Correlation of imaging techniques to histopathology in patients with diabetic foot syndrome and clinical suspicion of chronic osteomyelitis. The role of high-resolution ultrasound. Diabetes Care 1999; 22(2):294–9.

41. Capriotti G, Chianelli M, Signore A. Nuclear medicine imaging of diabetic foot infection: results of meta-analysis. Nucl Med Commun 2006;27(10): 757–64.

42. Kumar R, Basu S, Torigian D, et al. Role of modern imaging techniques for diagnosis of infection in the era of 18F-fluorodeoxyglucose positron emission tomography. Clin Microbiol Rev 2008;21(1):209–24.

43. Jay PR, Michelson JD, Mizel MS, et al. Efficacy of three-phase bone scans in evaluating diabetic foot ulcers. Foot Ankle Int 1999;20(6):347–55.

44. Sella EJ, Grosser DM. Imaging modalities of the diabetic foot. Clin Podiatr Med Surg 2003;20(4): 729–40.

45. Larcos G, Brown ML, Sutton RT. Diagnosis of osteomyelitis of the foot in diabetic patients: value of 111In-leukocyte scintigraphy. AJR Am J Roentgenol 1991;157(3):527–31.

46. Termaat MF, Raijmakers PG, Scholten HJ, et al. The accuracy of diagnostic imaging for the assessment of chronic osteomyelitis: a systematic review and

meta-analysis. J Bone Joint Surg Am 2005;87(11): 2464–71.

47. Schauwecker DS. The scintigraphic diagnosis of osteomyelitis. AJR Am J Roentgenol 1992;158(1): 9–18.

48. Poirier JY, Garin E, Derrien C, et al. Diagnosis of osteomyelitis in the diabetic foot with a 99mTc-HMPAO leucocyte scintigraphy combined with a 99mTc-MDP bone scintigraphy. Diabetes Metab 2002;28(6 Pt 1):485–90.

49. Rubello D, Casara D, Maran A, et al. Role of antigranulocyte Fab' fragment antibody scintigraphy (LeukoScan) in evaluating bone infection: acquisition protocol, interpretation criteria and clinical results. Nucl Med Commun 2004;25(1):39–47.

50. Delcourt A, Huglo D, Prangere T, et al. Comparison between leukoscan (sulesomab) and gallium-67 for the diagnosis of osteomyelitis in the diabetic foot. Diabetes Metab 2005;31(2):125–33.

51. Sugawara Y, Braun DK, Kison PV, et al. Rapid detection of human infections with fluorine-18 fluorodeoxyglucose and positron emission tomography: preliminary results. Eur J Nucl Med 1998; 25(9):1238–43.

52. Bleeker-Rovers CP, de Kleijn EM, Corstens FH, et al. Clinical value of FDG PET in patients with fever of unknown origin and patients suspected of focal infection or inflammation. Eur J Nucl Med Mol Imaging 2004;31(1):29–37.

53. Giurato L, Uccioli L. The diabetic foot: Charcot joint and osteomyelitis. Nucl Med Commun 2006;27(9): 745–9.

54. Keidar Z, Militianu D, Melamed E, et al. The diabetic foot: initial experience with 18F-FDG PET/CT. J Nucl Med 2005;46(3):444–9.

55. Hopfner S, Krolak C, Kessler S, et al. Preoperative imaging of charcot neuroarthropathy in diabetic patients: comparison of ring PET, hybrid PET, and magnetic resonance imaging. Foot Ankle Int 2004;25(12):890–5.

56. Basu S, Chryssikos T, Houseni M, et al. Potential role of FDG PET in the setting of diabetic neuroosteoarthropathy: can it differentiate uncomplicated charcot's neuroarthropathy from osteomyelitis and soft-tissue infection? Nucl Med Commun 2007; 28(6):465–72.

57. Gold RH, Hawkins RA, Katz RD. Bacterial osteomyelitis: findings on plain radiography, CT, MR, and scintigraphy. AJR Am J Roentgenol 1991;157(2):365–70.

58. Chandnani VP, Beltran J, Morris CS, et al. Acute experimental osteomyelitis and abscesses: detection with MR imaging versus CT. Radiology 1990; 174(1):233–6.

59. Riebel TW, Nasir R, Nazarenko O. The value of sonography in the detection of osteomyelitis. Pediatr Radiol 1996;26(4):291–7.

60. Kapoor A, Page S, Lavalley M, et al. Magnetic resonance imaging for diagnosing foot osteomyelitis: a meta-analysis. Arch Intern Med 2007;167(2): 125–32.

61. Fry DE, Marek JM, Langsfeld M. Infection in the ischemic lower extremity. Surg Clin North Am 1998; 78(3):465–79.

62. Sumpio BE. Foot ulcers. N Engl J Med 2000; 343(11):787–93.

63. Deo A, Fogel M, Cowper SE. Nephrogenic systemic fibrosis: a population study examining the relationship of disease development to gadolinium exposure. Clin J Am Soc Nephrol 2007;2(2):264–7.

64. Broome DR, Girguis MS, Baron PW, et al. Gadodiamide-associated nephrogenic systemic fibrosis: why radiologists should be concerned. AJR Am J Roentgenol 2007;188(2):586–92.

65. Sadowski EA, Bennett LK, Chan MR, et al. Nephrogenic systemic fibrosis: risk factors and incidence estimation. Radiology 2007;243(1):148–57.

66. US Food and Drug Administration. Gadolinium-based contrast agents for magnetic resonance imaging (marketed as Magnevist M, Omniscan, OptiMARK, ProHance). Available at: http://www.fda.gov/cder/drug/InfoSheets/HCP/gcca_200705HCP.pdf. Accessed July 30, 2008.

67. Kanal E, Barkovich AJ, Bell C, et al. ACR guidance document for safe MR practices: 2007. AJR Am J Roentgenol 2007;188(6):1447–74.

68. Birke JA, Franks BD, Foto JG. First ray joint limitation, pressure, and ulceration of the first metatarsal head in diabetes mellitus. Foot Ankle Int 1995; 16(5):277–84.

69. Birke JA, Patout CA Jr, Foto JG. Factors associated with ulceration and amputation in the neuropathic foot. J Orthop Sports Phys Ther 2000;30(2):91–7.

70. Ledermann HP, Morrison WB, Schweitzer ME. MR image analysis of pedal osteomyelitis: distribution, patterns of spread, and frequency of associated ulceration and septic arthritis. Radiology 2002; 223(3):747–55.

71. Mueller MJ, Minor SD, Diamond JE, et al. Relationship of foot deformity to ulcer location in patients with diabetes mellitus. Phys Ther 1990;70(6): 356–62.

72. Boulton AJ. The pathogenesis of diabetic foot problems: an overview. Diabet Med 1996;13(Suppl 1): S12–16.

73. Pitei DL, Foster A, Edmonds M. The effect of regular callus removal on foot pressures. J Foot Ankle Surg 1999;38(4):251–5 [discussion: 306].

74. Levin ME. Foot lesions in patients with diabetes mellitus. Endocrinol Metab Clin North Am 1996; 25(2):447–62.

75. Morrison WB, Schweitzer ME, Bock GW, et al. Diagnosis of osteomyelitis: utility of fat-suppressed

contrast-enhanced MR imaging. Radiology 1993; 189(1):251–7.

76. Morrison WB, Schweitzer ME, Batte WG, et al. Osteomyelitis of the foot: relative importance of primary and secondary MR imaging signs. Radiology 1998;207(3):625–32.

77. Ledermann HP, Morrison WB, Schweitzer ME. Pedal abscesses in patients suspected of having pedal osteomyelitis: analysis with MR imaging. Radiology 2002;224(3):649–55.

78. Schweitzer ME, Morrison WB. MR imaging of the diabetic foot. Radiol Clin North Am 2004;42(1):61–71, vi.

79. Tomas MB, Patel M, Marwin SE, et al. The diabetic foot. Br J Radiol 2000;73(868):443 50.

80. Moore TE, Yuh WT, Kathol MH, et al. Abnormalities of the foot in patients with diabetes mellitus: findings on MR imaging. AJR Am J Roentgenol 1991; 157(4):813–6.

81. Chatha DS, Cunningham PM, Schweitzer ME. MR imaging of the diabetic foot: diagnostic challenges. Radiol Clin North Am 2005;43(4):747–59, ix.

82. Ledermann HP, Schweitzer ME, Morrison WB. Non-enhancing tissue on MR imaging of pedal infection: characterization of necrotic tissue and associated limitations for diagnosis of osteomyelitis and abscess. AJR Am J Roentgenol 2002;178(1):215–22.

83. Weber MA, Krix M, Delorme S. Quantitative evaluation of muscle perfusion with CEUS and with MR. Eur Radiol 2007;17(10):2663–74.

84. Panchbhavi VK, Hecox SE. All that is gas is not gas gangrene: mechanical spread of gas in the soft tissues. A case report. J Bone Joint Surg Am 2006; 88(6):1345–8.

85. Brower AC. Septic arthritis. Radiol Clin North Am 1996;34(2):293–309, x.

86. Karchevsky M, Schweitzer ME, Morrison WB, et al. MRI findings of septic arthritis and associated osteomyelitis in adults. AJR Am J Roentgenol 2004; 182(1):119–22.

87. Graif M, Schweitzer ME, Deely D, et al. The septic versus nonseptic inflamed joint: MRI characteristics. Skeletal Radiol 1999;28(11):616–20.

88. Goodwin DW, Salonen DC, Yu JS, et al. Plantar compartments of the foot: MR appearance in cadavers and diabetic patients. Radiology 1995; 196(3):623–30.

89. Ledermann HP, Morrison WB, Schweitzer ME, et al. Tendon involvement in pedal infection: MR analysis of frequency, distribution, and spread of infection. AJR Am J Roentgenol 2002;179(4):939–47.

90. Boutin RD, Brossmann J, Sartoris DJ, et al. Update on imaging of orthopedic infections. Orthop Clin North Am 1998;29(1):41–66.

91. Sella EJ, Barrette C. Staging of charcot neuroarthropathy along the medial column of the foot in the diabetic patient. J Foot Ankle Surg 1999;38(1):34–40.

92. Morrison WB, Ledermann HP. Work-up of the diabetic foot. Radiol Clin North Am 2002;40(5): 1171–92.

93. Marcus CD, Ladam-Marcus VJ, Leone J, et al. MR imaging of osteomyelitis and neuropathic osteoarthropathy in the feet of diabetics. Radiographics 1996;16(6):1337–48.

94. Yuh WT, Corson JD, Baraniewski HM, et al. Osteomyelitis of the foot in diabetic patients: evaluation with plain film, 99mTc-MDP bone scintigraphy, and MR imaging. AJR Am J Roentgenol 1989; 152(4):795–800.

95. Clouse ME, Gramm HF, Legg M, et al. Diabetic osteoarthropathy. Clinical and roentgenographic observations in 90 cases. Am J Roentgenol Radium Ther Nucl Med 1974;121(1):22–34.

96. Brower AC, Allman RM. Pathogenesis of the neurotrophic joint: neurotraumatic vs. neurovascular. Radiology 1981;139(2):349–54.

97. Ahmadi ME, Morrison WB, Carrino JA, et al. Neuropathic arthropathy of the foot with and without superimposed osteomyelitis: MR imaging characteristics. Radiology 2006;238(2):622–31.

98. Tan PL, Teh J. MRI of the diabetic foot: differentiation of infection from neuropathic change. Br J Radiol 2007;80(959):939–48.

99. Gold GE, Suh B, Sawyer-Glover A, et al. Musculoskeletal MRI at 3.0 T: initial clinical experience. AJR Am J Roentgenol 2004;183(5): 1479–86.

100. Ruhl KM, Katoh M, Langer S, et al. Time-resolved 3D MR angiography of the foot at 3 T in patients with peripheral arterial disease. AJR Am J Roentgenol 2008;190(6):W360–364.

101. Chomel S, Douek P, Moulin P, et al. Contrast-enhanced MR angiography of the foot: anatomy and clinical application in patients with diabetes. AJR Am J Roentgenol 2004;182(6):1435–42.

102. Regatte RR, Schweitzer ME. Ultra-high-field MRI of the musculoskeletal system at 7.0T. J Magn Reson Imaging 2007;25(2):262–9.

103. Shapiro EM, Borthakur A, Dandora R, et al. Sodium visibility and quantitation in intact bovine articular cartilage using high field (23)Na MRI and MRS. J Magn Reson 2000;142(1):24–31.

104. Borthakur A, Shapiro EM, Beers J, et al. Sensitivity of MRI to proteoglycan depletion in cartilage: comparison of sodium and proton MRI. Osteoarthritis Cartilage 2000;8(4):288–93.

105. Borthakur A, Mellon E, Niyogi S, et al. Sodium and T1rho MRI for molecular and diagnostic imaging of articular cartilage. NMR Biomed 2006;19(7): 781–821.

106. Lin CC, Ding HJ, Chen YW, et al. Usefulness of thallium-201 muscle perfusion scan to investigate perfusion reserve in the lower limbs of Type 2

diabetic patients. J Diabetes Complications 2004; 18(4):233–6.

107. Nuutila P, Kalliokoski K. Use of positron emission tomography in the assessment of skeletal muscle and tendon metabolism and perfusion. Scand J Med Sci Sports 2000;10(6):346–50.

108. Goh V, Halligan S, Hugill JA, et al. Quantitative assessment of tissue perfusion using MDCT: comparison of colorectal cancer and skeletal muscle measurement reproducibility. AJR Am J Roentgenol 2006;187(1):164–9.

109. Duerschmied D, Maletzki P, Freund G, et al. Analysis of muscle microcirculation in advanced diabetes mellitus by contrast enhanced ultrasound. Diabetes Res Clin Pract 2008;81(1):88–92.

110. Thompson RB, Aviles RJ, Faranesh AZ, et al. Measurement of skeletal muscle perfusion during postischemic reactive hyperemia using contrast-enhanced MRI with a step-input function. Magn Reson Med 2005;54(2):289–98.

111. Lutz AM, Weishaupt D, Amann-Vesti BR, et al. Assessment of skeletal muscle perfusion by contrast medium first-pass magnetic resonance imaging: technical feasibility and preliminary experience in healthy volunteers. J Magn Reson Imaging 2004; 20(1):111–21.

112. Boss A, Martirosian P, Claussen CD, et al. Quantitative ASL muscle perfusion imaging using a FAIR-TrueFISP technique at 3.0 T. NMR Biomed 2006;19(1):125–32.

113. Noseworthy MD, Bulte DP, Alfonsi J. BOLD magnetic resonance imaging of skeletal muscle. Semin Musculoskelet Radiol 2003;7(4):307–15.

114. Galbraith SM, Lodge MA, Taylor NJ, et al. Reproducibility of dynamic contrast-enhanced MRI in human muscle and tumours: comparison of quantitative and semi-quantitative analysis. NMR Biomed 2002;15(2):132–42.

115. Li Y, Hazarika S, Xie D, et al. In mice with type 2 diabetes, a vascular endothelial growth factor (VEGF)-activating transcription factor modulates VEGF signaling and induces therapeutic angiogenesis after hindlimb ischemia. Diabetes 2007; 56(3):656–65.

# Index

Note: Page numbers of article titles are in **boldface** type.

## A

Abscess
  and diabetic pedal osteomyelitis, 1111–1112
Absent middle facet sign
  and subtalar coalition, 1022–1023
Absent sesamoid
  and hallucal sesamoid complex, 1086
Achilles tendon, 1029–1030
Adhesive capsulitis
  clinical symptoms and physical findings of,
    991
  and imaging, 991–992
  pathophysiology of, 991
  prevalence and epidemiology of, 990
  treatment of, 992
Adventitial bursa, 1093–1094
Adventitial bursitis
  anatomy involved in, 1074
  clinical examination of, 1074
  imaging of, 1076
  pathology of, 1074
  treatment of, 1076
Aneurysm
  of the hindfoot or midfoot, 1040
Ankle arthroplasty
  complications of, 1009–1014
  and component subsidence and migration,
    1011–1012
  and delayed syndesmotic union, 1013
  and implant design, 1003–1007
  indications for, 1003
  and ligament balancing, 1012–1013
  and malleolar fractures, 1009–1010
  and osteolysis, 1010–1011
  and postoperative imaging, 1007–1009
  and syndesmotic nonunion, 1013–1014
  and wound healing, 1010
Ankle impingement, 957–969
  anterior, 957–959, 983–984
  anterolateral, 959–960, 982–983
  anteromedial, 960–963
  and bony spurs, 957–969
  and magnetic resonance arthrography, 960,
    962, 981–992
  and magnetic resonance imaging, 958, 960–962,
    964, 967
  medial, 984
  posterior, 965–969, 984–986
  posteromedial, 963–965
  and ultrasound, 960, 964, 966–967
Ankle impingement syndromes, **957–971**
Ankle joint
  pathology of, 1037–1038
Ankle masses, 1038–1039
Anteater sign
  and calcaneonavicular coalition, 1024
Anterior ankle impingement, 983–984
  anatomy and pathophysiology of, 957–958
  clinical features of, 958
  and imaging, 958
  and magnetic resonance arthrography, 984
  and magnetic resonance imaging, 984
  pathophysiology of, 983
  prevalence and epidemiology of, 983
  treatment of, 958–959
Anterior tendons, 1036
Anterior tibialis tendon, 1036
Anterolateral ankle impingement, 982–983
  anatomy and pathophysiology of, 959
  clinical features of, 960
  and imaging, 960
  and magnetic resonance arthrography, 982–983
  and magnetic resonance imaging, 982
  management of, 960
  pathophysiology of, 982
  prevalence and epidemiology of, 982
Anteromedial ankle impingement
  anatomy and pathophysiology of, 960–961
  clinical features of, 961
  and imaging, 961–962
  management of, 962–963
Arthritis
  and hallucal sesamoid complex, 1085
Athletic injury
  and ankle impingement, 957–969
  and Lisfranc joints, 1049–1050
  and the metatarsophalangeal joints, 1082–1084,
    1086–1089
ATT. See Anterior tibialis tendon.
Avascular necrosis
  and hallucal sesamoid complex, 1084–1085
  versus osteochondral lesions, 1001
AVN. See Avascular necrosis.

Radiol Clin N Am 46 (2008) 1125–1129
doi:10.1016/S0033-8389(08)00201-7
0033-8389/08/$ – see front matter © 2008 Elsevier Inc. All rights reserved.

**B**

Bony spurs
    and ankle impingement, 957–969

**C**

C-sign
    and subtalar coalition, 1020
Calcaneonavicular coalition
    and anteater sign, 1024
    and computed tomography, 1024–1025
    and elongated navicular sign, 1024
    and magnetic resonance imaging, 1024–1025
    and radiography, 1024
Cellulitis
    and diabetic pedal osteomyelitis, 1111–1112
Coalitions of multiple bones, 1025
Computed tomography
    and calcaneonavicular coalition, 1024–1025
    and diabetic pedal osteomyelitis, 1107–1108
    and subtalar coalition, 1023–1024
Current concepts in imaging diabetic pedal
    osteomyelitis, **1105–1124**
Cystic tumor-like lesions, 1093–1094

**D**

Deltoid ligament sprains, 980–981
    anatomy of, 980–981
    and magnetic resonance arthrography, 981
    and magnetic resonance imaging, 981
    pathophysiology of, 981
Diabetes
    and pedal osteomyelitis, 1105–1120
Diabetic pedal osteomyelitis
    and computed tomography, 1107
    and gangrene, 1112
    and high field imaging, 1118–1119
    and imaging appropriateness criteria, 1118
    and magnetic resonance imaging, 1107–1108
    magnetic resonance imaging protocol for,
        1108
    versus neuropathic arthropathy, 1116
    nuclear medicine evaluation of, 1106–1107
    pathogenesis of, 1105–1106
    radiography of, 1106
    and septic arthritis, 1114–1115
    and skin callus, 1108–1109
    and soft tissue swelling, cellulitis, and abscess,
        1111–1112
    and spread of infection, 1115–1116
    and tissue perfusion and viability, 1120, 1119
    and ulceration and sinus tract, 1109–1110
    and ultrasound, 1107
Dysmorphic sustentaculum tali
    and subtalar coalition, 1020–1021

**E**

Elongated navicular sign
    and calcaneonavicular coalition, 1024

**F**

FDL. See *Flexor digitorum longus tendon.*
FHL. See *Flexor hallucis longus tendon.*
Flexor digitorum longus tendon, 1034–1035
Flexor hallucis longus tendon, 1035
Foot masses, 1038–1039
Forefoot
    and adventitial bursitis, 1074–1076
    anatomy of, 1065
    bones of, 1065–1068
    and Freiberg infarction, 1067–1068
    and intermetatarsal bursitis and fibrosis,
        1072–1074
    joints of, 1068–1071
    stress fractures of, 1065–1067
    and tendinopathy, 1071–1072
Foreign bodies
    in the foot, 1040–1041
Freiberg infarction
    clinical examination of, 1067
    history of, 1067
    imaging of, 1067–1068
    treatment of, 1068

**G**

Gadolinium
    in imaging diabetic patients, 1108
Ganglia, 1093
Ganglion cysts, 1039
Gangrene
    and diabetic pedal osteomyelitis, 1112
Giant cell tumor of tendon sheath, 1099
Gout, 1096

**H**

Hallucal sesamoid complex
    and absent sesamoid, 1086
    anatomy of, 1079–1081
    and arthritis, 1085
    and avascular necrosis, 1084–1085
    and infection, 1085–1086
    and nerve impingement, 1086
    pain in, 1081–1086
    and sesamoid trauma, 1083–1084
    and sesamoiditis, 1081–1083
Hindfoot
    infection of, 1039
    normal imaging findings in, 1017–1018
    and tarsal coalition, 1017–1025
    tendons of, 1027–1028

**I**

Imaging of Lisfranc injury and midfoot sprain, **1045–1060**
Imaging of painful conditions of the hallucal sesamoid complex and plantar capsular structures of the first metatarsophalangeal joint, **1079–1092**
Imaging of soft tissue lesions of the foot and ankle, **1093–1103**
Imaging of tarsal coalition, **1017–1026**
Intermetatarsal bursitis and fibrosis
 anatomy involved in, 1072–1073
 clinical examination of, 1073
 imaging of, 1073–1074
 pathology of, 1073
 treatment of, 1074
Intra-articular loose bodies
 and magnetic resonance arthrography, 990


**L**

Lateral collateral ligament complex
 anatomy of, 977
 and magnetic resonance arthrography, 977–978
 and magnetic resonance imaging, 977
 treatment of, 978
Leiomyosarcoma, 1102
Ligamentous constraints
 and Lisfranc joint injuries, 1047–1048
Ligamentous injuries
 deltoid ligament sprains, 980–981
 lateral collateral ligament complex, 977–978
 and magnetic resonance arthrography, 976–981
 syndesmosis, 978–980
Ligaments, 1036–1037
Lipomas, 1039–1040, 1099-1100
Lisfranc joint
 anatomy of, 1045–1049
 imaging of, 1050–1058
 and injury classification, 1050
 and injury mechanism, 1049
 and ligamentous constraints, 1047–1048
 and magnetic resonance imaging, 1055–1058
 and multidetector computed tomography, 1055
 radiography of, 1050–1054
 and radionuclide bone scans, 1054


**M**

Magnetic resonance arthrography
 of the ankle, 973–992
 and ankle impingement, 960, 962, 981–992
 and deltoid ligament sprains, 981
 direct, 973–975
 indications for, 976–992
 indirect, 975–976
 and intra-articular loose bodies, 990
 and lateral collateral ligament complex, 977–978
 and ligamentous injuries, 976–981
 and osteochondral and cartilage lesions of the talus, 989
 and syndesmosis, 980
Magnetic resonance imaging
 and ankle impingement, 958, 960–962, 964, 967
 and calcaneonavicular coalition, 1024–1025
 and deltoid ligament sprains, 981
 and diabetic pedal osteomyelitis, 1107–1108
 and lateral collateral ligament complex, 977
 of Lisfranc joint, 1055–1058
 and metatarsalgia, 1061–1069, 1072–1074, 1076
 and osteochondral lesions, 988–989, 997–1001
 and subtalar coalition, 1023–1024
and syndesmosis, 980
MDCT. See *Multidetector computed tomography.*
Medial ankle impingement, 984
Medial tendons, 1033–1035
Metatarsalgia, 1061–1076
 and imaging protocols, 1061
 and magnetic resonance imaging, 1061–1069, 1072–1074, 1076
 and proton density imaging, 1061, 1063, 1069–1070, 1072, 1076
 treatment of, 1065
 and ultrasound, 1061–1066, 1072–1074, 1076
Metatarsophalangeal joints
 anatomy of, 1061–1062, 1068–1069, 1079–1081
 clinical examination of, 1062
 imaging of, 1062–1065
 instability of, 1061–1065
 mechanism of injury, 1062
 and synovitis, 1069–1071
Middle facet sign
 absent in subtalar coalition, 1022–1023
Midfoot
 infection of, 1039
 sprain of, 1045–1059
 tendons of, 1027–1028
Morton's neuroma, 1073–1074, 1094
MR arthrography of the ankle: Indications and technique, **973–994**
MR imaging and ultrasound of metatarsalgia—The lesser metatarsals, **1061–1078**
MTP joints. See *Metatarsophalangeal joints.*
Multidetector computed tomography
 of Lisfranc joint, 1055
 and osteochondral lesions, 997, 999–1000


**N**

Nerve impingement
 and hallucal sesamoid complex, 1086
Nerve sheath tumors, 1039

Neuropathic arthropathy
    versus diabetic pedal osteomyelitis, 1116
    superimposed infection in, 1116–1118
Noncystic tumor-like lesions, 1094–1095
Nuclear medicine evaluation
    of diabetic pedal osteomyelitis, 1106–1107


O

OCL. See *Osteochondral lesions,*
Osteochondral and cartilage lesions of the talus,
    986–990
    clinical symptoms and physical findings of, 988
    and imaging cartilage repair, 990
    and magnetic resonance arthrography, 989
    and magnetic resonance imaging, 988–989
    pathophysiology of, 988
    prevalence and epidemiology of, 986–988
    treatment of, 989–990
Osteochondral lesions, 995–1002
    versus avascular necrosis and osteoarthritis, 1001
    imaging of, 997–1001
    and magnetic resonance imaging, 997–1001
    and multidetector computed tomography, 997,
        999–1000
    staging system for, 999
    treatment of, 1001–1002
Osteochondral lesions about the ankle, **995–1002**
Osteomyelitis
    diabetic pedal, 1105–1120
    of the sesamoids, 1085–1086


P

Pedal osteomyelitis
    and diabetes, 1105–1120
    and evaluation of diabetic patients, 1106
Peroneal tendons, 1030–1033
    subluxation and dislocation of, 1032–1033
Pigmented villonodular synovitis, 1096
Plantar fasciitis, 1038
Plantar fibromatosis, 1098–1099
Plantar plate
    anatomy of, 1061–1062, 1081
    disruption of, 1061–1065
    injuries to, 1086–1090
Posterior ankle impingement, 984–986
    anatomy and physiology of, 965–966
    clinical features of, 966
    and imaging, 966–967
    magnetic resonance arthrography of, 986
    and magnetic resonance imaging, 986
    management of, 967, 969
    pathophysiology of, 985–986
    prevalence and epidemiology of, 984
    and the Steida process, 965

Posterior tibialis tendon, 1033–1036
Posteromedial ankle impingement
    anatomy and pathophysiology of, 963
    clinical features of, 963
    and imaging, 963–964
    management of, 964–965
Postoperative imaging of the total ankle arthroplasty,
    **1003–1015**
Proton density imaging
    and metatarsalgia, 1061, 1063, 1069–1070, 1072,
        1076
PTT. See *Posterior tibialis tendon.*


R

Radiography
    and calcaneonavicular coalition, 1024
    and diabetic pedal osteomyelitis, 1106
    of Lisfranc joint, 1050–1054
    and subtalar coalition, 1019–1023
Rheumatoid nodules, 1094


S

Sarcoma
    synovial, 1100
    undifferentiated pleomorphic, 1100–1102
Septic arthritis
    and diabetic pedal osteomyelitis, 1114–1115
Sesamoiditis, 1081–1083
Skin callus
    and diabetic pedal osteomyelitis, 1108–1109
    on the foot, 1095
Soft tissue chondroma, 1100
Soft tissue infection
    and diabetic pedal osteomyelitis, 1105–1120
Steida process
    and posterior ankle impingement, 965
Stress fractures
    clinical examination of, 1066
    history of, 1065–1066
    imaging of, 1066–1067
    treatment of, 1067
Subtalar coalition
    and absent middle facet sign, 1022–1023
    and blunted lateral process of talus, 1021
    and C-sign, 1020
    and computed tomography, 1023–1024
    and dysmorphic sustentaculum tali, 1020–1021
    and magnetic resonance imaging, 1023–1024
    and radiography, 1019–1023
    and talar beak, 1021–1022
Syndesmosis
    anatomy of, 978–979
    and magnetic resonance arthrography, 980
    and magnetic resonance imaging, 980

pathophysiology of, 979–980
Synovial-based processes, 1095–1096
Synovial chondromatosis, 1095–1096
Synovial cysts, 1093
Synovial sarcoma, 1100
Synovitis
    clinical examination of, 1069
    history of, 1069
    imaging of, 1069
    pigmented villonodular, 1096
    primary, 1069–1070
    secondary, 1070–1071
    treatment of, 1071


T

Talar beak
    and subtalar coalition, 1021–1022
Talus
    blunted lateral process of, 1021
    osteochondral lesions of, 995–1002
Tarsal coalition
    imaging of, 1017–1025
Tarsometatarsal joint
    injury to, 1045–1059
Tendinopathy
    anatomy involved in, 1071–1072
    clinical examination of, 1072
    imaging of, 1072

treatment of, 1072
Tendinosis, 1072
Tendons
    Achilles, 1029–1030
    anterior, 1036
    of the hindfoot and midfoot, 1027–1028
    medial, 1033, 1035
    peroneal, 1030–1033
Tenosynovitis, 1072
Tumor-like lesions, 1093–1096
Tumors
    of the foot and ankle, 1096–1102
Turf toe, 1086–1090
    clinical presentation of, 1087–1089
    imaging of, 1089–1090
    mechanism of injury, 1087
    treatment of, 1090


U

Ulceration
    and diabetic pedal osteomyelitis, 1109–1110
Ultrasound
    and ankle impingement, 960, 964, 966–967
    and diabetic pedal osteomyelitis, 1107
    and metatarsalgia, 1061–1066, 1072–1074, 1076
Ultrasound of the hindfoot and midfoot, **1027–1043**
Undifferentiated pleomorphic sarcoma,
    1100–1102

# Moving?

## Make sure your subscription moves with you!

To notify us of your new address, find your **Clinics Account Number** (located on your mailing label above your name), and contact customer service at:

**E-mail: elspcs@elsevier.com**

**800-654-2452 (subscribers in the U.S. & Canada)**
**314-453-7041 (subscribers outside of the U.S. & Canada)**

**Fax number: 314-523-5170**

**Elsevier Periodicals Customer Service**
11830 Westline Industrial Drive
St. Louis, MO 63146

*To ensure uninterrupted delivery of your subscription, please notify us at least 4 weeks in advance of move.

**United States Postal Service**

## Statement of Ownership, Management, and Circulation
### (All Periodicals Publications Except Requestor Publications)

**1. Publication Title**
Radiologic Clinics of North America

**2. Publication Number**
5 9 6 - 5 1 1 0

**3. Filing Date**
9/15/08

**4. Issue Frequency**
Jan, Mar, May, Jul, Sep, Nov

**5. Number of Issues Published Annually**
6

**6. Annual Subscription Price**
$290.00

**7. Complete Mailing Address of Known Office of Publication** (Not printer) (Street, city, county, state, and ZIP+4)

Elsevier Inc.
360 Park Avenue South
New York, NY 10010-1710

**Contact Person**
Stephen Bushing

**Telephone** (Include area code)
215-239-3688

**8. Complete Mailing Address of Headquarters or General Business Office of Publisher** (Not printer)

Elsevier Inc., 360 Park Avenue South, New York, NY 10010-1710

**9. Full Names and Complete Mailing Addresses of Publisher, Editor, and Managing Editor** (Do not leave blank)

**Publisher** (Name and complete mailing address)

John Schrefer , Elsevier, Inc. , 1600 John F. Kennedy Blvd. Suite 1800, Philadelphia, PA 19103-2899

**Editor** (Name and complete mailing address)

Barron Dudlick, Elsevier, Inc., 1600 John F. Kennedy Blvd. Suite 1800, Philadelphia, PA 19103-2899

**Managing Editor** (Name and complete mailing address)

Catherine Bewick, Elsevier, Inc., 1600 John F. Kennedy Blvd. Suite 1800, Philadelphia, PA 19103-2899

**10. Owner** (Do not leave blank. If the publication is owned by a corporation, give the name and address of the corporation immediately followed by the names and addresses of all stockholders owning or holding 1 percent or more of the total amount of stock. If not owned by a corporation, give the names and addresses of the individual owners. If owned by a partnership or other unincorporated firm, give its name and address as well as those of each individual owner. If the publication is published by a nonprofit organization, give its name and address.)

| Full Name | Complete Mailing Address |
|---|---|
| Wholly owned subsidiary of | 4520 East-West Highway |
| Reed/Elsevier, US holdings | Bethesda, MD 20814 |

**11. Known Bondholders, Mortgagees, and Other Security Holders Owning or Holding 1 Percent or More of Total Amount of Bonds, Mortgages, or Other Securities. If none, check box** ☐ None

| Full Name | Complete Mailing Address |
|---|---|
| N/A | |

**12. Tax Status** (For completion by nonprofit organizations authorized to mail at nonprofit rates) (Check one)
The purpose, function, and nonprofit status of this organization and the exempt status for federal income tax purposes:
☐ Has Not Changed During Preceding 12 Months
☐ Has Changed During Preceding 12 Months (Publisher must submit explanation of change with this statement)

PS Form 3526, September 2006 (Page 1 of 3 (Instructions Page 3)) PSN 7530-01-000-9931 **PRIVACY NOTICE:** See our Privacy policy in www.usps.com

---

**13. Publication Title**
Radiologic Clinics of North America

**14. Issue Date for Circulation Data Below**
May 2008

**15. Extent and Nature of Circulation**

| | | Average No. Copies Each Issue During Preceding 12 Months | No. Copies of Single Issue Published Nearest to Filing Date |
|---|---|---|---|
| a. Total Number of Copies (Net press run) | | 6767 | 6300 |
| b. Paid Circulation (By Mail and Outside the Mail) | (1) Mailed Outside-County Paid Subscriptions Stated on PS Form 3541. (Include paid distribution above nominal rate, advertiser's proof copies, and exchange copies) | 3479 | 3238 |
| | (2) Mailed In-County Paid Subscriptions Stated on PS Form 3541 (Include paid distribution above nominal rate, advertiser's proof copies, and exchange copies) | | |
| | (3) Paid Distribution Outside the Mails Including Sales Through Dealers and Carriers, Street Vendors, Counter Sales, and Other Paid Distribution Outside USPS® | 2239 | 1985 |
| | (4) Paid Distribution by Other Classes Mailed Through the USPS (e.g. First-Class Mail®) | | |
| c. Total Paid Distribution (Sum of 15b (1), (2), (3), and (4)) | ▲ | 5718 | 5223 |
| d. Free or Nominal Rate Distribution (By Mail and Outside the Mail) | (1) Free or Nominal Rate Outside-County Copies Included on PS Form 3541 | 87 | 79 |
| | (2) Free or Nominal Rate In-County Copies Included on PS Form 3541 | | |
| | (3) Free or Nominal Rate Copies Mailed at Other Classes Mailed Through the USPS (e.g. First-Class Mail) | | |
| | (4) Free or Nominal Rate Distribution Outside the Mail (Carriers or other means) | | |
| e. Total Free or Nominal Rate Distribution (Sum of 15d (1), (2), (3) and (4)) | ▲ | 87 | 79 |
| f. Total Distribution (Sum of 15c and 15e) | ▲ | 5805 | 5302 |
| g. Copies not Distributed (See instructions to publishers #4 (page #3)) | ▲ | 962 | 998 |
| h. Total (Sum of 15f and g) | ▲ | 6767 | 6300 |
| i. Percent Paid (15c divided by 15f times 100) | | 98.50% | 98.51% |

**16. Publication of Statement of Ownership**

☐ If the publication is a general publication, publication of this statement is required. Will be printed in the **November 2008** issue of this publication.
☐ Publication not required

**17. Signature and Title of Editor, Publisher, Business Manager, or Owner**

*[signature]*

Stephen Fanucci - Executive Director of Subscription Services

**Date**
September 15, 2008

I certify that all information furnished on this form is true and complete. I understand that anyone who furnishes false or misleading information on this form or who omits material or information requested on the form may be subject to criminal sanctions (including fines and imprisonment) and/or civil sanctions (including civil penalties).

PS Form 3526, September 2006 (Page 2 of 3)